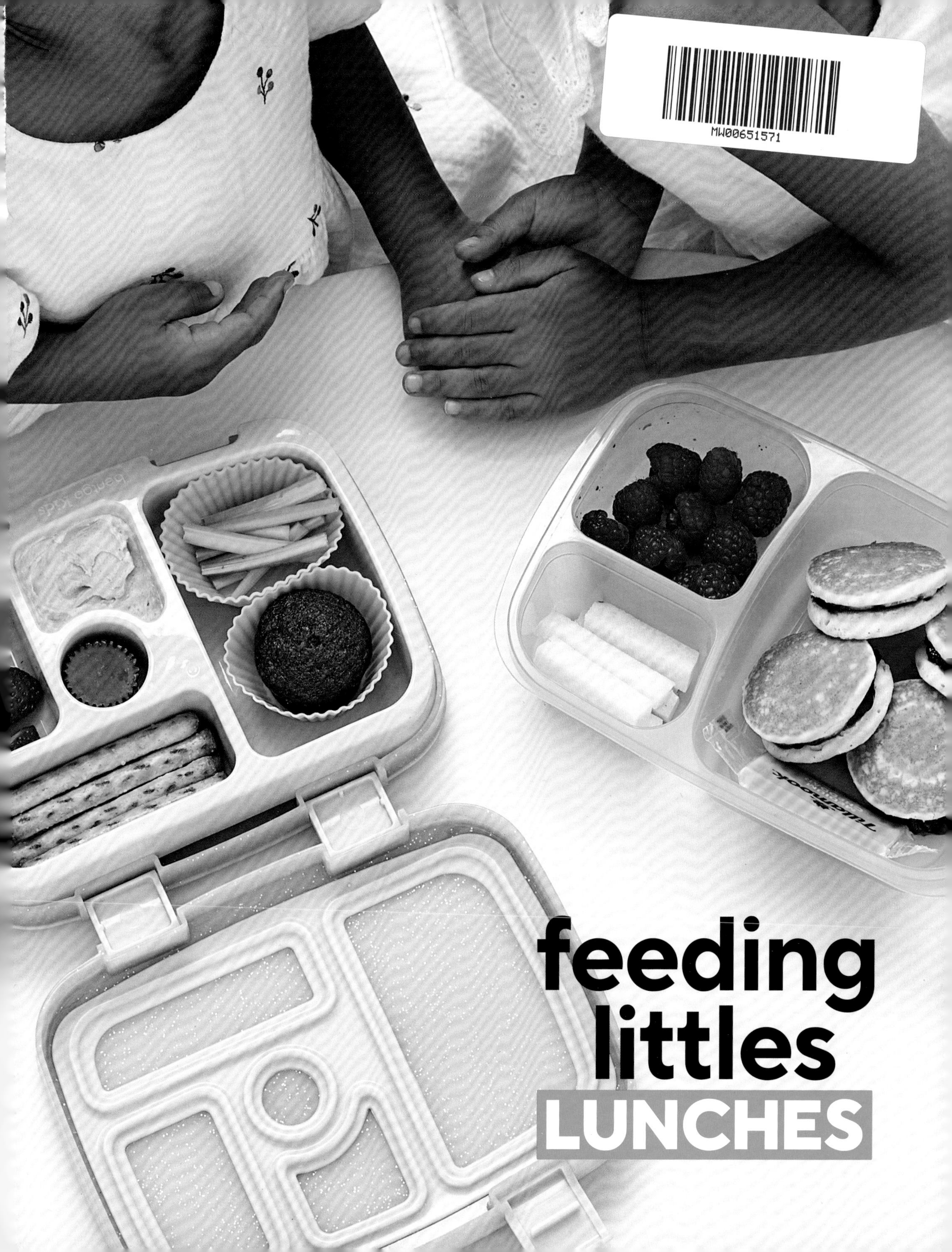

feeding littles LUNCHES

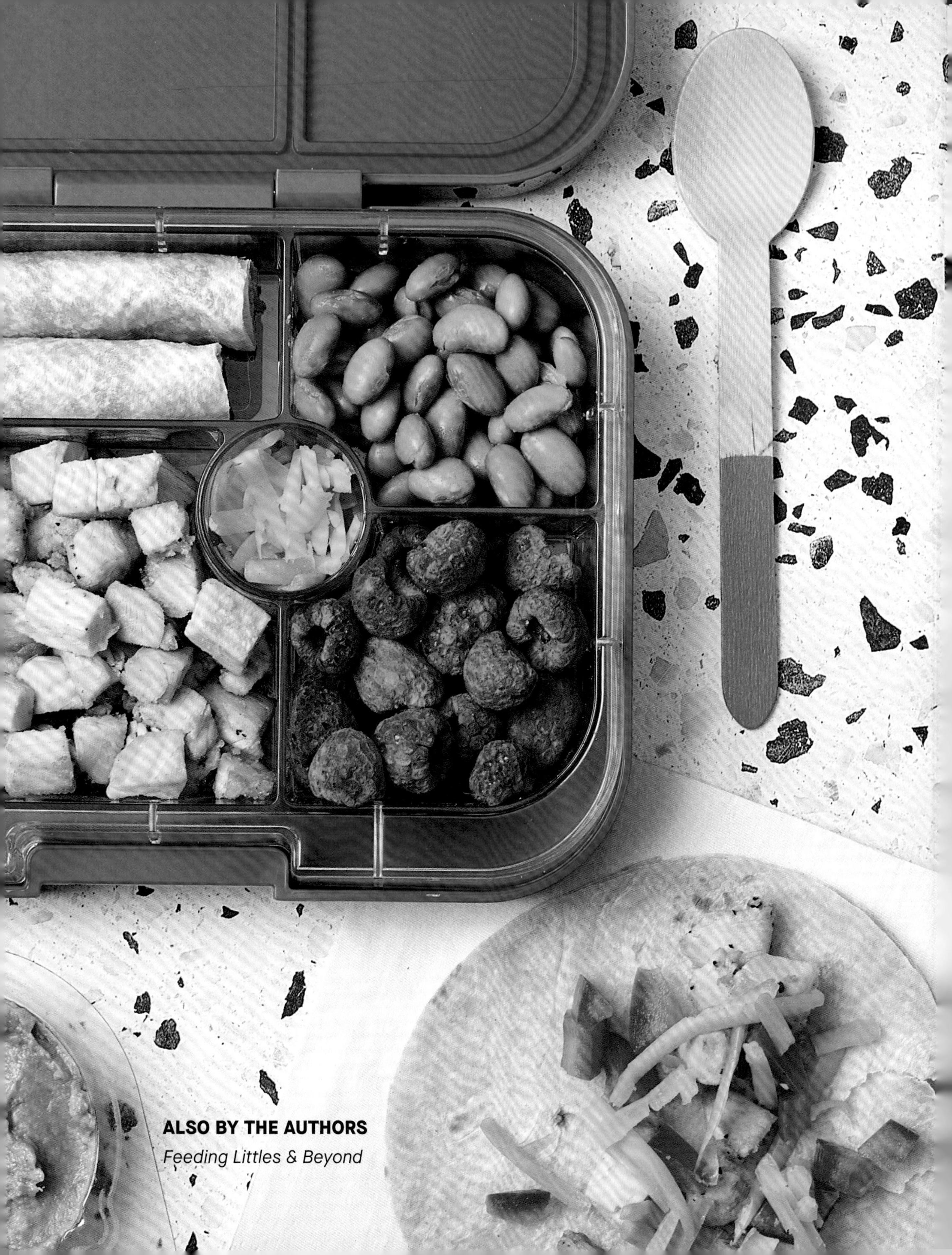

ALSO BY THE AUTHORS

Feeding Littles & Beyond

75+
No-Stress
Lunches
Everyone Will
Love

feeding littles LUNCHES

Megan McNamee, MPH, RDN
AND
Judy Delaware, OTR/L, CLC
PHOTOGRAPHS BY CARLA CHOY

RODALE
New York

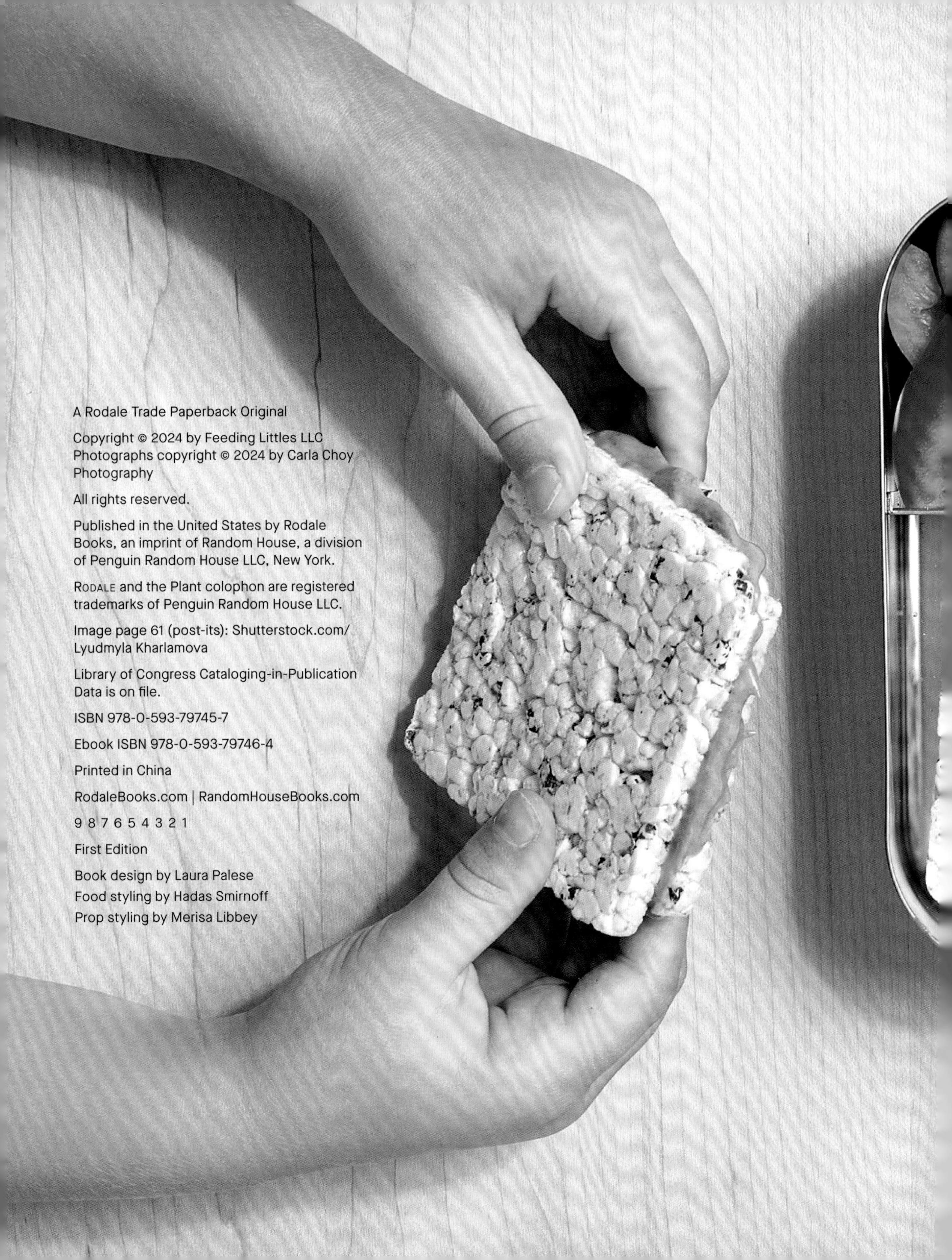

A Rodale Trade Paperback Original

Published in the United States by Rodale Books, an imprint of Random House, a division of Penguin Random House LLC, New York.

RODALE and the Plant colophon are registered trademarks of Penguin Random House LLC.

Image page 61 (post-its): Shutterstock.com/ Lyudmyla Kharlamova

Library of Congress Cataloging-in-Publication Data is on file.

ISBN 978-0-593-79745-7

Ebook ISBN 978-0-593-79746-4

Printed in China

RodaleBooks.com | RandomHouseBooks.com

9 8 7 6 5 4 3 2 1

First Edition

Book design by Laura Palese
Food styling by Hadas Smirnoff
Prop styling by Merisa Libbey

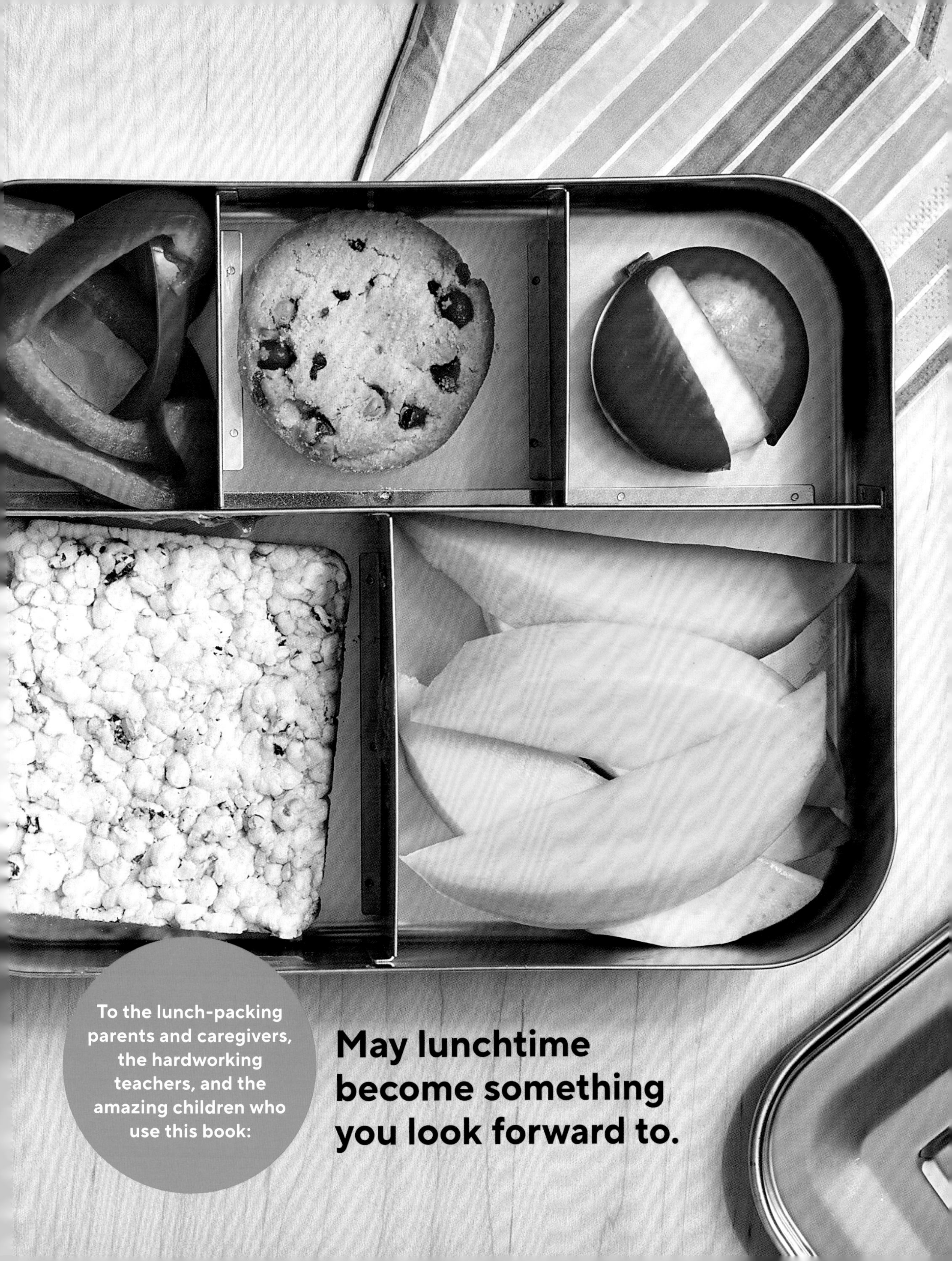

To the lunch-packing parents and caregivers, the hardworking teachers, and the amazing children who use this book:

May lunchtime become something you look forward to.

Contents

THE INTR

"I can't believe I have to pack my kid's lunch again." Sound familiar? If lunch packing makes your eyes roll to the back of your head, please know that you're not alone. You've come to the right place.

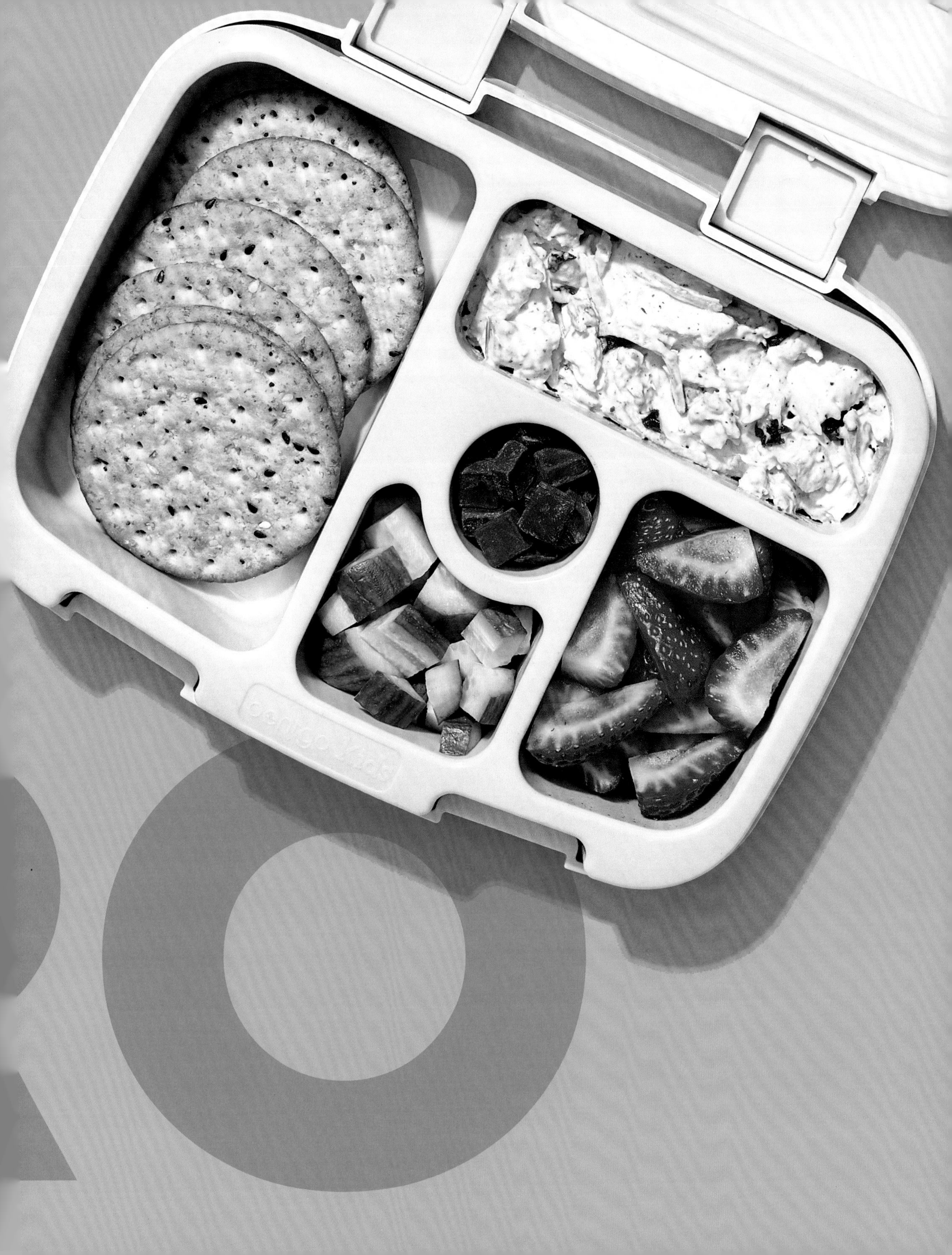

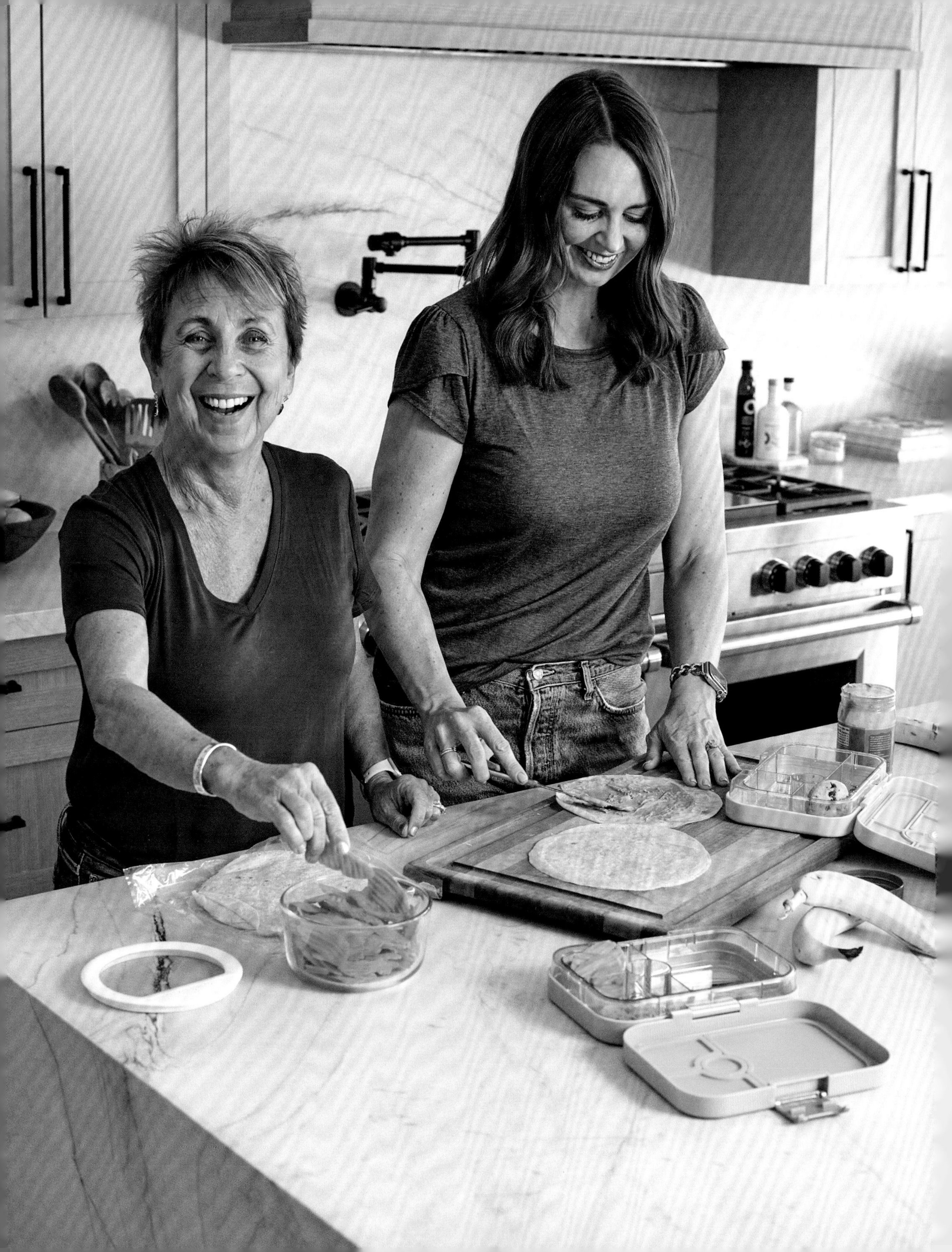

Meet Feeding Littles

Many of our clients have told us that packing lunch is one of their least favorite things about parenting.

It's constant, it's annoying, and their kids might not eat it anyway. Plus, when we're uninspired and out of ideas, it can feel really tedious.

Social media doesn't help either. We see images of gorgeous lunch boxes filled with every color of the rainbow, and we feel like we're a failure if we don't follow suit. We know our kids would probably love to find animal shapes complete with candy eyeballs when they open their lunch boxes, but our capacity for that on a daily basis is almost non-existent. We're either putting in a lot of effort, or we're doing it "wrong."

It doesn't have to be like this, friends. Promise.

We're Megan and Judy, and as feeding and nutrition professionals, we *definitely* understand how hard it is to feed kids. Here's the good news: Packing lunches can be *easy* when you have a good formula in your head and a bunch of simple ideas at your fingertips. No need to spend a ton of money, time, or effort, and certainly no candy eyeballs involved.

Before we get to these easy lunch ideas, we want to tell you a little bit about ourselves. Judy is an occupational therapist, specializing in feeding therapy and sensory processing, in Louisville, Colorado. Megan is a registered dietitian nutritionist, specializing in maternal/child nutrition and eating disorder prevention, in Scottsdale, Arizona.

We started Feeding Littles in 2014 as a way to bring our professional expertise to the world via social media content and online courses. Today we have the privilege of reaching millions of parents who are seeking nutrition, feeding, and parenting support—without all the judgment typically found online. Our goal is to help families all over the world raise adventurous, intuitive eaters.

While Judy's kids are young adults who (thankfully) pack their own lunches for work, Megan is still in the throes of packing school lunch most days. Her older daughter was just a year old when Feeding Littles began, and Megan has been sharing lunch box inspo ever since.

The formula has always been pretty straight-forward, independent of kids' ages: a starch, a protein, a vegetable, and a fruit. Add a dip, chips, or a dessert if you want. Offer simple, easy-to-assemble foods that you can pack in just a few minutes, utilizing leftovers and convenience items. Don't make it complicated.

As the Feeding Littles audience grew, so did the appreciation for our lunch content. Our followers loved seeing realistic, easy options that didn't require specific recipes or hours of prep to put together.

After years of evolving our approach, listening to our audience, and testing out tons of lunch ideas, we finally have a spot to compile all our inspiration and encouragement—and that's the book you're reading now. *Thank you* for supporting our work. We hope this book becomes a beloved resource for your whole family.

From our hearts (and kitchens) to yours,

Megan and Judy

First and Foremost . . .

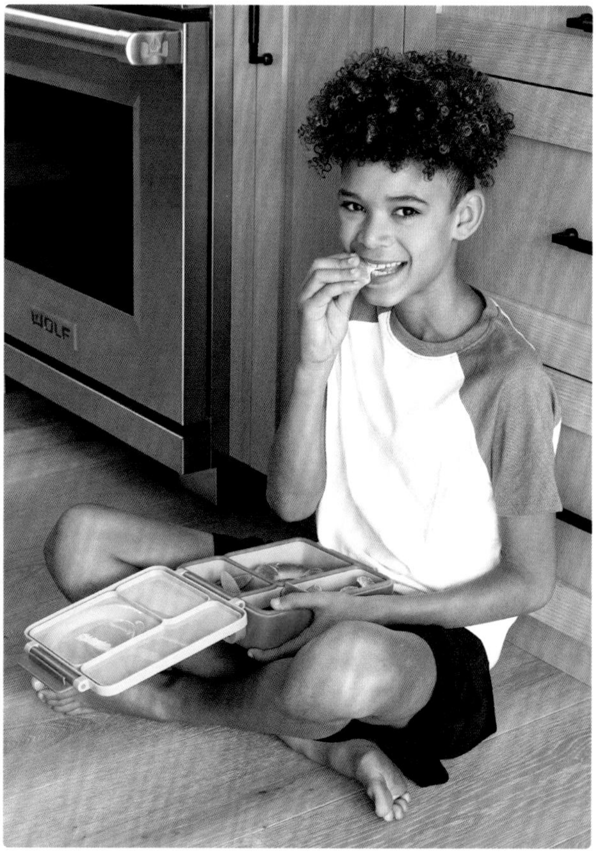

Thank you for your support of our tiny, women-owned company. We never dreamed of writing this, our second book, and we hope you find it valuable.

We hope this book helps you get out of your lunch rut and feel confident packing a nourishing lunch for your toddler, preschooler, or big kid while they're at school.

This is *not* a recipe book. You won't find any recipes in here because most of our audience has reported that they don't want to follow recipes specifically for lunch. In the allergy section you will find a QR code to recipes with allergy-friendly products, but this book itself is not meant to be a cookbook. If you do find you need recipes, check out our cookbook *Feeding Littles & Beyond,* co-authored by Ali Maffucci.

Instead, we're here to offer creative yet simple ways to use store-bought items or leftovers in your child's lunch. If a lunch idea calls for cooked pasta, it assumes that you already cooked pasta for another meal and are using leftovers for lunch. We are trying to make your life *easier,* not harder!

You'll notice in this book that we include all types of foods and a lot of convenience items. This is different from many lunch resources available. We wanted to show you realistic foods your child would actually want to eat while also offering delicious ways to add more nutrition to their lunch. Yes, nutritious food matters, and we want to help you build a lunch that meets your child's needs. However, it's not the *only* thing that matters. Taste, familiarity, culture, tradition, and enjoyment all play a part in eating, so in this book you'll find lots of different types of foods and ideas.

Will your child eat everything in here? Probably not. That's OK. Just as you would with a cookbook, you likely won't use every single idea presented in these pages, but the goal is to break you out of your rut and give you new and delicious ideas that you might not have thought of before.

Will you feel comfortable buying everything in this book (or even have access to it)? Again, probably not. If you have a young toddler, you might not be ready to send them out of the house with a cookie in their lunch box. This book is adaptable to all ages, and we hope you take what works for you and leave the rest.

If you're new to Feeding Littles, here are some philosophies we hope you'll keep in mind when making lunch (or any meal) for your children.

- **You know your child best.** We hope to offer guidance and inspiration, but only *you* know what works for your family. Never forget that.

- **We eat for many reasons.** Health and nutrition are just some of them. It's OK to have a balance of foods that nourish the body and foods that nourish the soul. All foods can fit, and enjoyment is a very important part of eating.

- **You provide; your child decides.** While you might make their lunch, the child gets to decide how much of it to eat. We don't recommend requiring bites or making kids finish certain foods before eating others. Why? We want kids to listen to their own internal cues to decide how much of any given food to eat (if they eat it at all). Only they know how much their body needs. This means that they might not eat the veggie you pack. This can be frustrating, but it's very common.

- **You won't adopt every idea in this book.** In fact, you might look through this entire book and decide that you're sticking with what's working right now. That's OK. Please do not feel guilty if you stick to the same trusted lunch every day. There's no judgment from us. We hope to take away some of your stress, not add to it.

- **Above all else,** kids need to get enough to eat and trust that they'll have adequate access to food. Sometimes we have to pack familiar, "safe" foods to make sure our kids get enough to eat while they're out of our care. What might seem "unhealthy" to one person is quite "healthy" to another, as the food is providing much-needed energy for growth and learning.

- **Kids don't always have control** over what goes in their lunch, and parents do their best to send foods they can afford and that they hope their kids will eat. This is especially true for picky eaters or kids with feeding challenges. It's also an issue for kids who bring their unique cultural foods to school. We can teach our kids to not "yuck on someone's yum," and we can communicate with teachers and cafeteria employees if our child—or what's in their lunch—is a target of negativity.

> **"You know your child best. We hope to offer guidance and inspiration, but only *you* know what works for your family.**

Most important, we hope that these ideas help you *enjoy* packing and eating lunches just a little bit more. Satisfaction and enjoyment are such an important part of eating, and if you find even a few new ideas that make your child's lunch (or your own lunch) that much more delicious, it's a win in our book.

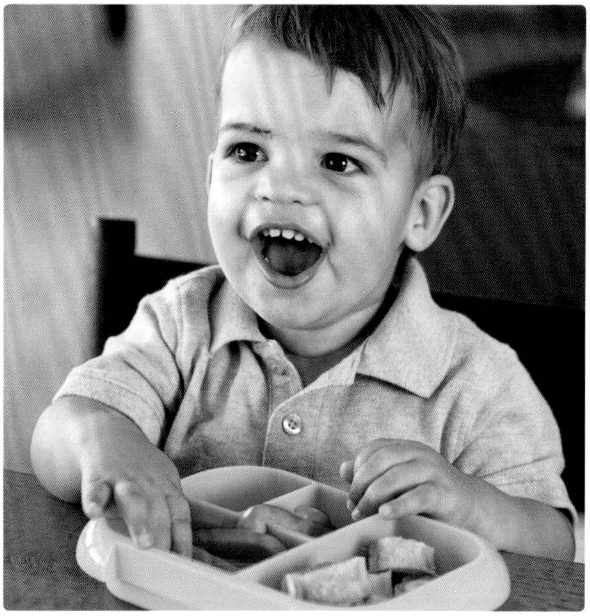

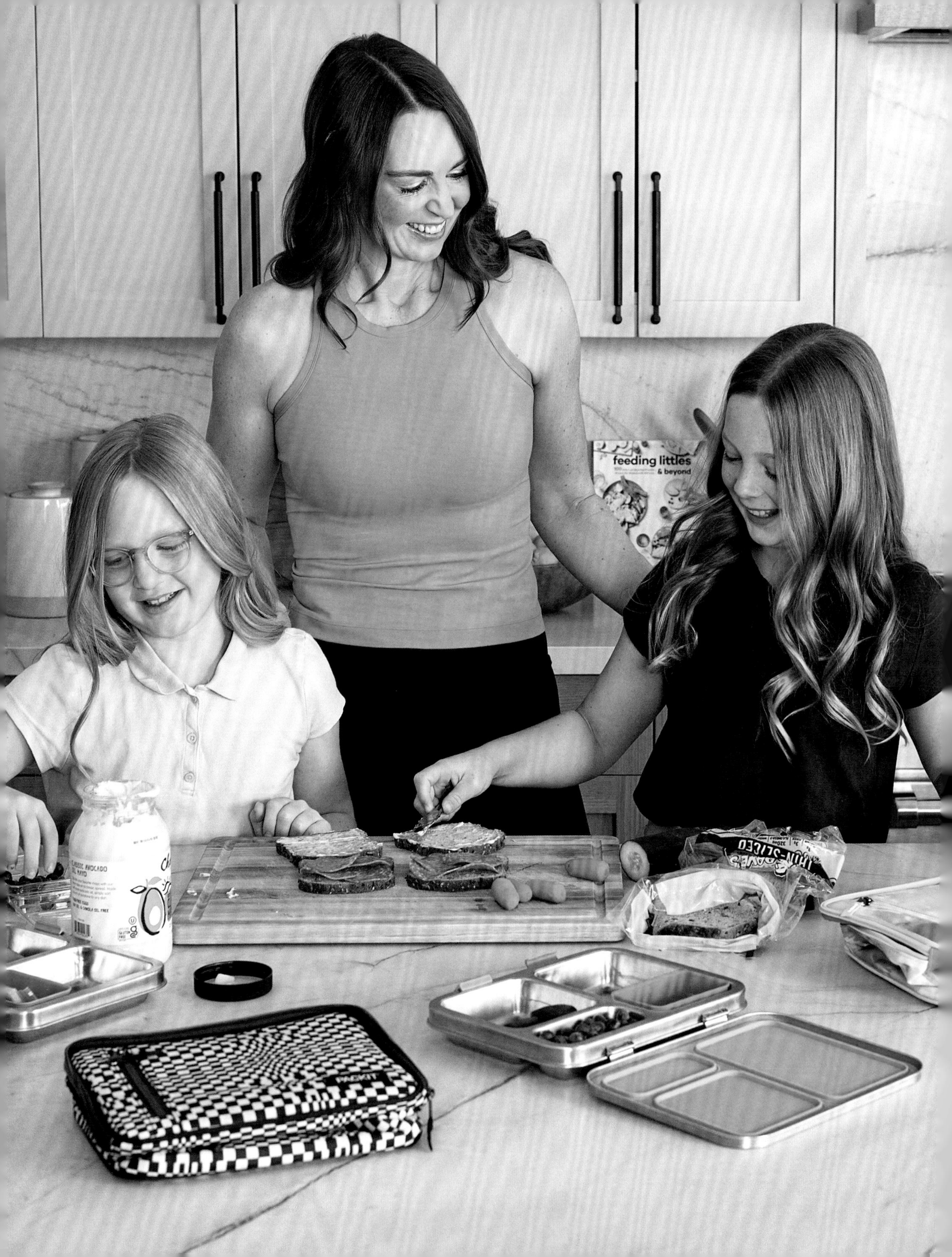
feeding littles
& beyond
PACKIT

What About Lunch Purchased at School?

While this is a lunch box book, it doesn't mean that we think lunches made at school are "bad" or "less healthy." Food insecurity is real. School lunches are essential for the health of millions of children across the globe—and they can be a godsend for busy parents. Eating a hot lunch at school can help kids branch out and try new foods, and at schools worldwide school lunch is the norm.

Yes, school lunches face a lot of challenges and absolutely need more funding, but they can also be the only access to nutrition that some kids have.

In some settings, school lunch carries a stigma. It can be seen as an option only for the kids who need a free or reduced-price lunch. For this reason, we think it's really important that all kids, independent of their economic status, consider getting lunch at school every so often if that's an option.

Alas, many kids don't have the option of school lunch or just don't want to eat it, and that's why this book was written.

How to Use This Book

We hope this book is something you'll refer to often for your kids in day care, preschool, elementary school, and beyond. It's meant to be functional and practical. Here are some ways it can be used:

- Go through it with your child to **pick out new ideas** or foods they want to try.
- Use the **index** at the back to look up certain ingredients you already have on hand and see how they're presented in new ways.
- Offer it as inspiration for your **older child** who is packing their own lunch.
- **Send it along** with your kids when they stay at someone else's house and their host asks what to pack them for lunch.
- Bring it with you to the **grocery store** to pick out a few fun new items.
- Use it to **inspire** your own packed lunches for work, school, or days out of the house.
- Keep it on your **kitchen counter** for easy reference.

NOTE "I Can't Even" is a term used throughout this book to define shortcuts or simple ideas for days when you just . . . can't even.

"Many kids don't have the option of school lunch or just don't want to eat it, and that's why this book was written.

The Feeding Littles Lunch Formula

Packed lunches don't have to be complicated. To break it down, we use this simple lunch formula:

- **starch or grain**
- **protein**
- **fruit**
- **vegetable**
- **dip, dessert, or chips**

NOTE You might not offer all these components in each lunch, and that's OK too.

Why This Formula?

Balance: A balance of nutrients helps kids feel more satisfied from their food. The protein, fat, and fiber found in these different food groups help more effectively regulate your child's blood sugar and offer longer-lasting satiety for growth, learning, and play.

Exposure: Kids learn to eat new foods by seeing them frequently in different ways. When they expect a variety of foods in their lunch box, they're more likely to eat a wider variety over time—even if they're not eating them yet. We include both a fruit and a vegetable in our formula because they can be more challenging foods for kids to eat, but with exposure they often learn to love them.

Enjoyment: Opening up a lunch box with a few different options, flavors, and textures can get kids excited about lunchtime. We all eat with our eyes, and kids look forward to a yummy lunch with foods they enjoy.

Nutrition: Different foods offer different nutrients. Protein is important for growth and satiety, while carbohydrate foods like grains and starches supply much-needed energy for learning and play. Fruits and veggies offer hydration, fiber, vitamins, and minerals. Your child might not eat all these foods at any given meal, but having them as an option helps ensure that they'll get their nutritional needs met over the course of a week.

What Could This Look Like?

Sunflower seed butter and jelly sandwich + blueberries + bell pepper slices + chocolate chips

Pita wedges + hummus + hard-boiled egg + cucumber + strawberries

Leftover meatballs + leftover cold penne pasta + marinara sauce + mandarin orange wedges + mini cinnamon graham crackers

NOTE Dietary fat is important for kids and adults, and we assume that it's inherent in the foods you're offering—for example, a sunflower seed butter sandwich with carrots, strawberries, and a cookie will have fat in the sunflower seed butter and the cookie.

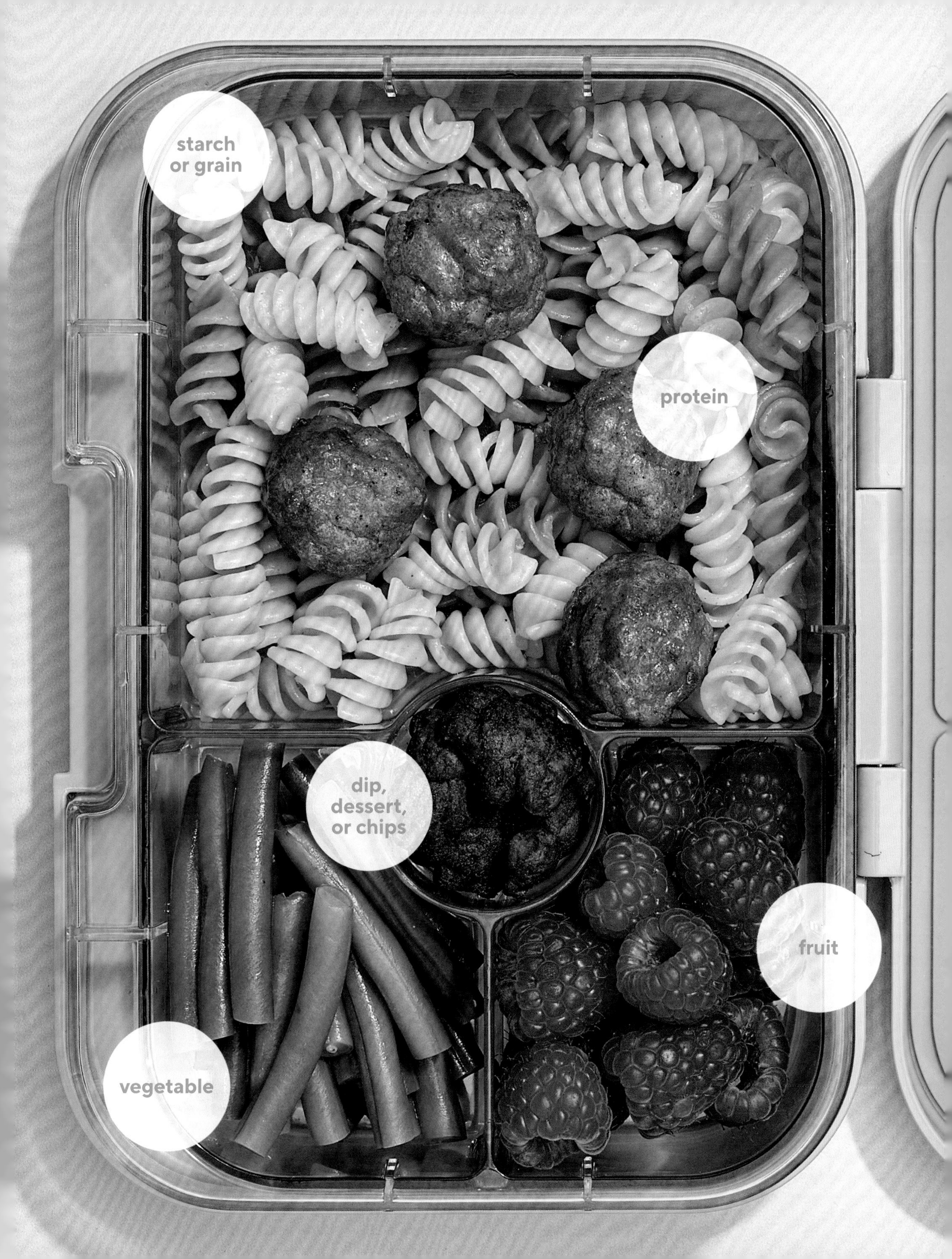
starch or grain
protein
dip, dessert, or chips
fruit
vegetable

Using This Book Based on Your Child's Age and Hunger Levels

Whether your child is eighteen months old or eighteen years old, we hope this book becomes a valuable resource when it's time to pack school lunch. Due to this wide age range, you'll notice a lot of variety in the types and sizes of food we feature. While some lunches may seem like they're just for "big kids," pretty much everything you see can be modified or substituted for your younger child—and vice versa. Similarly, a "toddler" lunch can be made for older kids just by adding more food. When appropriate, we notate each lunch with tips for modifying it for different ages.

Serving Sizes

Knowing how much food to send to school is tricky. Your kid might eat a lot one day and very little the next, or maybe they decide that they want only one or two of the components of their lunch. It will take some time to figure out how much food your child needs. If you find that they continuously eat everything, you might have to send more food; if they rarely eat it all, you might want to send less.

The serving sizes shown in this book are just estimates, and we purposefully didn't include specific ages or food quantities for that reason. There's no "right amount" to send, and there's nothing "wrong" if your kid eats more or less than what's shown. We want kids to follow their hunger and fullness patterns, not eat based on serving sizes.

If you're pretty certain your child won't eat something, consider sending a very small amount of it—think two slices of cucumber. They're still getting exposed to that food—and they might surprise you and eat it, especially if there are only a few unassuming cucumber slices in their lunch.

"Can My Kid Eat That?"

Some of the foods in this book require a little more skill to eat. For example, your toddler might not be ready for a wrap or sandwich, but maybe you can send a deconstructed version by separating the bread and filling.

Throughout this book you'll find tips for making foods easier for your younger kiddo to eat, as well as modifications for choking hazards. Our goal is for you to be able to send the same lunch with all your kids simply by making easy modifications for your younger eaters.

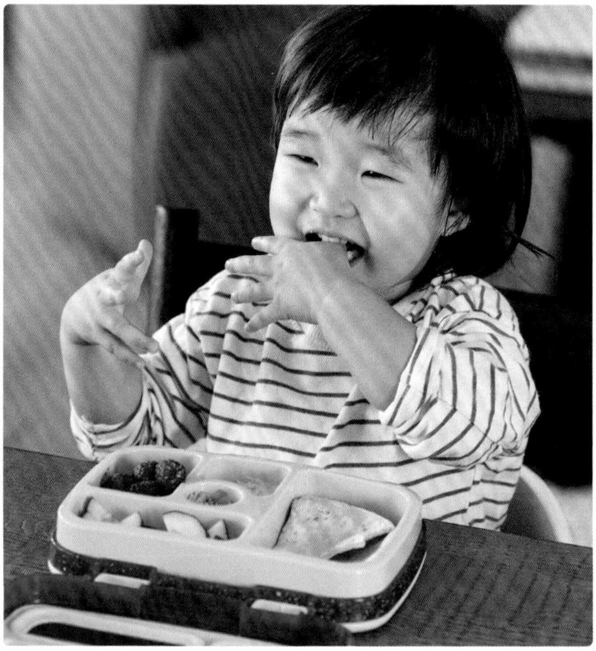

“Do I Need to Send a Dessert with Their Lunch?”

It’s up to you! If your child is a young toddler, they might not even eat desserts or sweets yet. Your day care or preschool might not allow sweets with lunch.

As your child gets older, they might notice that other kids get sweets for lunch. A small dessert or sweet food might be something they look forward to at lunchtime. We want our kids to see sweets as just another food—not something “special” or something to be earned with good behavior. When we make sweets or sugary foods something to be earned, our kids actually want them more because these foods feel off-limits. We recommend serving sweets or desserts periodically as your child gets older, as long as it feels comfortable to you and is allowed by their school.

For that reason, you’ll see desserts in many of the lunches here. You can omit them if desired.

When Megan’s girls were in preschool, she served desserts a few times a week with lunch. Now that they’re in elementary and middle school, they get something sweet with each school lunch, just like most of their peers.

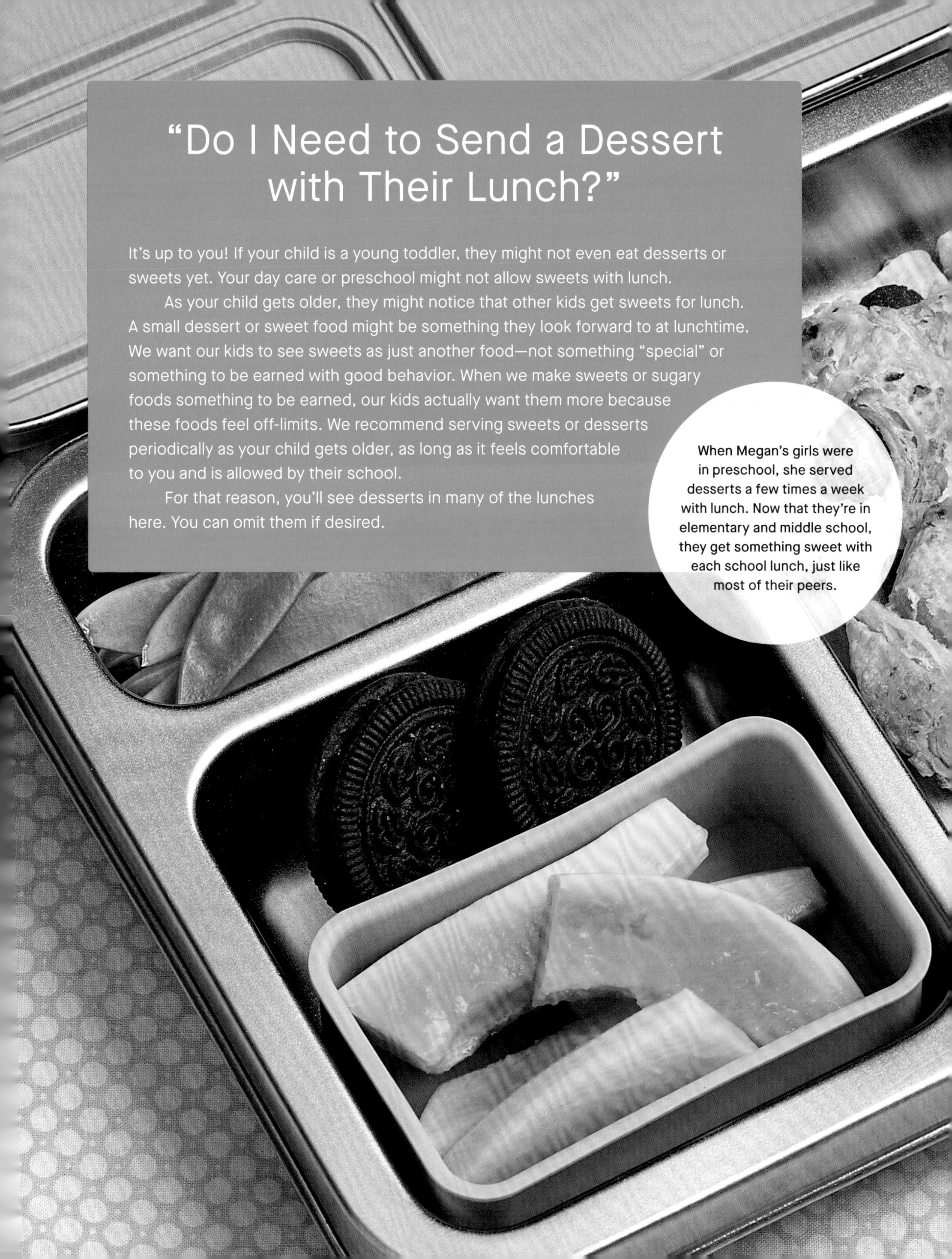

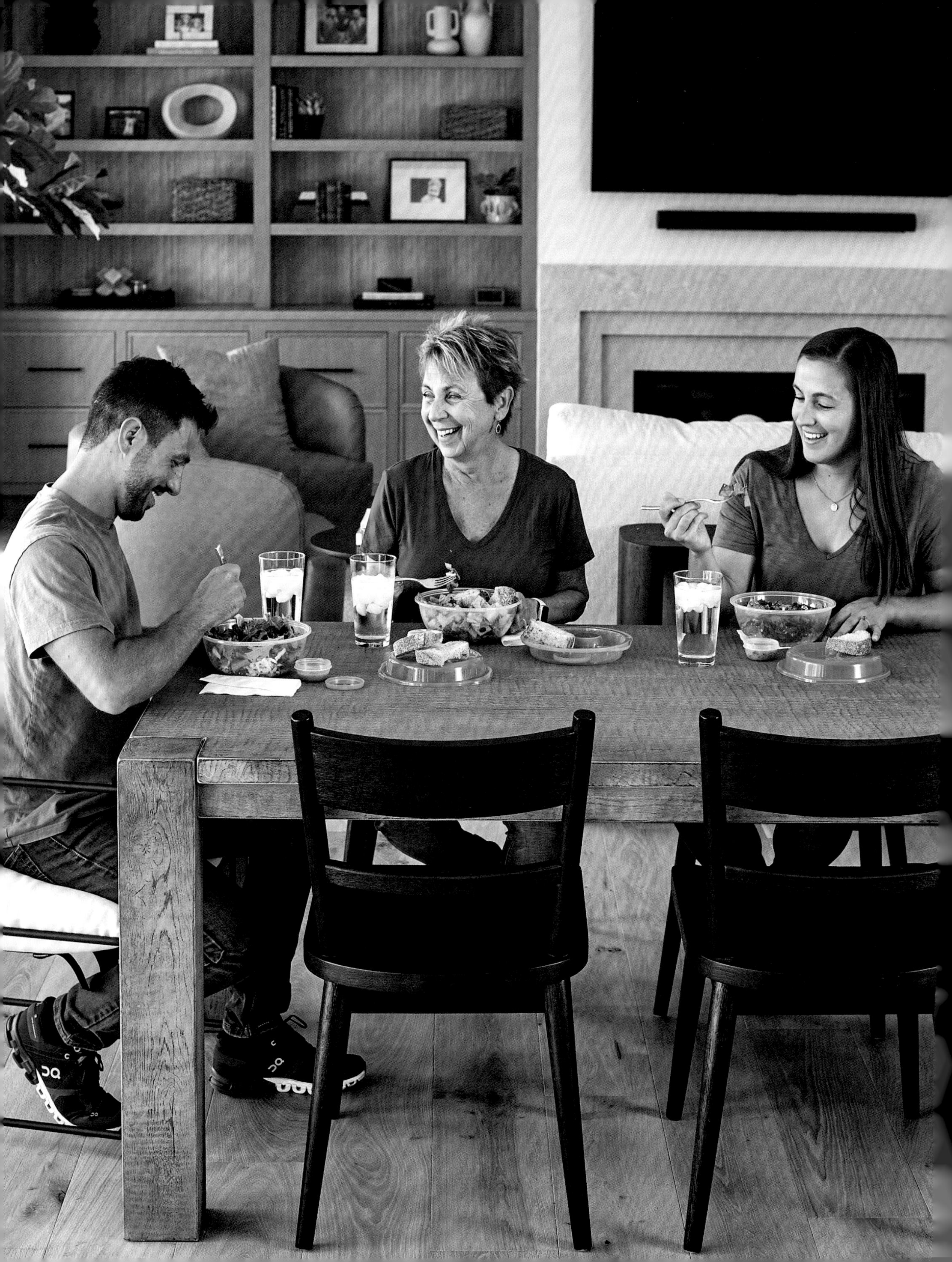

Our Top Lunch Box Tips

- **Pack the night before!** This saves so much time on busy, chaotic school mornings. Megan tends to pack lunch after school right after cleaning out her children's lunch boxes. Some foods like sliced banana, avocado, or apple might brown too much to pack the night before, but if refrigerated in a leakproof container, most foods will stay fresh until lunch the next day.

- **Leftovers** are *so easy* to send in packed lunches. Put them directly in your child's lunch box as you clean up after dinner.

- Similarly, if you're **prepping ingredients** for dinner, save some of them for your kiddo's lunch. For example, if you're cutting up carrots for a soup or pasta dish, slice a few extra for lunch the next day.

- Don't get nervous about sending **cold food.** Many kids love cold pizza, quesadillas, sliced chicken, or pasta. When we polled our audience, more than 70 percent of them send cold food all the time, and another 20 percent send cold food "often." You won't know until you try it!

- **Perishable food** needs to be kept refrigerated or sent with two ice sources. Check out page 34 for more food safety tips.

- **There is no "right" amount** of food to send with kids, as they are pretty unpredictable in how much they'll eat. Go with your gut and adjust as you see what your child eats. If they're consistently finishing all or most of their food, you might want to pack more.

- It is *so normal* for your child to **eat differently** at school than at home. Furthermore, they might not touch foods at home that they normally enjoy while at school. This is super common. The school cafeteria experience (or the preschool classroom) is very different from any other environment.

- Send a **labeled water bottle** to school every day. You might remember drinking water only from the water fountain at school, but today's kids tend to keep water with them throughout the school day. Hydration is important to help kids stay mentally focused at school and is critical for joint and circulatory health, so regular access to water is key. This is especially important if your child is an athlete or you live in a warm climate. Talk to your child (or their teachers) about how they can fill up their water if they run out. If they're too young to ask for more water, make sure their teachers check their bottles regularly. You don't have to send a separate beverage for lunch if they have their water bottle, but you can if you'd like.

- Have your child get **hot lunch** at school if it's available to you (and your child will eat it). Some families opt for it 100 percent of the time, while others choose which day their child will eat it. It helps kids eat new foods, can take the pressure off parents for packing daily lunches, and can help destigmatize school-made lunches.

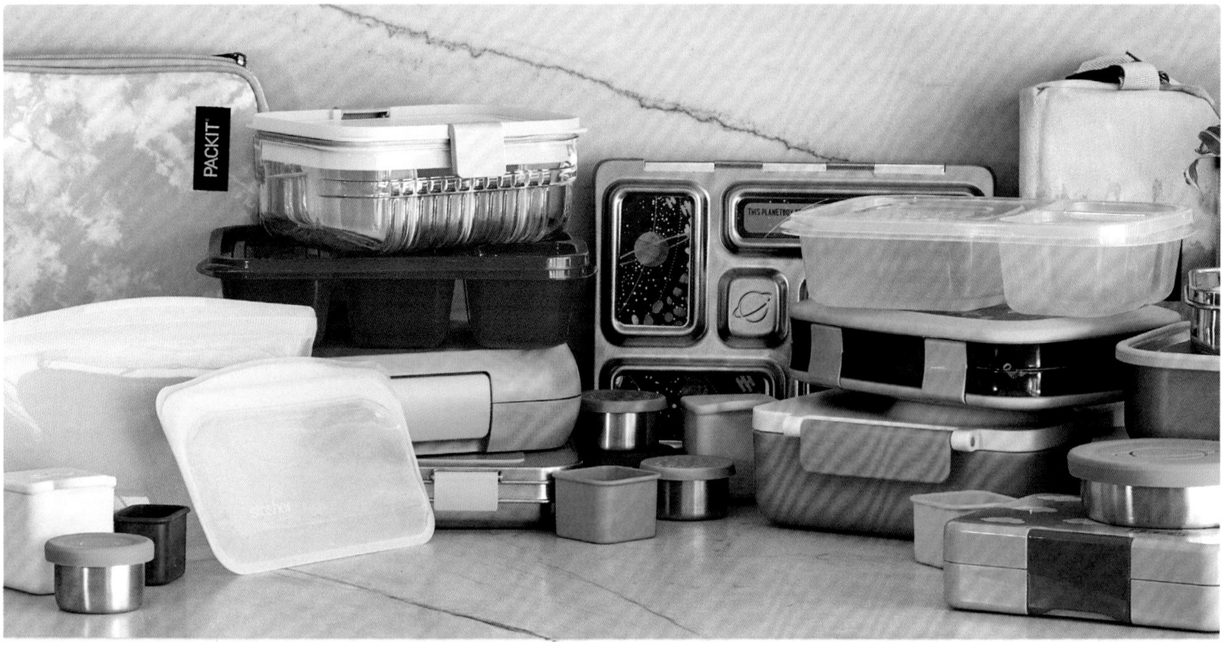

Containers

In this book you'll see a variety of reusable lunch boxes and containers that can be purchased at varying price points. We hope to normalize packing lunches in reusable containers for both environmental and cost reasons, and our goal is to show you how to use them successfully for kids of all ages.

However, we recognize that for some families disposable lunches might be the only option. We do have some examples of this throughout the book. *Please know that you do not need to use fancy or expensive containers to make a delicious, satisfying lunch.* For example, the Bentgo Easyboxes (formerly EasyLunchboxes brand) are featured heavily in this book and cost about $4 each.

Many of the containers you'll see feature multiple compartments that fully seal when closed. This prevents leaking and allows food to stay fresh as it jumbles around in your child's backpack during the day. Leakproof containers are key: There's nothing worse than opening up your lunch to find that raspberry juice has spilled into your turkey sandwich!

NOTE ***One important note about containers:*** **Make sure your child can open and close them before heading off to school. Many day-care and preschool teachers help students open containers, but kids are usually on their own once they get to elementary school. Practice opening and closing their lunch box with them before school starts. If you're sending a yogurt tube, prepackaged string cheese, a drink box, or other food in a package, make sure they know how to open it or ask for help. The same goes for any fruit that needs peeling.**

USE THIS QR CODE for discounts on the products used in this book.

https://sites.prh.com/feedinglittleslunches
Penguin Random House collects and processes your personal information. See our Notice at Collection and Privacy Policy at prh.com/notice.

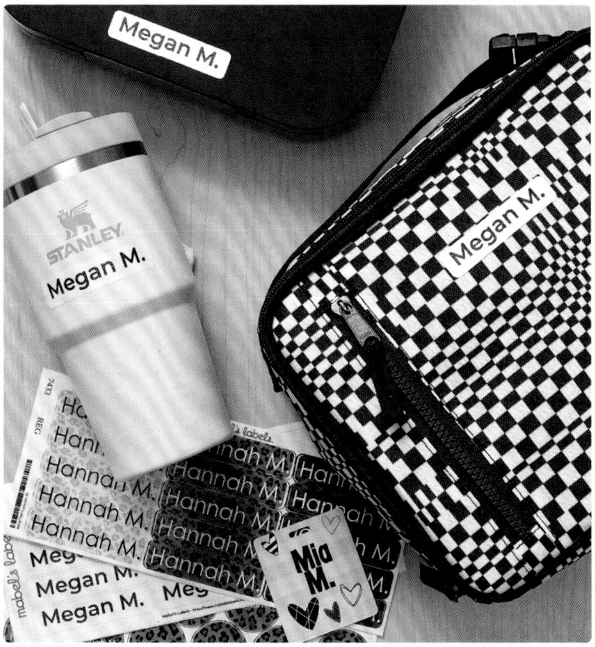

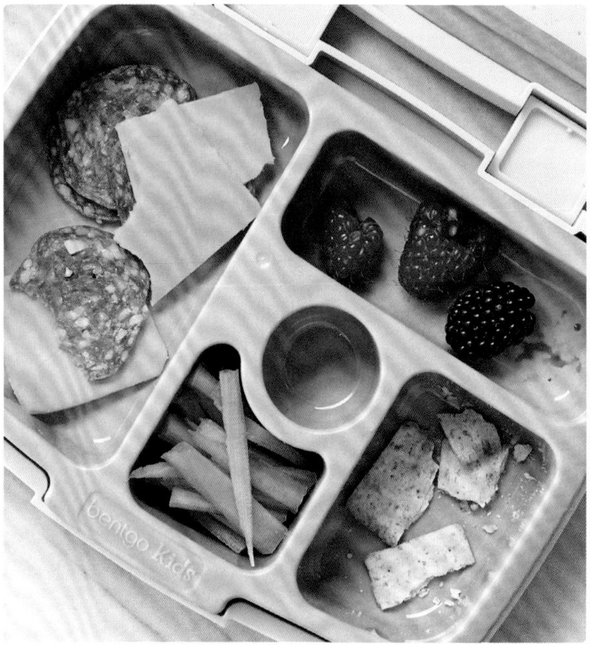

Labels

Kids lose stuff at school, period. Even though they might love their new water bottle, three of their buddies might have the same one. Make sure to label all their lunch gear, including their lunch box, lunch bag, any ice packs, utensils, and water bottles. We have used and loved Mabel's Labels since 2015 and are always impressed by their durability.

USE THIS QR CODE to check out exclusive product discounts.

https://sites.prh.com/feedinglittleslunches
Penguin Random House collects and processes your personal information. See our Notice at Collection and Privacy Policy at prh.com/notice.

What About Food Waste?

It's so frustrating when kids come home with a full lunch box. This is a reality for many families because the school lunch environment can be distracting and overwhelming. Unfortunately, food waste can be an inherent part of feeding kids. There are no guarantees that they'll eat their lunch, even if you send all their favorite foods.

If your child usually throws away uneaten food, it's OK to ask them to keep it in their lunch box and bring it home. This can help you understand which foods they're enjoying and which ones they're struggling with.

If you want to eat or repurpose uneaten lunch food, make sure it's a safe temperature when it comes home. Food should be below 41 degrees Fahrenheit to be safe to eat. When kids don't have time to finish their lunch, they may like to eat it after school as a snack—just make sure it has maintained a safe temperature.

Lunch Box Cleaning Tips

One of the worst parts about making lunches in reusable containers is cleaning them up afterward. Small compartments can be difficult to clean effectively, and it gets tedious doing it day in and day out. Here are our favorite tips:

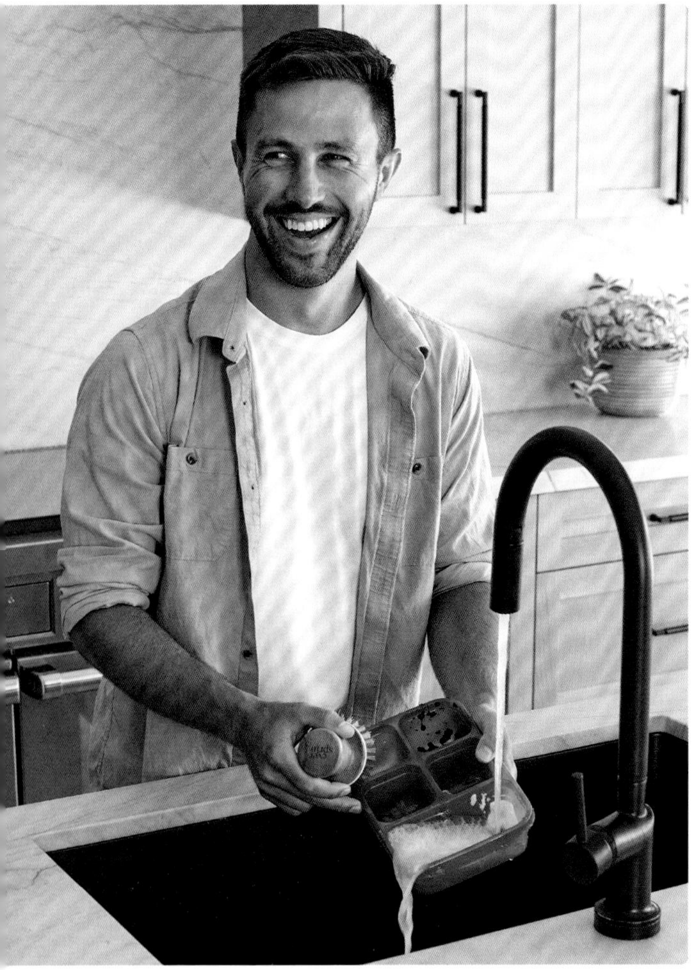

1. If you have a **leakproof or fully sealed container** like Bentgo brand, store it slightly opened or disassembled after you wash it until you know it is completely dry. If there is any liquid inside, it can grow into mold if you leave it closed for a prolonged period, just like any other fully sealed container with moisture inside.

2. If possible, **buy more than one lunch box** so you don't have to hand-wash each box every day and can rely on the dishwasher (if appropriate for the box you purchased).

3. **Take the box apart** before cleaning, if possible. It's easier to clean, and food or water won't get trapped inside it.

4. **Wash your child's lunch box** when you're cleaning up after dinner. You already have soap and water—what's one more container?

5. Use a brush, sponge, or scrubber to **get into the crevices** of your child's lunch box, especially if it has a lot of compartments. Many lunch boxes are thankfully dishwasher-safe.

6. **To clean insulated lunch bags,** use mild soap and water and follow the manufacturer's instructions. Many lunch bags look brand-new with a little cleaning.

Tips for Making Packed Lunches More Affordable

- **YOU DON'T NEED TO BUY** *every single thing* you see in this book. Quite the contrary, actually. Pick a few fruits and a few veggies each week, and alternate through a few different protein/starch options. This adds some natural variety without costing a lot of money.
- **VEGETARIAN SOURCES OF PROTEIN CAN BE LESS EXPENSIVE** than meat-based ones. Try beans, lentils, nut/seed butters, tofu, or hard-boiled eggs.
- **BUY SEASONALLY WHEN YOU CAN.** It's generally less expensive and tastes better.
- **TAKE ADVANTAGE OF LEFTOVERS.** Extra cooked pasta can be turned into a cold pasta salad for lunch the next day. Leftover shredded chicken is awesome in a quesadilla or as a chicken salad wrap.
- **BUYING FRESH FOOD IN BULK IS GREAT TO MINIMIZE COST,** but if you can't eat it before it goes bad, it's a waste of money. Check online for produce storage guides to maximize the life of your fruits and veggies. We love to do a vinegar soak on berries—simply soak them in one part white vinegar, three parts water for a few minutes, and then rinse and dry completely before storing them in the original container lined on the bottom with a paper towel. Strawberries last more than a week this way!
- **IF POSSIBLE, USE A REUSABLE LUNCH CONTAINER.** The cost of disposable plastic sandwich bags adds up over time.
- **USE CANNED OR JARRED FRUITS AND VEGGIES.** They'll stay in your pantry for a long time and are great options when you don't have anything fresh. Plus, they're cheaper than fresh produce.
- **KEEP PORTIONS SMALL,** especially for foods your child doesn't eat a ton of. It's OK to put two slices of cucumber in their lunch if they rarely touch their veggies. You're still exposing them to that vegetable without overwhelming them. Bonus: They are more likely to eat it if it's just a piece or two anyway.

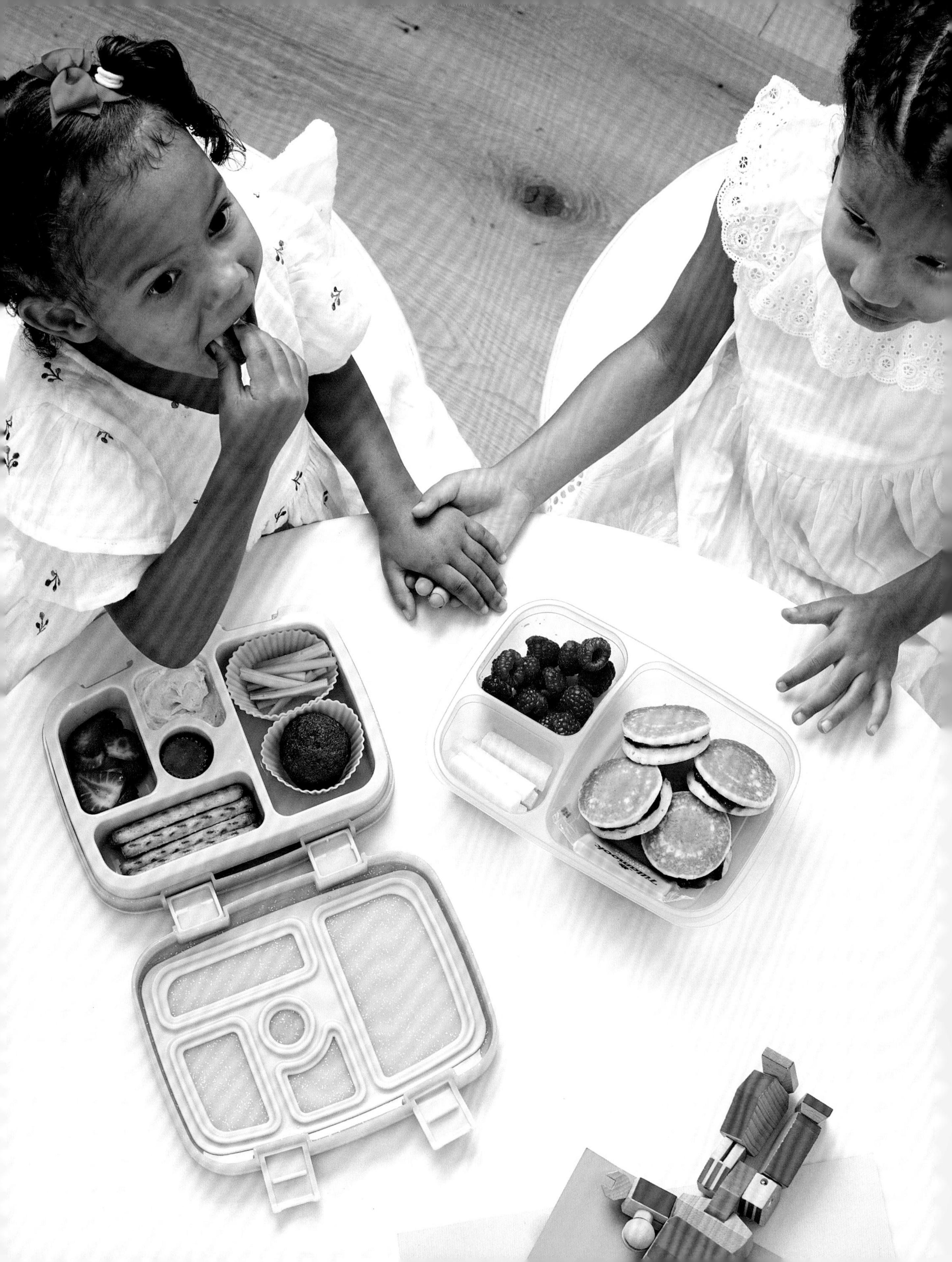

The Cafeteria Social Experience

You might not remember the food that you ate at school, but you probably have vivid memories of things that happened in the school cafeteria. School lunch is a very social experience, one that can significantly affect how your child eats. Even the most easygoing kids can struggle with lunchtime because of the behavioral and social challenges the lunchroom presents.

We want you to know that it's very, *very* common for kids to eat differently at school than at home. There are many social, environmental, and behavioral factors at play—it's no wonder kids come home with full lunch boxes, even if you send their favorite foods.

Here are a few reasons why lunch at school might be different than lunch at home:

- **Many schools schedule only twenty minutes to eat,** which go by quickly when kids also need to buy food or want to socialize.
- **Oftentimes recess is scheduled after lunch,** so kids who are itching to get outside eat the bare minimum before packing it all up.
- **Lunch might be the only time your child has to socialize** with certain friends. This can distract them from the important job of eating.
- **Conversely, lunch might be a difficult social experience** if your child is struggling to make friends or get along with classmates, or is experiencing bullying.
- Sometimes lunch is scheduled at a time when **your child might not be hungry.** At Megan's kids' school, lunch in kindergarten starts at 10:15 a.m.
- **Food shaming or pressure** from teachers can affect how much your child eats.

If you ever get a chance to volunteer in your child's lunchroom, take it. You'll be fascinated to see how much this unique environment—with all its social challenges—affects your kid's eating habits. How can you help your child if they're not eating well at school?

- **If your child is verbal, ask them what's up.** "I noticed that you're not eating much of your lunch. Can you tell me why?" You might be surprised by their response.
- **Let your child help you pack their lunch** (depending on their age). Offer choices—"Strawberries or blueberries?"—and let them assemble food when possible. When they're involved in making the choice, they're more likely to eat their food.
- **Read children's books about kids overcoming adversity at lunchtime.** We love *Carla's Sandwich* by Debbie Herman, *Lailah's Lunchbox* by Reem Faruqi, and *The Invisible Boy* by Trudy Ludwig, but there are so many great books available.
- **Talk to their teachers or lunchroom workers,** especially if your child is getting pressured to eat or if they're experiencing bullying for the types of food in their lunch box. They likely have very important insights on what's happening.

SCAN THIS QR CODE to access a free printable you can give to your child's teachers or lunchroom staff that addresses some common issues.

https://sites.prh.com/feedinglittleslunches

Five Tips Teachers Want Parents to Know About School Lunch

BY SUSIE ALLISON, EdM, @BUSYTODDLER

School cafeterias are a happening place, buzzing with midday kid energy. Getting kids to eat during all that fun and excitement is critical to their school-day health. Whether your child has been in day care, in preschool, or at home, the school cafeteria is something else, something big, and something new. Setting up kids for success in this new eating environment is key.

Since it may have been a few years since you last ate in a school cafeteria (wink), here are five lunchroom tips, tricks, and things you need to know.

BUT FIRST, READ THIS: Your child's lunchtime may be shorter than you remember or expect, or what your child is used to. Between walking kids to the cafeteria, finding their seat, opening the lunch box, and cleaning up for dismissal at the end, the actual time for eating gets shrunk down big-time. Sometimes students have only ten to fifteen minutes of actual dedicated eating time. It's important to note this as you consider your child's at-school lunch.

1. Don't let yourself (or your child) be startled by this short time for lunch. Talk to school officials, current students, or their parents about the lunchroom. Find out approximately how much time kids have to actually eat, and plan accordingly.

2. Practice eating lunch at home using a lunch you plan to send before the school year begins. Think of this as a dress rehearsal (but practice often). See how long it takes your child to eat the food you pack for them. Adjust what you plan to pack, if needed.

3. Make sure your child can feed themselves the lunch you pack and clean it up at the end. During your trial run of lunches, check that your child is able to scoop, cut, or pour (for example) the food you send; can use any packed utensils on their own; and is able to clean up and repack the lunch box at the end.

4. Lunchrooms are supervised and staffed by a limited number of adults and *usually not the classroom teacher.* This means there aren't enough adults to assist each child with their lunch. Although these adults want to help, a child waiting for assistance from them wastes valuable eating time. (Note: In preschool settings, teachers are usually able to help kids with their lunch, so this applies more to an elementary school cafeteria.)

5. Expect lunches to come home with leftover food, especially on the first few days of school as kids adjust and you adjust to what they need, will eat, or have time to eat. Make sure to bring a snack to pickup or have one ready at home. Kids come back from a day at school next-level hungry.

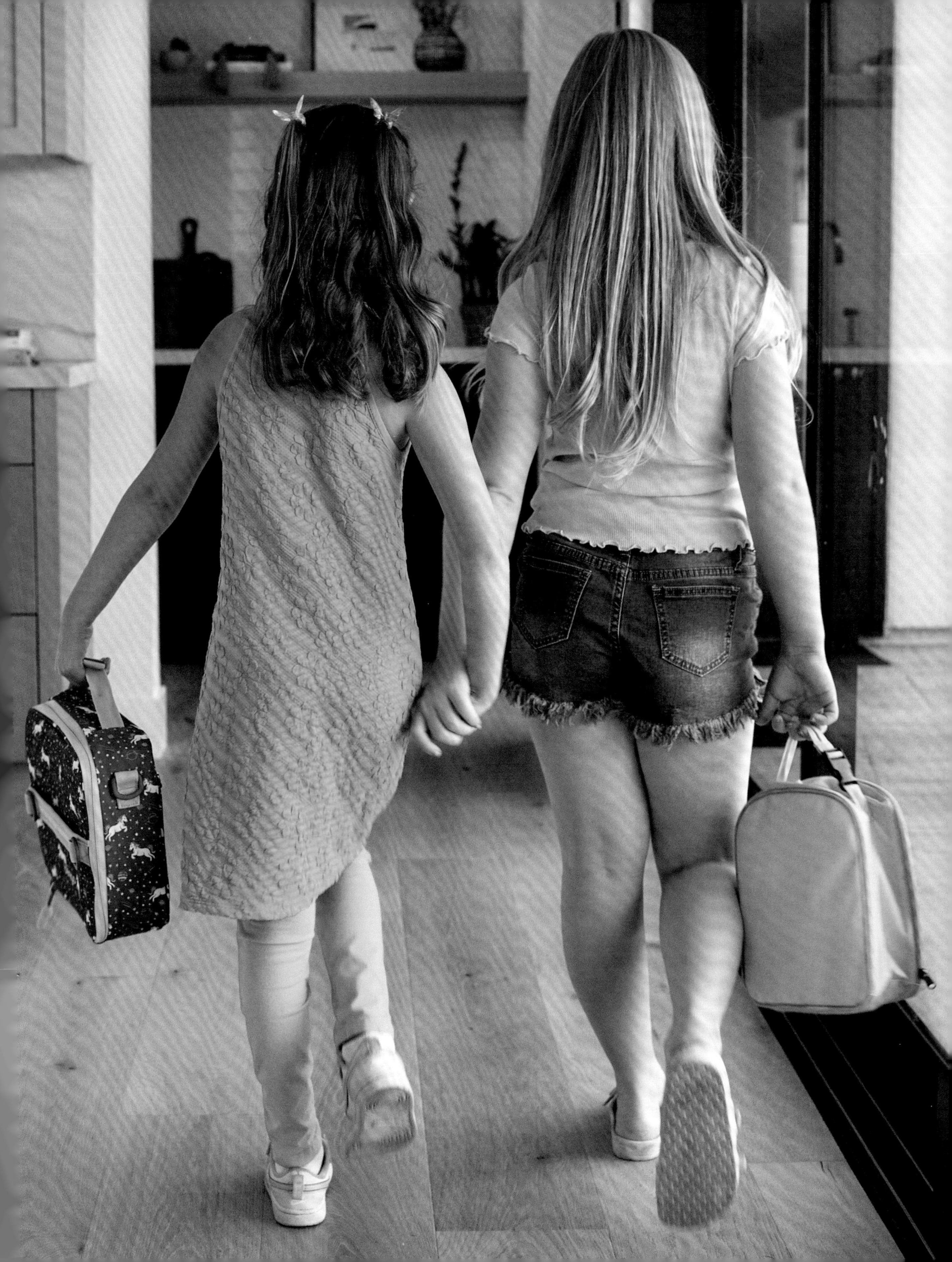

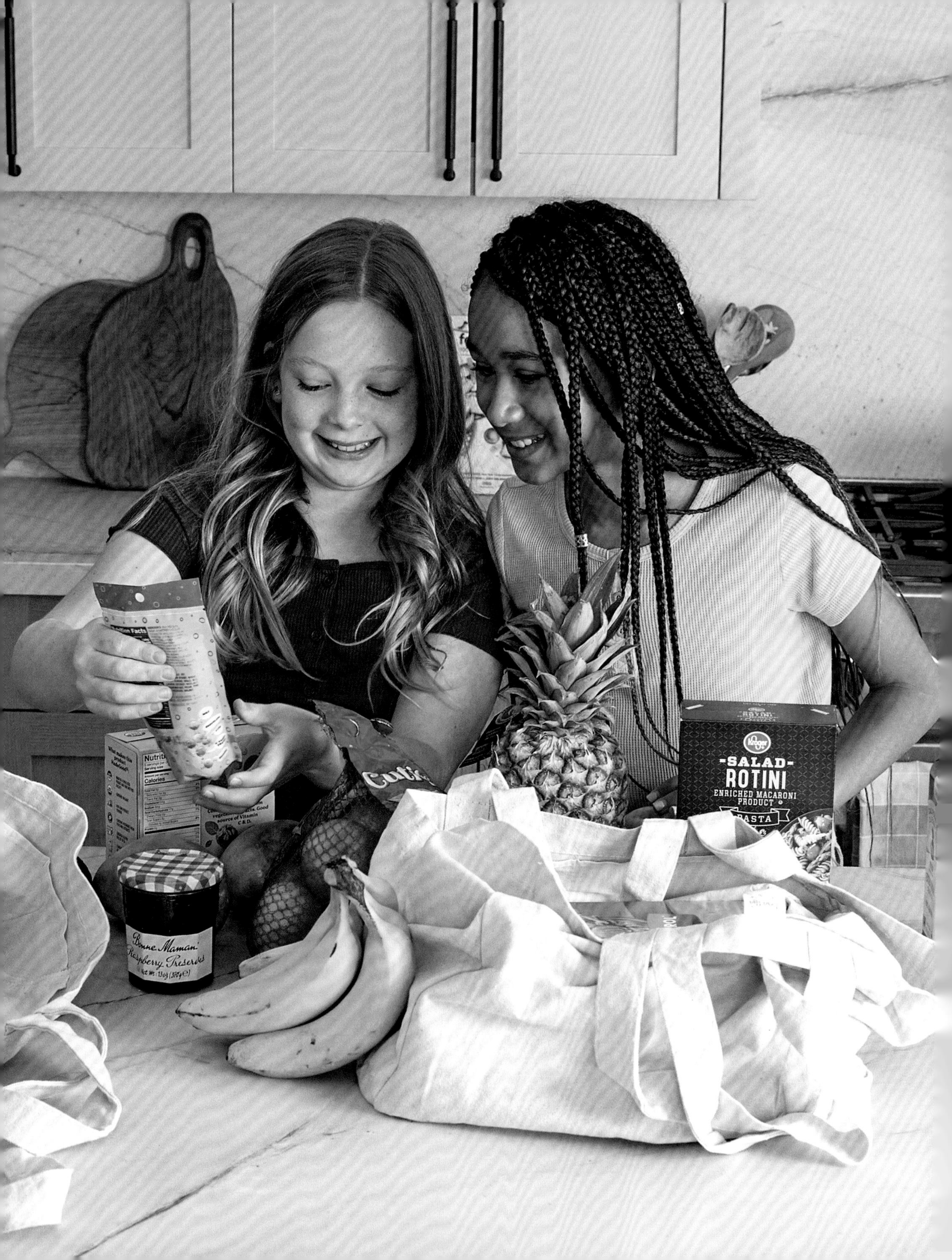
-SALAD-
ROTINI
ENRICHED MACARONI PRODUCT
PASTA
Bonne Maman
Raspberry Preserves

Lunches at Home

Is your child at home for lunch every day? These lunch ideas can still be useful. Whether your kids are too young for school or you're homeschooling, we all need to eat midday. If you're eating at home, simply serve these ideas on a plate.

However, packing a lunch can still be helpful even if your kids aren't going off to school or day care. It's nice to have food ready and waiting when you come home from a morning outing, especially if your toddler needs to take a nap quickly. Many of our homeschooling friends pack lunches every morning to allow more flexibility in their day. During the COVID-19 pandemic, Megan packed lunches for her virtual learners. It kept them in the lunchtime routine and saved time during the school day.

"Can My Kids Pack Their Own Lunch?"

Depending on your child's age and skill level, you might want them to pack their own lunch. This saves you time, helps them learn an important skill, and increases the likelihood that they'll eat their lunch.

In teaching kids to pack their own lunch, it helps to emphasize the Feeding Littles Lunch Formula: a starch, a protein, a fruit, and a veggie. Add a dessert, dip, and/or chips if you'd like. To help your kids visualize this, check out the QR code for a free printable you can customize and hang in your kitchen.

https://sites.prh.com/feedinglittleslunches

ADDITIONAL TIPS FOR KIDS WHO WANT TO PACK THEIR OWN LUNCH

1. If the idea of your kid packing their own lunch makes you cringe **because it would take an hour and cause a huge mess in the kitchen, you can instead have them help with something small. It doesn't have to be all-or-nothing. Give them a choice of what fruit to pack, or let them pick out their dessert. If your child is still working on knife skills or cannot safely use a kitchen knife, they can still participate in packing their own lunch. Let them wash and dry produce, assemble sandwiches, pick out a dessert, or place food in their lunch box.**

2. Decide if you want to let your child pick every part of their lunch **or if you want to make some decisions too. You can say, "We're going to include carrots—which dip do you want?" or "Here are the carrots for your lunch. How should we cut them?"**

3. To make this process more streamlined **for younger kids, line up all the components on the countertop so your child can focus on getting lunch prepped and in their lunch box. As they get older, they'll get more efficient at knowing where to find and put away food.**

4. This gets easier with time and practice. **In a few years, your child will be able to make a balanced, delicious lunch all by themselves, especially if they have been helping you do it all along!**

CHECK OUT THE QR CODE on the left for a free, fun printable you can customize to help your child pack their own nutritious, delicious lunch.

Picky Eaters

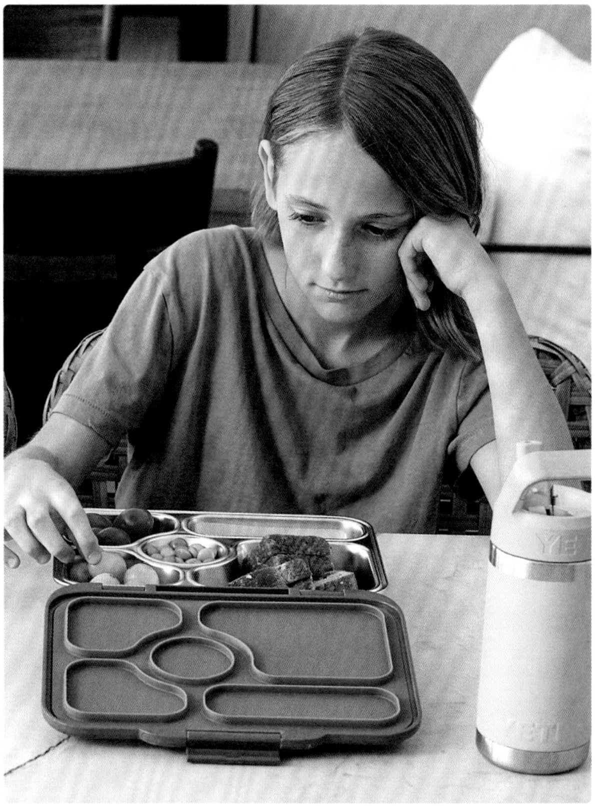

Does your child shun entire food groups or refuse new foods? You're definitely not the only one dealing with this. Research suggests that somewhere between 20 and 50 percent of kids can be described as picky eaters.

Picky eating can be typical behavior to some extent in childhood. Many kids go through phases where they gravitate toward one type of food (like beige, crunchy foods) or don't love trying new things. This often starts in toddlerhood and can come in waves. You might notice that your child loves tomatoes today and rejects them tomorrow. This is considered expected behavior.

Some researchers think that picky eating is actually a biological protective mechanism. Picky eating usually begins when toddlers become more mobile and able to wander off on their own. If they did not have an inherent skepticism of new foods, they might willingly eat the poisonous berry or mushroom while wandering through the forest. Their picky eating could be what keeps them safe.

Of course, this skepticism of new foods might not be necessary in the modern world, but it's helpful to know that some level of selective eating is likely hardwired in our kids.

For some children, picky eating is more than a nuisance—it affects every aspect of their life. When kids become extremely limited in what they will eat; when they continue to drop previously accepted foods; when they struggle to chew or swallow; when they refuse to touch certain textures; or when they have medical, neurological, or developmental issues affecting eating, it might be time to seek help. Judy recommends an evaluation for kids who eat less than a total of twenty foods. (She counts Cheerios and crispy rice cereal, for example, as two separate foods.) Our Toddler & Kid course, found at feedinglittles.com, can be a great first step for picky eating, and we recommend talking to your health-care provider about a feeding evaluation by a trained professional.

One key technique we use with picky eaters? *Exposure.* Some kids need to see and touch a new food ten to fifteen-plus times before they'll want to eat it. (Annoying, right?) The more a child sees a food, the closer they come to eating it eventually.

This doesn't mean that we have to obsess about new foods or count exposures. It also doesn't mean that our kids will like every food we offer them. For many kids, eating new foods takes time and requires seeing food a lot before they actually eat it.

The concept of exposure is why our Feeding Littles Lunch Formula has a starch, a protein, a veggie, *and* a fruit—it gives us a chance to expose our kids to multiple different foods at each lunch.

Tips for Picky Eaters at Lunchtime

Keeping in mind that (1) picky eating is pretty common in childhood, (2) exposure is important, and (3) the hectic school lunch environment can really throw off your kid, here are some tips when you're dealing with picky eating:

- **OFFER A PREFERRED FOOD WITH EACH MEAL** so they have something they enjoy eating while at school or in day care. If everything in their lunch box is new, they might not have enough to eat at lunchtime.
- **ADD VARIETY GRADUALLY.** If you have been serving the same exact lunch every day, changes might feel overwhelming to your kid. Consider starting small. Maybe you swap out the strawberries for blueberries, or you buy a different brand of bagel. Once your child gets used to seeing a little variety in their lunch, they'll come to expect more variety over time.
- **TALK TO YOUR CHILD WHEN THEY DON'T EAT MUCH LUNCH.** Did they not enjoy their food, or were there other factors involved that prevented them from eating it? Was socializing more of a priority? Did they struggle to access their food because the containers were too difficult for them to open? If your child cannot verbalize these ideas, ask their teacher or lunchroom monitor.
- **GET THEM INVOLVED IN PACKING THEIR LUNCH.** Give them a few choices ("Vanilla yogurt or lemon yogurt?") and let them put food in their own lunch box. When kids participate and share ownership in the process, they're more likely to eat their meal.
- **HAVE A SUBSTANTIAL SNACK READY AT PICKUP.** Most kids are hungry at school pickup, no matter what time you pick them up or what they ate for lunch, and it's especially helpful to have a hearty snack after school if your child struggles at lunchtime.
- **STAY PATIENT.** Learning to eat a variety of foods takes time. Try not to get frustrated when your child doesn't eat *all the things*. They're not being purposefully difficult or disrespectful to your cooking (or the money spent on food)—they might be struggling with textures or flavors. Instead of labeling them as a "picky eater," you could say they're "learning to love new foods" on their own terms.

NOTE **Even very adventurous eaters come home with full lunch boxes from time to time. No matter what you serve, sometimes the school lunch environment keeps kids from eating well at lunchtime.**

Safety

Safety is twofold when it comes to packed lunches:

- Is the food a **safe temperature?**
- Is this food a **choking hazard** for my child?

Food Safety

You might have eaten warm bologna and cheese sandwiches at school as a kid, but there are actually pretty specific guidelines about food safety and packed lunch. It's recommended to send all perishable foods with *two* sources of ice in an insulated bag. This helps maintain a safe temperature (below 40 degrees Fahrenheit) until it's time to eat.

"What does this look like?" Place an ice pack above and below your child's lunch container and put them all in an insulated bag, if possible. You can also use a lunch bag with built-in ice packs or use a frozen beverage as one of your child's ice sources. Conversely, some schools store all lunches in refrigerators, so you don't have to send your child's lunch with ice packs.

"How do I know if foods are perishable and need to be kept cold?" According to the USDA, "Items that don't require refrigeration include whole fruits and vegetables, hard cheese, canned meat and fish, chips, breads, crackers, peanut butter, jelly, mustard, and pickles."* So, if you send any cut-up produce, dairy, meat, poultry, or fish, it must be kept cold to stay safe. Megan tends to err on the side of caution and adds ice packs to every lunch she sends.

Check out page 66 for non-perishable lunch ideas that can be sent on field trips or when your child will be unable to keep their lunch cold.

"What about sending hot food?" An insulated container designed for hot food is a must.

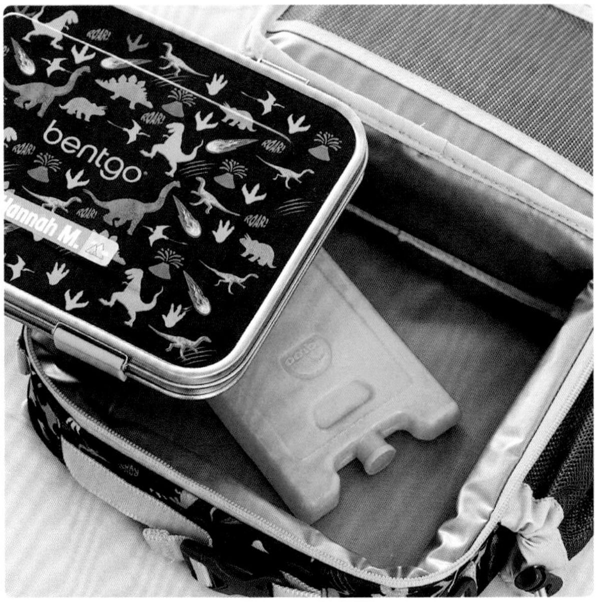

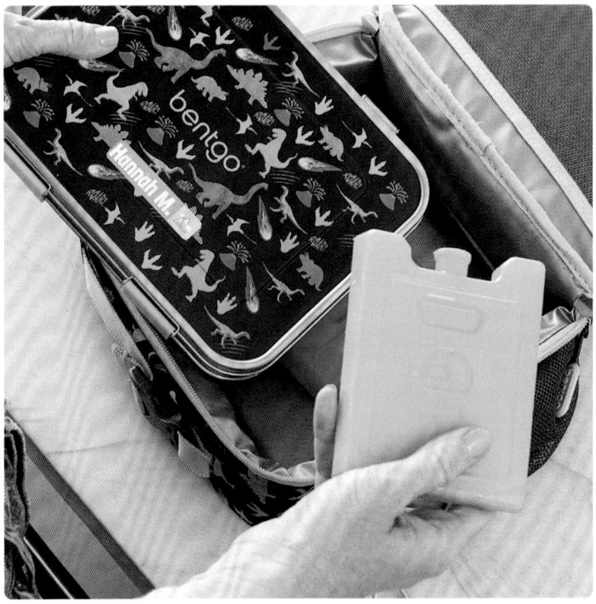

According to the USDA, fill your insulated container with boiling water and let it stand for a few minutes. Pour the water out of the container, then add piping-hot food. To stay warm, the food needs to be saucy. Think soup, stew, oatmeal, casseroles, pasta with sauce, chili, or curry. Foods like chicken nuggets, rice, plain pasta, or eggs won't stay hot even if you put them in a warmed container.

* "Keeping 'Bag' Lunches Safe," FSIS, USDA, www.fsis.usda.gov/food-safety/safe-food-handling-and-preparation/food-safety-basics/keeping-bag-lunches-safe.

NOTE We have not tested lunch containers to guarantee that they stay hot enough (above 140 degrees Fahrenheit) until lunchtime. If you are sending hot food, you might want to test out how long your container keeps that food hot.

"What if my school can heat up my child's lunch in the microwave?" Awesome! We recommend microwaving in glass or another material labeled Microwave Safe. Some schools even remove food from its container to put on a plate and microwave. Avoid using single-use plastics in the microwave, as chemicals in the plastic can leach into food. If you microwave in plastic, make sure it's labeled for microwave-oven use.

The majority of our audience sends cold lunches all or most of the time, so in this book you'll see many options for cold lunch. However, we have included a number of items that can be served hot or cold.

Choking Hazards

Choking hazards are foods that have a higher risk of blocking a child's airway and making it difficult or impossible to breathe. These foods are considered hazards until kids are age four, but if your child has any oral-motor challenges or a history of choking, you might want to modify foods beyond that age.

The following lists include choking-hazard foods compiled from various sources. The sources differ in their guidance on certain foods (specifically chips, celery, carrots, and apples), but since we've seen many issues with these foods in practice, we have included them in our list.

In the end, you know your kid best and must decide which foods you feel comfortable sending to school. Remember that your child might not be as closely supervised at school as they are at home, so choking hazards are especially important to pay attention to. We have also noted choking hazards throughout the lunch ideas in this book.

CHOKING-HAZARD FOODS

Modify these foods until age four:

- Hot dogs or sausage links—cut into small pieces (not rounds)
- Whole nuts—offer as thinly spread (not spoonful of) nut butter or as ground nuts
- Whole grapes, cherries, or cherry tomatoes—cut into quarters lengthwise
- Large hard carrots or celery—soften by cooking until fork-tender, grate, or cut into thin pieces
- Whole apples—soften by cooking, grate, or cut into thin pieces
- Hard pears—soften by cooking, grate, or cut into thin pieces
- Hard dried fruit—soften by cooking (put in oatmeal, baked goods)
- Whole olives—cut into quarters lengthwise
- Marshmallows—bake into foods
- Large chunks of hard meat or hard cheese—cut into smaller pieces

Avoid these foods until age four:

- Whole large seeds
- Popcorn
- Hard candy
- Gummy bear candy
- Sticky candy—taffy, fruit leather
- Chewing gum
- Hard chips (potato chips, tortilla chips)

Modifying Choking Hazards

Many popular lunch foods are choking hazards for kids under four. To keep these foods safe for your toddler, we recommend making these modifications:

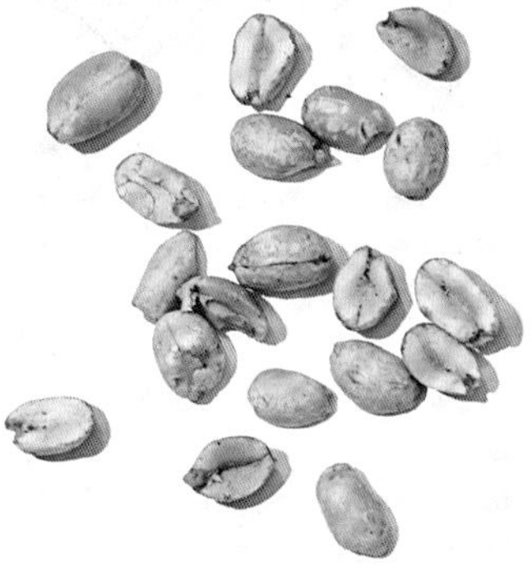
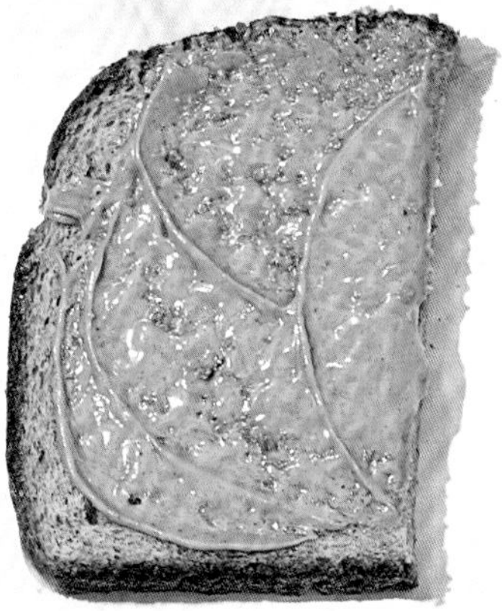

whole nuts, peanuts, or large seeds → thinly spread nut butter, peanut butter, or seed butter

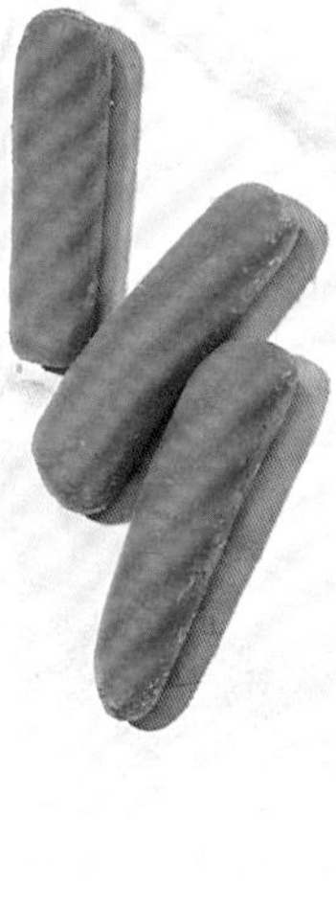
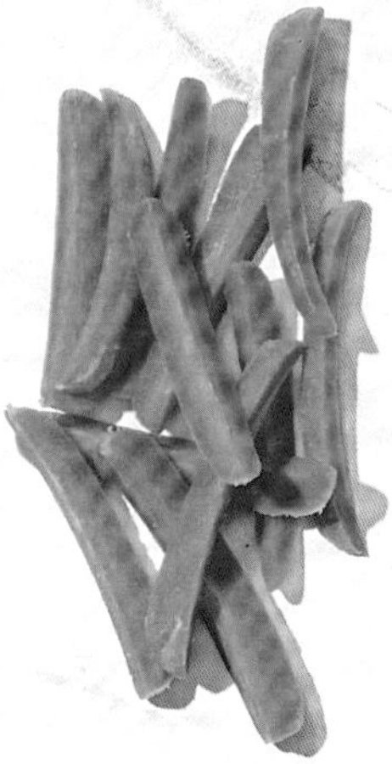
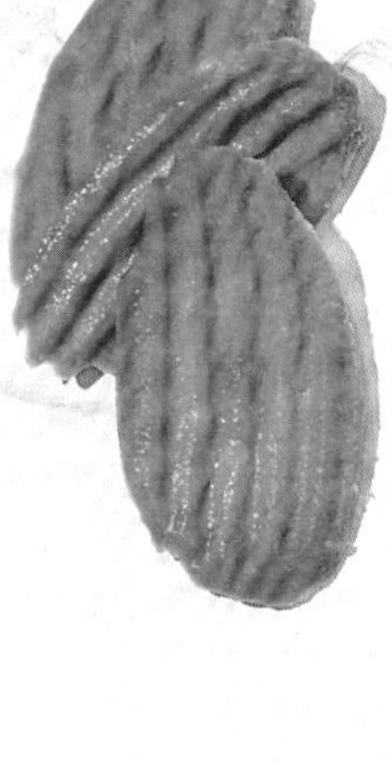
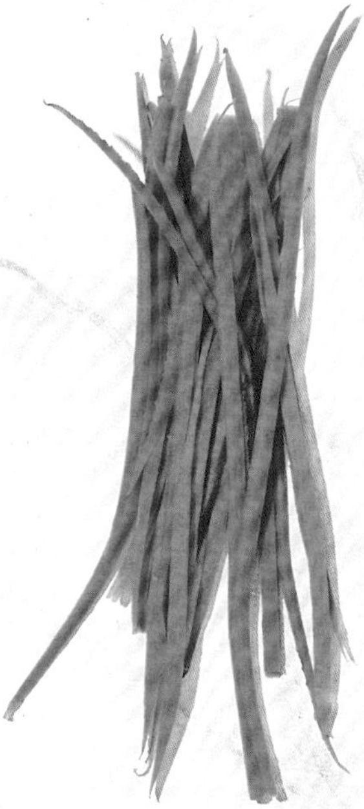

raw baby carrots → thinly cut carrots/carrot chips/shredded carrots

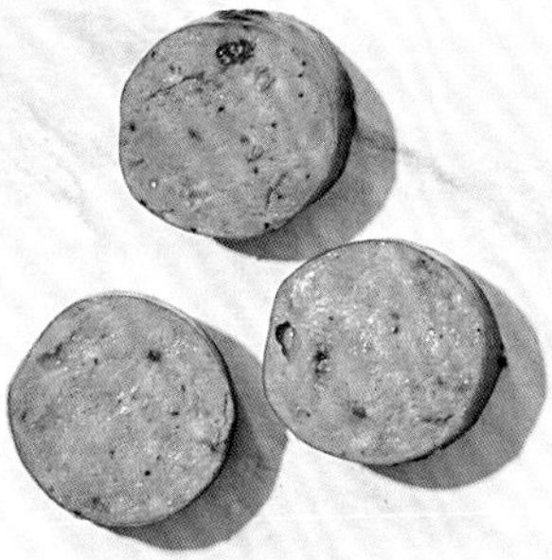

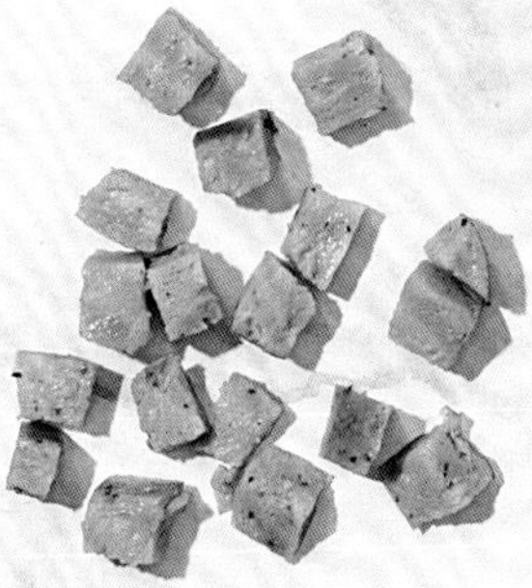

sausage cut into coins → diced sausage

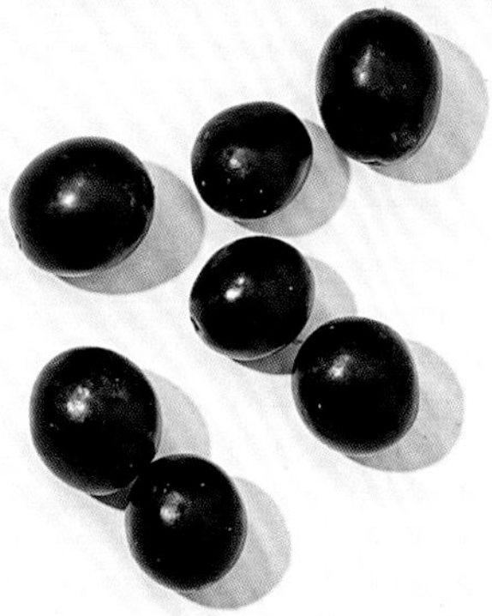

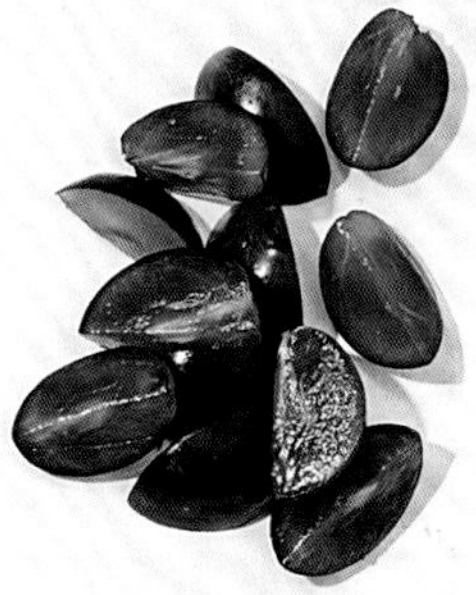

whole grapes → grapes quartered lengthwise

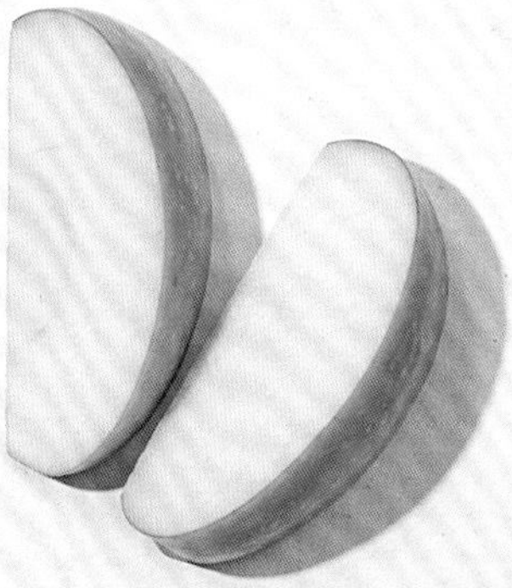

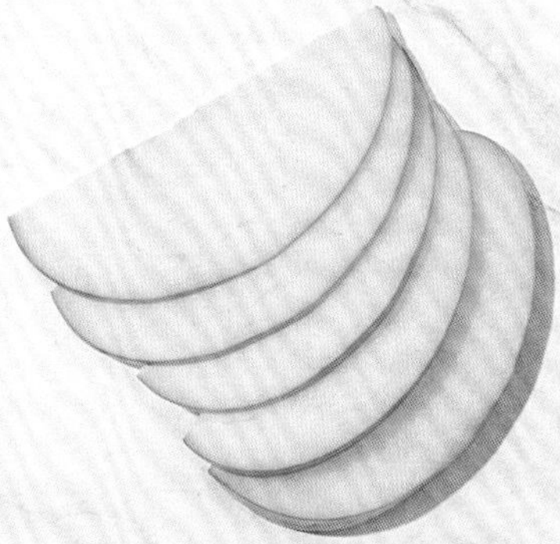

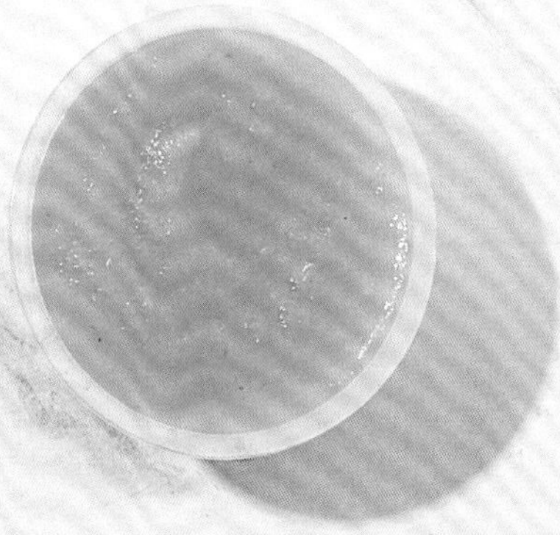

thick apple slices → thin apple slices/applesauce

Food Allergies

Food allergies can be so difficult, and we want this book to be a resource both for allergy families and for parents who need guidance on what *not* to pack, based on allergy restrictions at their school.

Kathlena, The Allergy Chef (@theallergychef), has collaborated with us on this section and has reviewed all the allergy swaps in the lunch ideas. We are enormously grateful for her contribution and expertise in this area.

One in every thirteen children in the United States has a food allergy. This translates to about two kids per standard-size classroom, according to Food Allergy Research and Education. For some kids, food allergy reactions are minor. For others, they're life-threatening.

Kids (and adults) can be allergic to any food. Judy, for example, is allergic to avocados, mangoes, strawberries, walnuts, and a host of other delicious things. Megan is allergic to eggplant. While allergies can be all over the board, the majority of food allergies (90 percent) are found in the top nine allergens.

NOTE **FOR OUR EUROPEAN FRIENDS: The list above refers to allergens as defined in the United States. In Europe, the list is much larger and encompasses what they define as the top fourteen allergens: cereals containing gluten (wheat, rye, barley, oat); crustaceans (for example, prawns, crab, lobster, crayfish); eggs; fish; peanuts; soybeans; milk; nuts; celery (including celeriac); mustard; sesame; sulfur dioxide/sulfites; lupin, which includes lupin seeds and flour (which can be found in some breads, pastries, and pasta); and mollusks (for example, clams, mussels, oysters, snails, and squid). For the purposes of this book, we reference the top nine allergens only.**

THE TOP NINE ALLERGENS

1. **Wheat**
2. **Milk**
3. **Egg**
4. **Soy**
5. **Peanuts**
6. **Tree nuts**
7. **Fish**
8. **Shellfish**
9. **Sesame**

Some schools do not have an allergy policy, and students are allowed to bring in any type of food. Other schools or individual classrooms have restrictions on certain allergens, the most common being peanuts and tree nuts.

If your school is "peanut-free," it means that whole peanuts, peanut butter, and all peanut products (like Bamba puffed snack) are not allowed.

Some schools go a step further and enforce a "no-nut" policy, which generally means no peanuts *and* no tree nuts. Tree nuts include almonds, cashews, pistachios, macadamia nuts, walnuts, pine nuts, etc., so when a school is entirely nut-free, parents have to be conscious of more than just peanuts. (For those in the know, peanuts are technically legumes, not nuts, but they're considered a nut when talking about "nut-free" policies. Confusing, right?)

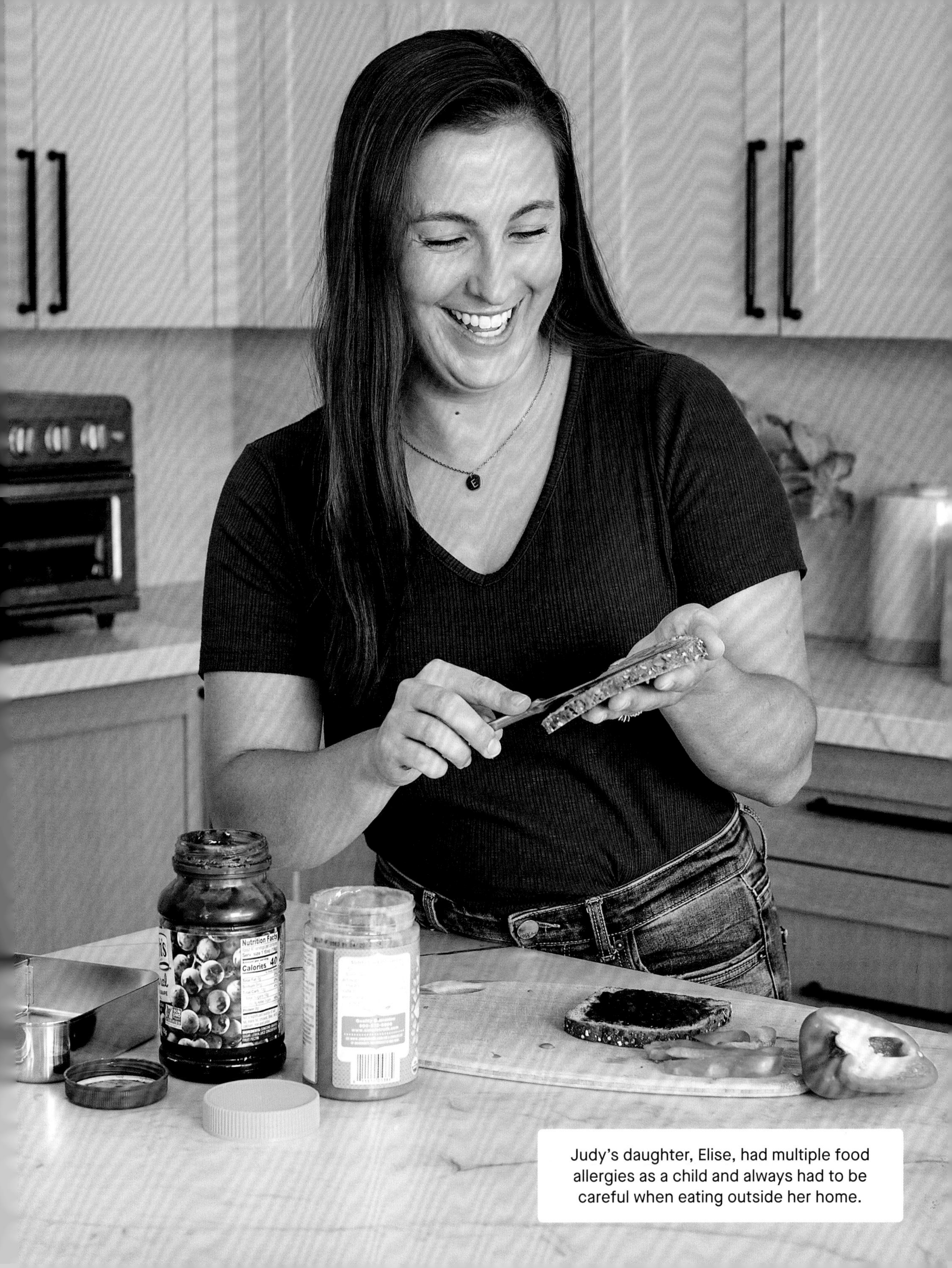

Judy's daughter, Elise, had multiple food allergies as a child and always had to be careful when eating outside her home.

Swaps for Food Allergens

Peanuts

PEANUT BUTTER: almond or other nut butter (if allowed), sunflower seed butter, granola butter, soy butter, chickpea butter, tiger nut butter (a tuber, NOT a tree nut)

Tree Nuts

ALMOND BUTTER: peanut butter (if allowed), sunflower seed butter, granola butter, soy butter, chickpea butter, tiger nut butter (a tuber, NOT a tree nut)

NUTELLA: chocolate sunflower seed butter, chocolate granola butter, chocolate chickpea butter

Wheat

BREAD PRODUCTS (WHOLE-GRAIN BREAD, BAGELS, OR ENGLISH MUFFINS): gluten-free bread products

PASTA: rice, quinoa, lentil, corn, or other gluten-free pasta

FLOUR TORTILLAS: corn tortillas, gluten-free tortillas, coconut tortillas, or cassava tortillas

Dairy

YOGURT: dairy-free yogurt (coconut yogurt, soy yogurt, oat yogurt, almond-based yogurt, if allowed)

CREAM CHEESE: dairy-free cream cheese or another sauce/spread like hummus (may contain sesame) or smashed avocado

CHEESE: dairy-free cheese or another sauce/spread like pesto (may contain nuts), marinara sauce, guacamole, hummus, or black bean spread

NOTE For those who are new to eating dairy-free, please don't rush into dairy-free cheese, especially if you *loved* cow's milk cheese. Dairy-free cheese has a very distinct taste, and it can be very off-putting in smell, taste, and texture for those with a point of reference to dairy. When you do choose a dairy-free cheese, if you can have tree nuts, start with a cashew-based cheese, as you may find that more enjoyable than a soy- or coconut-based cheese. You might also like specialty brands that create artisan-style, dairy-free cheese. When you're just starting out on the dairy-free path, lean into guacamole and hummus as a cheese replacement. It takes time to get used to dairy-free cheese, although many kids don't know the difference if they've been eating it their whole life.

Egg

HARD-BOILED EGG: cubed turkey or chicken, cubed tofu or beans (chickpeas, black beans)

Soy

EDAMAME: kidney beans, garbanzo beans, black beans

TERIYAKI SAUCE: soy-free teriyaki sauce or coconut aminos

Finned Fish

CANNED TUNA OR SALMON SALAD: chicken or egg salad, chickpea salad, leftover cooked chicken, deli meat

> **School can be scary for parents whose kids have food allergies, especially if their reaction to a given food is severe.**

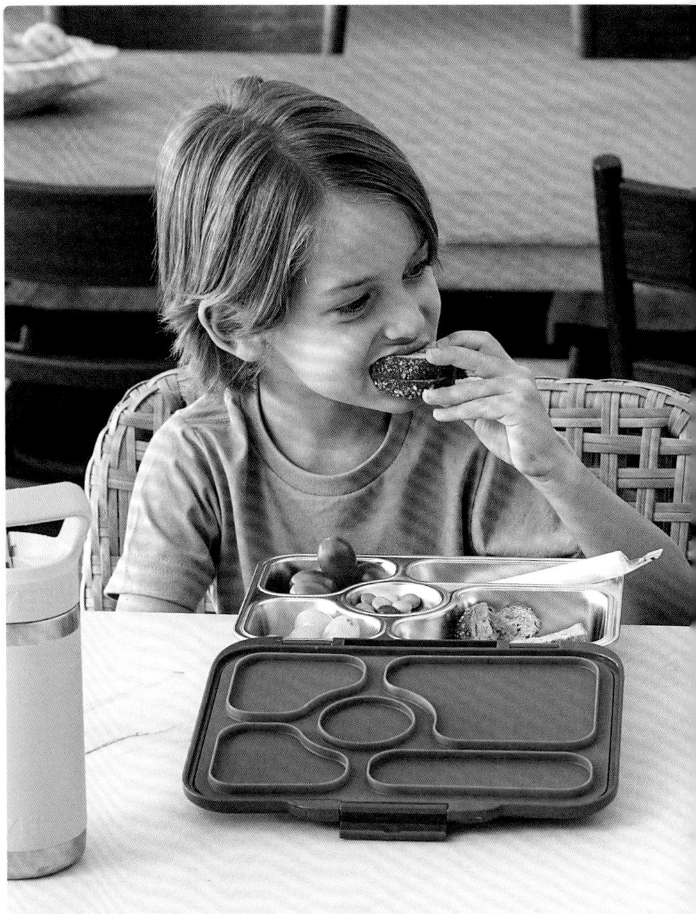

Your school might have an allergy policy that depends on the students in attendance. For example, if your child is in preschool and they eat all their meals and snacks in a classroom where no allergies are present, they might be able to bring anything to lunch. However, if a child with a peanut allergy enrolls, the school might ask parents not to send peanuts.

To err on the safe side, ask your school for clarification. If they're using the blanket term *nuts,* ask if they're referring to both tree nuts and peanuts. You might be able to send more foods than you expected.

School can be scary for parents whose kids have food allergies, especially if their reaction to a given food is severe. When classrooms or entire schools enforce allergy policies, it's for good reason—they're trying to keep vulnerable kids safe.

Not every school is allergy-friendly or nut-free, and, in some schools, kids with allergies are advised to sit at a "nut-free table" if they cannot be around peanut or tree nut products. There are pros and cons to this approach—sure, it's nice for kids who want to bring a PB&J, but it can be socially isolating for kids with allergies.

While food allergy policies help keep allergic kids safe, they can also be really challenging for families dealing with picky eating. Sometimes a peanut butter and jelly sandwich is all a kid wants to eat, and parents of picky eaters may feel frustrated that their child cannot enjoy a preferred food at school. However, the safety of everyone at school is of the utmost importance, and schools have a difficult task in managing food allergies *and* food preferences.

Throughout this book we will include alternatives to common allergens in every lunch featured. You'll see swaps for bread products, hard-boiled eggs, cheese or yogurt, soy sauce, hummus (which usually contains sesame), and more. We hope that it helps allergy families use this book effectively.

However, it is impossible to account for all allergens present in every packaged food, since a

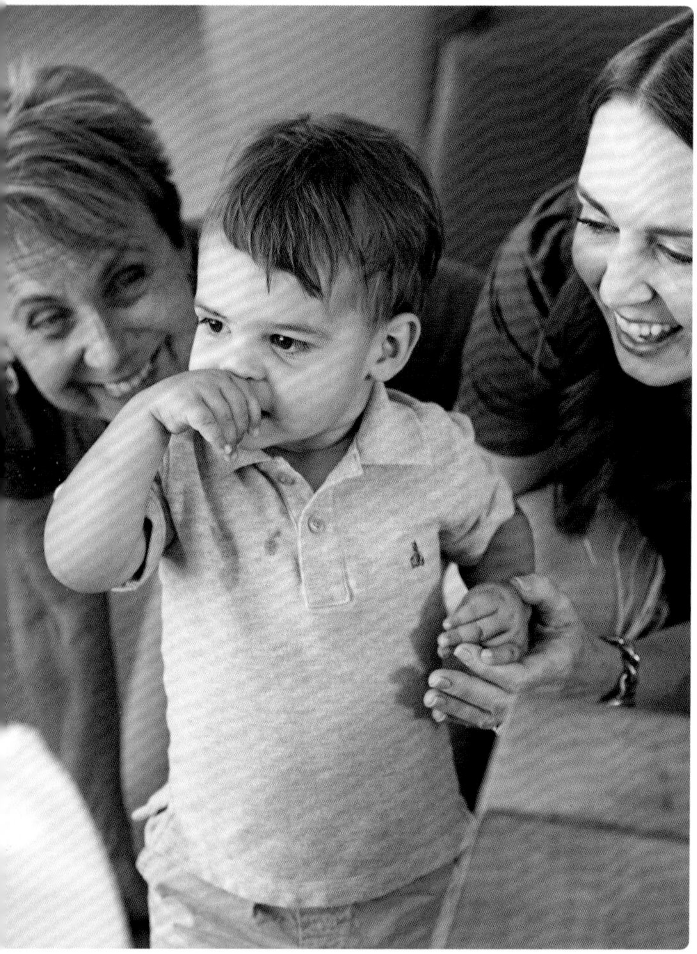

WHAT ABOUT GLUTEN?

Celiac disease means a person must avoid gluten, a protein found in wheat, rye, and barley. In the United States, oats are not considered a gluten-containing grain. In other countries, they are. Oats contain a protein called avenin, which causes reactions in approximately 25 percent of those with celiac disease.

On the other hand, a wheat allergy means a person avoids only wheat, which is what they have an allergic reaction to. They can consume rye, barley, and oats, as long as they're not processed with wheat (which is common). This means it's possible to purchase a "wheat-free" product that still contains gluten.

In this book, we offer swaps for those with a wheat allergy that are often appropriate for those avoiding gluten. As with any allergy, sensitivity, or intolerance, carefully read labels before purchasing any products. Sometimes gluten-free products still contain wheat starch.

lot of these products are purchased at your local store and are region-dependent. For example, soy and sesame are commonly present in many bread products, crackers, and snack foods. We assume that parents of kids with soy and sesame allergies already carefully review ingredient lists of everything they buy. We do not include a caveat on every lunch that soy, sesame, or another allergen might be present in certain store-bought foods—if we did, we'd be repeating ourselves for every single lunch.

Instead, we're identifying allergens when they are obviously present. For example, if a lunch features hummus, which contains sesame in the form of tahini, we offer a swap for the hummus. We just don't say, "Also check your pita bread for sesame" since we hope you're already doing that if you have allergies in your family.

While you might not be able to make every single lunch in this book, we hope that many of them are safe for your child and add some variety to their usual lineup. For those managing multiple allergies, some of the swaps we suggest may not be possible. Use products that are safe for you where you can and build on the lunch from there. Be sure to check out the Allergy Guide QR code for product ideas, a few base recipes, and additional resources.

https://sites.prh.com/feedinglittleslunches

Teachers, School Staff, and Their Role in Lunches

Before we start this section, we want to emphasize one important thing: Teachers and school staff are *angels*. They are incredible humans who give so much of their time, heart, and energy to raising the next generation of humans. They foster curiosity and a love of learning. They guide our kids from childhood into adulthood with so much care and attention.

Thank you, teachers and school staff, for your incredible contribution to our world. We know that your job is very difficult.

Preschool teachers and school cafeteria staff can have a big impact on how or what your child eats at school. They have the difficult task of ensuring that a bunch of kids safely eat their lunches so they can return to playing and learning, and with so many different personalities and eating styles, it can be tough.

To further complicate this, in some preschools parents ask teachers to "make sure" their kids eat. This puts teachers in a difficult position, because not all families abide by this philosophy.

Sometimes preschool teachers or cafeteria staff will pressure kids to eat their "growing foods" before their "fun foods." They might not let kids eat desserts or sweet foods until they finish all their protein foods or vegetables. This instruction comes from a good place—they want kids to be fueled for their day and not act out due to hunger, and oftentimes this philosophy "works" in this setting because kids tend to obey their teachers or other authority figures at school.

If you've been part of the Feeding Littles community for a while, you probably know that we recommend letting your child decide how much to eat from what you serve. Yes, you're in charge of what goes in the lunch box, but they're in charge of what goes in their body. This allows kids to listen to their hunger and fullness cues, and it also takes into account the fact that kids don't always like—or feel good eating—what's in their lunch box. Only they know what foods feel the best to them. This is an important skill we want kids to practice well into adulthood: knowing how much—and what—to eat when their parents are no longer in charge of their meals.

When we make dessert or sweets dependent on other foods eaten, we teach kids that dessert is "special" or something to be earned. We put it on a pedestal. You know what humans do when they think something is off-limits? They fixate on it. The same goes with kids. When dessert is the prize, kids want it even more. In efforts to help kids eat "healthier," we teach them to obsess over "treats" and sugary foods.

Think about it this way: Making a child finish a food they're not hungry for to earn their dessert (which usually is small and not very filling) can teach them to eat more than they need. We are asking kids to eat more food to get more food. Rest assured, if they're not hungry for the last few bites of sandwich but want to eat their piece of chocolate, it's OK.

"Thank you, teachers and school staff, for your incredible contribution to our world. We know that your job is very difficult.

> **If your child isn't eating their lunch and only wants their dessert, talk to them.**

What if a child wants to eat their dessert before anything else in their lunch? Well, they were going to eat it anyway, right? Why does the order matter? When we allow kids to choose the quantity of food and the order to eat it in, we're trusting that they know what their body needs and they're learning about what foods feel good to them.

If your child isn't eating their lunch and only wants their dessert, talk to them. Did they not have enough time? Is there a social issue or a time factor involved? Is their lunch period too early for them to be hungry? So many factors can be at play, and sometimes kids just eat a little bit of their lunch and need a big snack (or lunch 2.0) at pickup. Let your child help pack their lunch and check out the picky eater tips on page 33 for more guidance.

Food Shaming from Teachers or Staff

Clients and followers frequently tell us that adults comment on their child's lunch at school. These comments are usually well meaning and are simply observations, but they can have a dramatic impact on kids and how they feel about lunchtime.

Children are not usually responsible for what goes in their lunch and can't control what food is available at home. Their parents or caregivers might not have access to enough food or the capacity to pack a balanced lunch.

Furthermore, many kids deal with significant picky eating, to the point where it's a win if they simply eat *anything*. This is not something you would know just by looking at a child or having them in your class. Kids can have difficulty chewing or feeling food appropriately in their mouth, or they might be dealing with a significant diagnosis that affects eating. While some people might see their lunches as "unhealthy," eating this food is actually quite healthy for these kids because it means they're eating *enough*.

When adults negatively comment on kids' lunches at school, kids might not want to eat what's packed. This can have a major impact on how or what they eat over time, and it happens much, much more commonly than people think—it has even happened to our Feeding Littles staff members' kids.

"What do I do if I don't agree with the food philosophies at my child's school?"

1. **Decide if it's something you need to address.** For example, if it doesn't bother your child or affect how they eat, it might be something you let slide. Kids quickly learn that there are different rules at different places. You can explain to them what *your* rules are and how you want your child to eat when they're away from you. For example, "You can choose how much to eat" or "It's OK if you eat the food in any order."

2. If it's something you need to bring up, **talk to the teacher or staff member directly first.** Remember, in elementary school and up, most teachers are not in the cafeteria—they probably don't know what's happening and you'll need to talk to the cafeteria staff instead. You might need to escalate your concerns to administration, but give the preschool teacher or cafeteria staff member a chance to discuss it with you first.

3. **Emphasize that you're coming from a spirit of collaboration.** This stuff is tricky, and everyone is trying to do their best for your child. Oftentimes, teachers or staff have food rules that they use because they aren't aware of any other way to handle kids who aren't eating their lunch or prioritizing their "healthy" food.

4. **Explain that you're trying to help your child learn to listen to their body when it comes to food.** You trust that they know how much to eat and ask that no one pressure them into eating a certain amount of food or in a certain order. If they must adhere to a "sweets last" policy, please make sure they do not force your child to eat a certain amount before eating their dessert.

5. For some people, the way food is handled at school is a deal-breaker, and they make **the difficult decision to switch schools.** Only you can decide if this is the step you need to take, but usually this decision is made only in extreme circumstances.

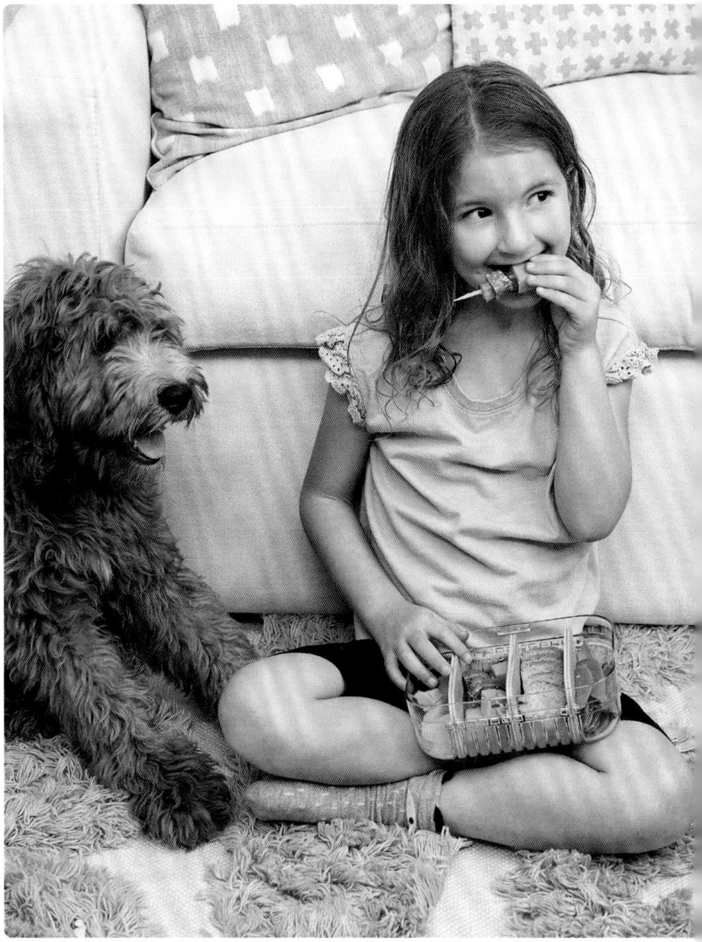

Megan has had to address food rules with teachers and staff at all her kids' schools. These discussions have always been productive and positive, and they usually lead to great dialogue and meaningful changes in the preschool classroom or lunchroom.

> "When adults negatively comment on kids' lunches at school, kids might not want to eat what's packed. This can have a major impact on how or what they eat over time.

SCAN THIS QR CODE to access a free printable and resources for teachers and cafeteria staff.

https://sites.prh.com/feedinglittleslunches

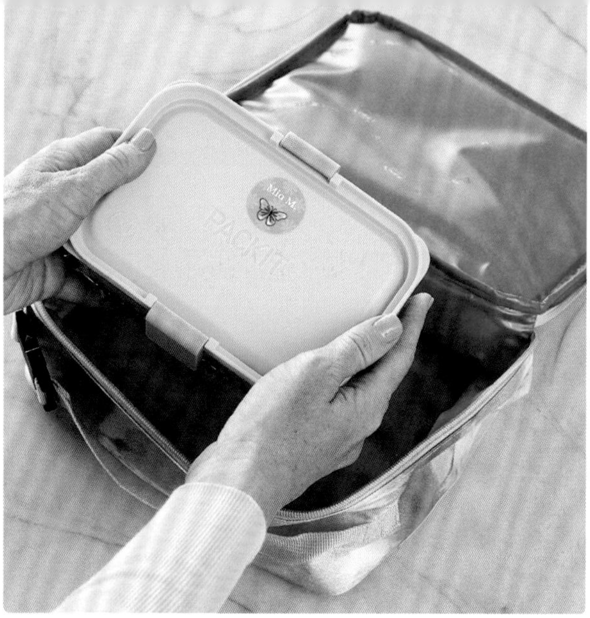

"I work in the lunchroom or at a preschool—how can I help kids eat without making them eat?"

1. This is tough because **kids come into school with really different types of lunches.** Some kids have a variety of foods packed every day—others have bags of candy with every meal. When you take into account the influence of parents and the child's behavior in the classroom, it makes your role very challenging. We absolutely get that.

2. We recommend **not commenting on the "healthfulness"** or worthiness of a child's meal. Again, they usually have no control over what goes into their lunch. If you want to mention something about their lunch, try to keep it positive: "Oh, I love those chips!" "The strawberries are so sweet right now!" "That looks delicious—how does it taste to you?"

3. **To encourage kids to eat enough, check in with them.** "How does your stomach feel?" "Are you full?" "Are you eating enough to have energy for the rest of the day?" Or try saying, "We only have five minutes left. Let's make sure we eat enough before packing up everything."

4. If you're a preschool teacher and you want to help your students eat a wider variety of food, **focus on certain qualities of the food.** Identifying the textures, colors, or flavors of food in their lunch can be a great learning experience, and when kids interact with food—especially with peers—they're more likely to eat it.

   - "Who has a type of fruit in their lunch today? Can you tell me what it's called? What color is it?"
   - "If you have a vegetable in your lunch, can you pick it up with me? If you want, let's take a bite together. Is it crunchy? Soft?"
   - If everyone has the same lunch: "Let's notice the colors on our plate. How many strawberries do we have? Let's count them!"
   - "Let's do a tummy check-in! Are we not full, a little full, all the way full? Too full? What is your tummy telling you right now?"

If you need more help with this, please reach out to us at @feedinglittles or feedinglittles.com.

A Word on Culture

This book was written in the United States and reflects foods commonly available and eaten by our families and clients. We recognize that this is not what lunch necessarily looks like for the rest of the world, or even in different parts of the United States. This book does not encompass lunches eaten by multiple different cultures or in different countries.

If you do not live in the United States or don't have access to these specific foods, you can still use this book to help inspire the foods you pack. Use the Feeding Littles Lunch Formula to build a balanced lunch with the foods you buy and enjoy.

Baby Jack

We promised no cutesy shapes or spelling out words in this book, but here and later in these pages you'll see the name Jack spelled out in alphabet soup. It's a special reminder of how we started. Judy and Megan met because of baby Jack back in 2014. Jack had spinal muscular atrophy (SMA), which at the time had no treatment or cures. His family spent his short life giving him all the experiences they could. They celebrated holidays early, took him sledding, and brought him all over the place to experience as much as possible, knowing his condition was terminal. He lived a big life and taught so many to be brave. To never give up.

Judy was Jack's feeding therapist during the short six months of his life; Megan was friends with his mom, Sarah. A few years after Jack's death on December 23, 2011, his mom introduced Megan and Judy. She knew they had to do something together, even though they lived in different states.

At Feeding Littles we try to honor Jack in all we do. This little boy, who never got to eat real food, is helping us inspire millions of families and walk them through their biggest mealtime challenges. He allows us to share intuitive eating and the importance of mealtime with so many people worldwide.

Feeding Littles donates a portion of every online course sold to the Gwendolyn Strong Foundation. GSF was instrumental in helping Jack's parents through his diagnosis, including accessing services and equipment needed as his body slowly lost the ability to swallow and breathe. We are grateful to our Feeding Littles family for giving us the chance to support this amazing organization.

Photos of Jack's siblings can be found on pages 32 and 41 of this book, and his mama is now an integral member of the Feeding Littles team. We wanted to make sure he was represented here too.

We love you, Jack Jack.

—Judy and Megan

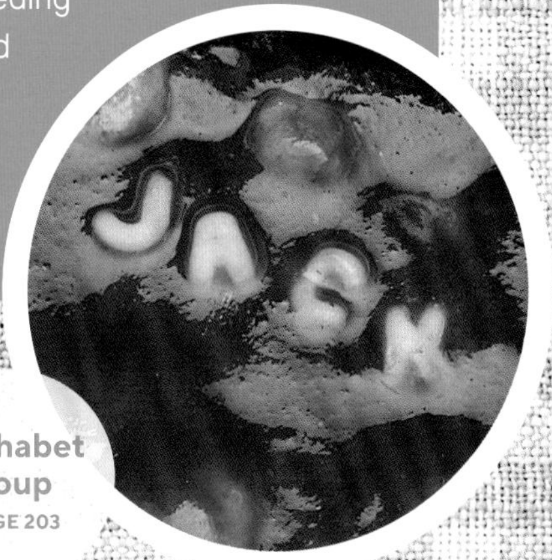

Alphabet Soup

PAGE 203

THE GU

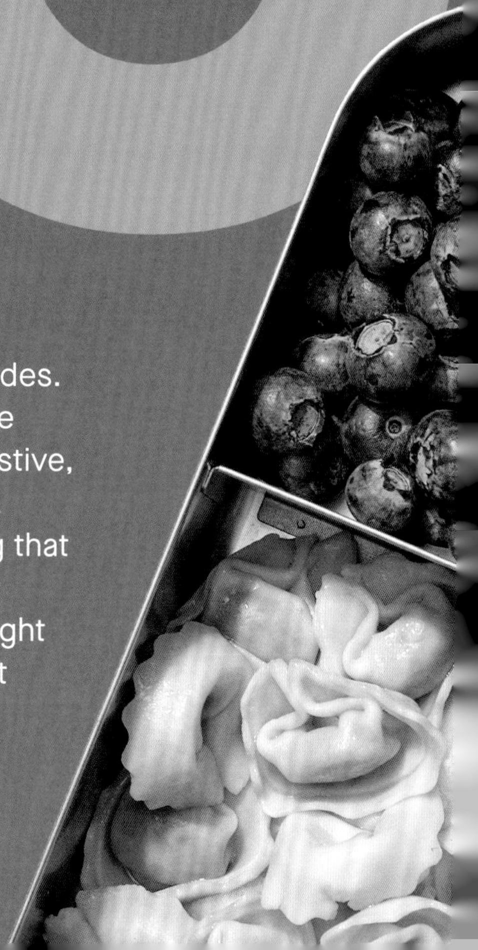

We hope the photos in this book will be helpful to you in packing lunches, but some people also love lists and guides. This section contains charts to help you add a little more variety to your kid's lunches. These guides are pretty exhaustive, and you wouldn't purchase all these foods at the store. Rather, the goal is to simply inspire you to try one new thing that you didn't buy the week before. These foods are more commonly available in the United States, although they might not be available at every store. You might have different foods available where you live.

IDES

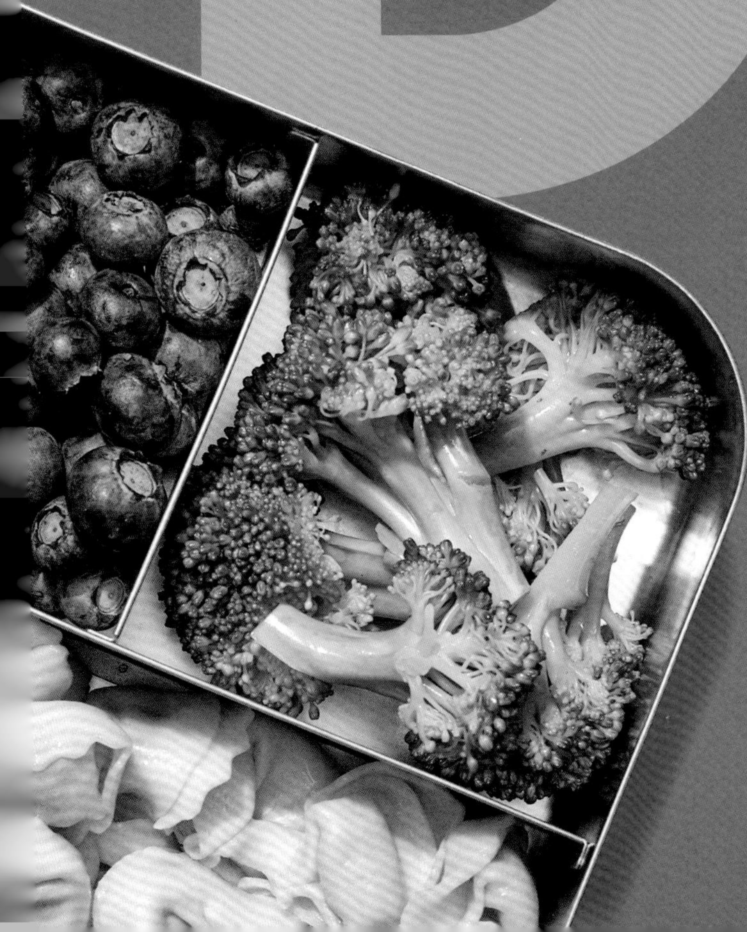

Starches/ Grains

Grains and carbohydrate foods give kids much-needed energy for growth, learning, and play. Many kids love starchy foods, and it makes sense—they have a predictable taste and texture and are delicious to eat. While carbohydrates come in many types of foods, a starch or grain food can be that "safe" or predictable food your child looks forward to eating when they sit down to lunch.

This list is, of course, not representative of *all* the starches you could send. Plus, some grains have so many choices—for example, tortillas. You can buy corn, flour, gluten-free, and grain-free (cassava or almond) tortillas at many grocery stores. Choose what your family enjoys and what you can afford, keeping in mind that **whole grains will offer extra nutrition** in the form of fiber, vitamins, and minerals. If your child is allergic to wheat or is gluten-intolerant, choose gluten-free grains.

Bread

Bagels

English muffins

Rice

Tortillas (soft, crunchy, or tortilla chips)

Waffles

Crackers

Pasta

Naan

Pita (soft or as pita chips)

Pretzels

Rice cakes

Sandwich rolls

Granola

Graham crackers

Cereal

Quinoa

Buckwheat

Millet

Couscous

Orzo

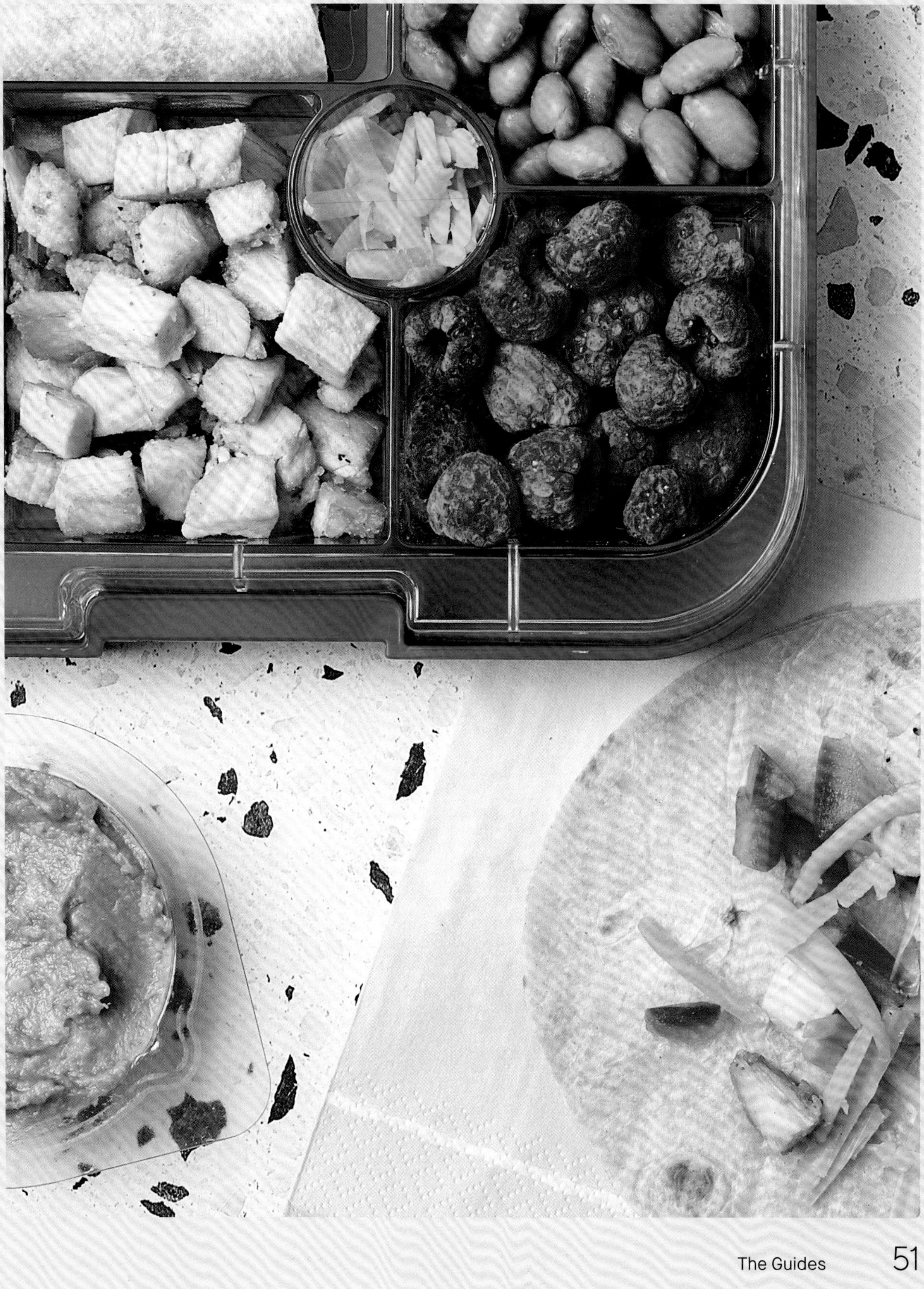

Proteins

Protein foods help your child build muscle, repair tissue, develop, and grow. You might have noticed that protein makes meals more satisfying to you—this is also true for kids! However, children don't have to eat a lot of protein to get enough. For example, estimated minimum protein needs are probably less than you think.

- **1–3 years: ~13 grams**
- **4–8 years: ~19 grams**
- **9–13 years: ~34 grams**
- **14–18 years: ~52 grams**

Given that one ounce of meat or poultry contains seven grams of protein, a cup of milk has eight grams, and one piece of whole-grain bread can have five grams, most kids get plenty of protein, despite what many parents assume. We don't worry about too much protein unless your child is getting it in supplemental forms in large quantities.

Protein doesn't have to come from an animal source—nut or seed butter, beans, tofu, and edamame are also good protein options!

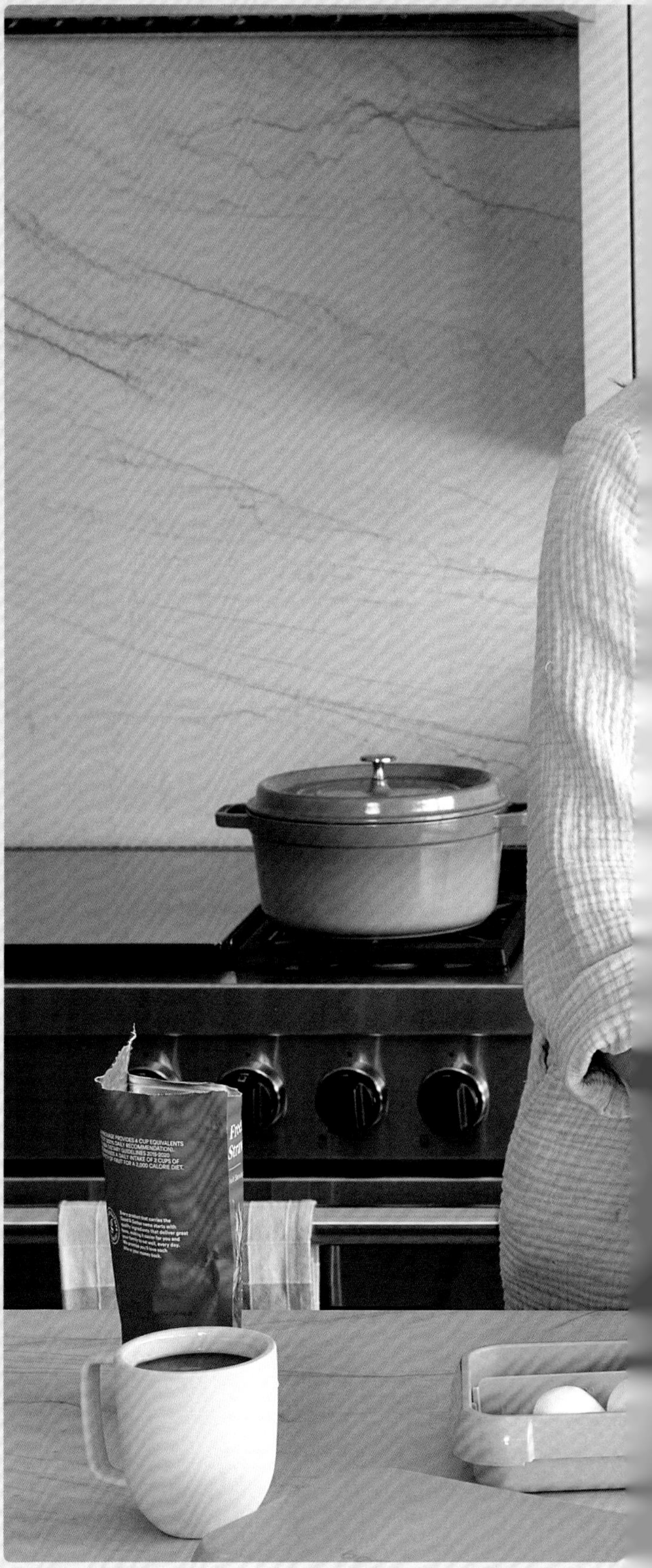

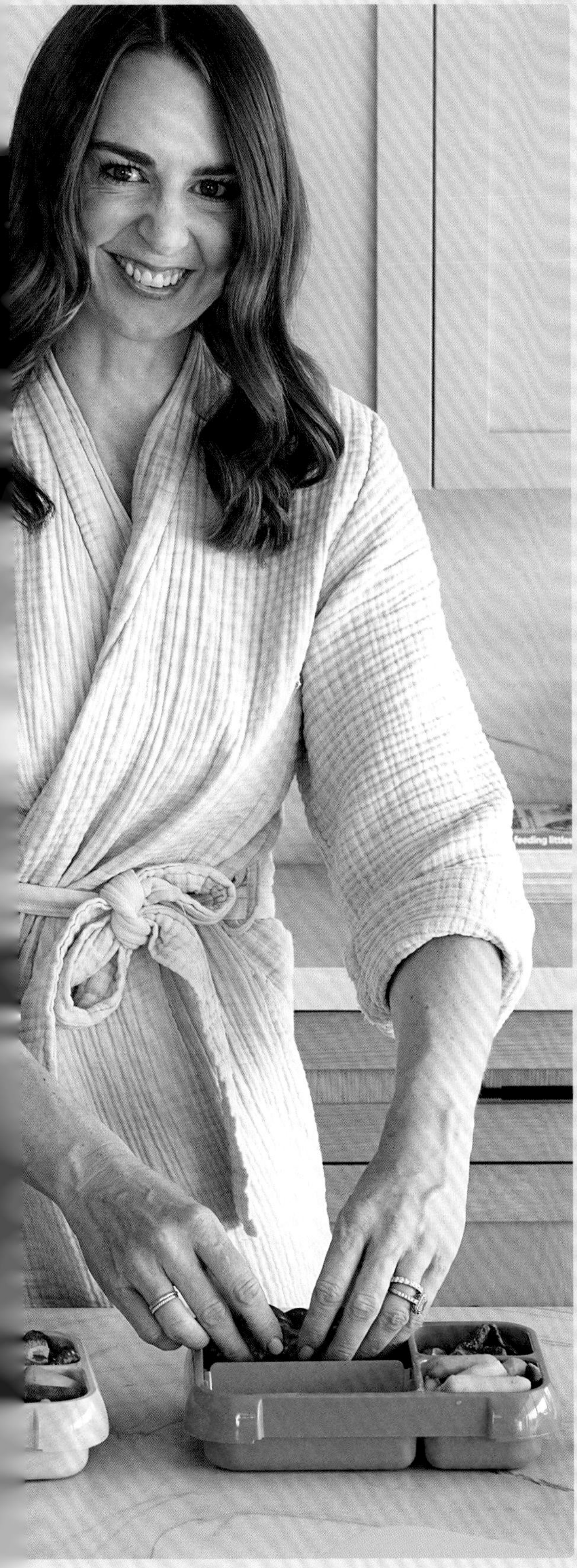

Hard-boiled eggs

Nut or seed butters

(peanut butter, almond butter, sunflower seed butter)

Whole nuts or seeds

(kids ages 4+)

Beans

(black, garbanzo, kidney, pinto)

Cheese

Yogurt

Chicken

Beef

Turkey

Deli meat

(turkey, chicken, salami, ham, roast beef, pepperoni—choose nitrate-/nitrite-free when possible)

Sausage or hot dogs

(choose nitrate-/nitrite-free when possible)

Hummus or black bean dip

Tuna salad

Tofu

Cottage cheese

Sunflower seeds

Meatballs

Lox

(smoked salmon)

Egg salad

Chicken salad

Energy bites/ energy bar

Tzatziki

Fruits

Fruits are an awesome source of vitamins, minerals, plant nutrients, and fiber. They can also help hydrate your child on days they're not drinking enough water. Many kids are what we lovingly call "fruit monsters"—they adore fruits and would eat them over almost anything else. This is great, especially if they're not quite into veggies just yet. Fruits can offer similar nutrients as vegetables and can help fill in nutritional gaps during picky eating phases.

One fruit option you'll see frequently in this book is freeze-dried fruit. Freeze-drying is a different process than what's used to make dried fruit. Freeze-drying removes almost all the moisture from food without dramatically changing the shape or nutrient profile of the food. It makes the fruit shelf-stable and is an awesome way to offer more crunch in your child's lunch. Freeze-dried fruits may be more expensive than fresh, dried, or canned fruits, but you'll see them periodically here because they're a kid-friendly option that has a longer shelf life than fresh fruit.

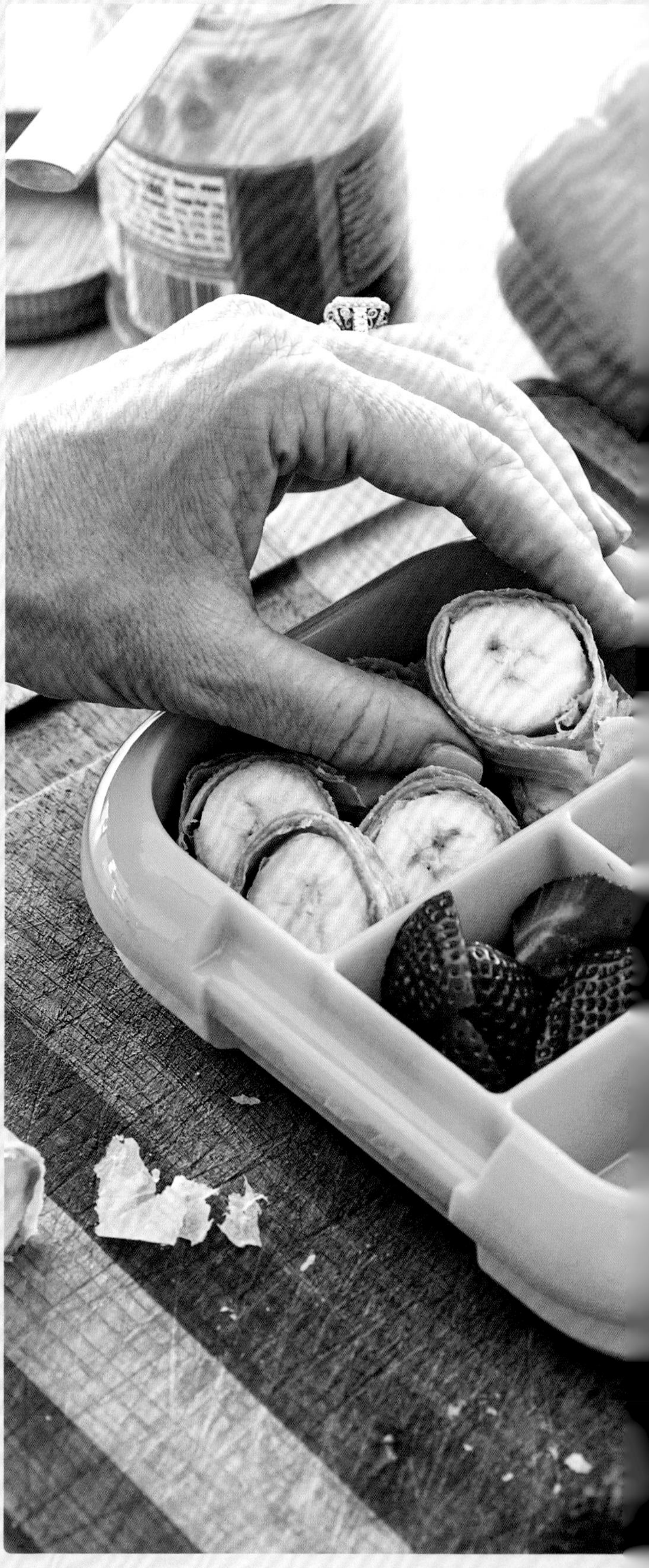

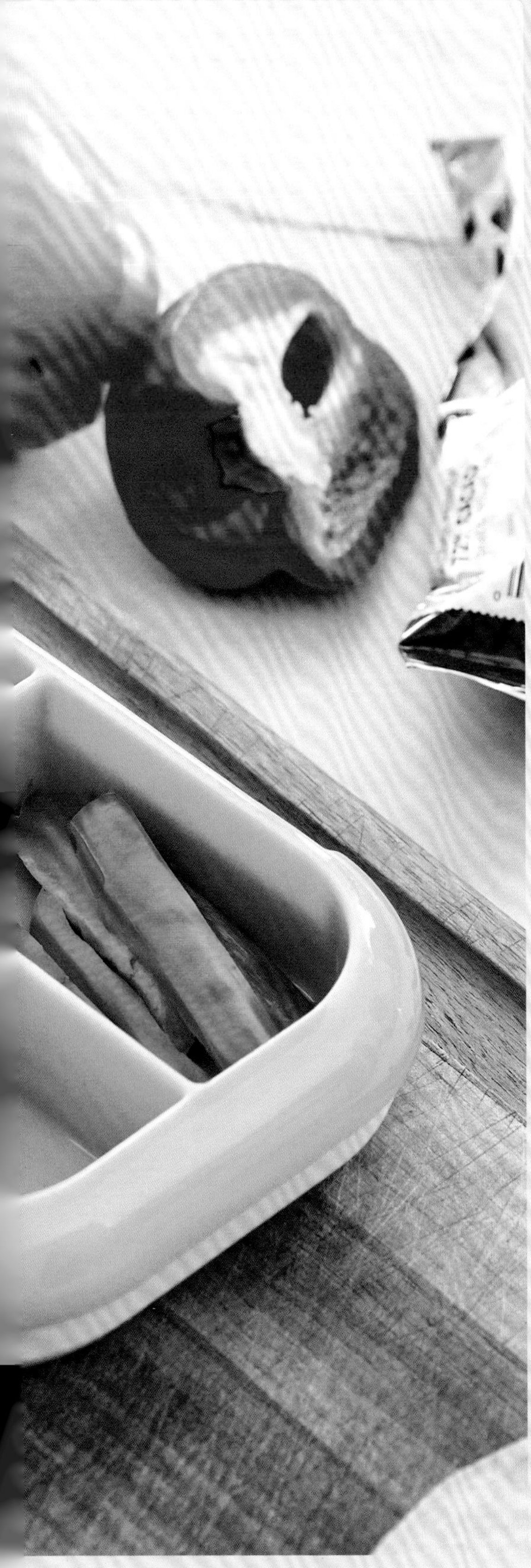

Strawberries
(fresh, dried, freeze-dried)

Blueberries
(fresh, dried, freeze-dried)

Apples
(fresh, dried, freeze-dried, applesauce)

Bananas
(fresh, dried, freeze-dried)

Oranges

Tangerines

Mandarin oranges
(fresh, canned/jarred)

Grapes
(fresh, dried as raisins)

Raspberries
(fresh, freeze-dried)

Pineapple
(fresh, dried, freeze-dried, canned/jarred)

Watermelon

Cantaloupe

Pomegranate seeds

Honeydew

Peaches
(fresh, freeze-dried, canned/jarred)

Pears
(fresh, canned/jarred)

Nectarines

Plums

Blackberries

Avocados

Cherries

Apricots
(fresh, dried)

Coconut
(fresh, dried)

Kiwi
(fresh, freeze-dried)

Papaya

Mango
(fresh, freeze-dried)

Grapefruit

Cranberries
(dried, freeze-dried)

Dragonfruit

Guava

Vegetables

Are vegetables a sore subject in your home? If you're like many of our clients, you're nodding your head in agreement. Why are veggies so tough for some kids? Well, they have strong flavors and unpredictable textures. Unlike fruit, they're generally not sweet. And sometimes they become ground zero for dinnertime battles—when kids sense that we're trying to get them to eat their veggies, they tend to resist them even more.

What's a parent (who wants their kid to love veggies) to do? Think *exposure*, not *intake*. Learning to love vegetables takes time. Some kids need to have them in their lunch over and over to love them one day.

Despite what we see on social media, kids don't *have* to eat vegetables to meet their nutritional needs, especially if they eat lots of fruits. Do we want them to love veggies one day? Absolutely. But they can grow and thrive without veggies too.

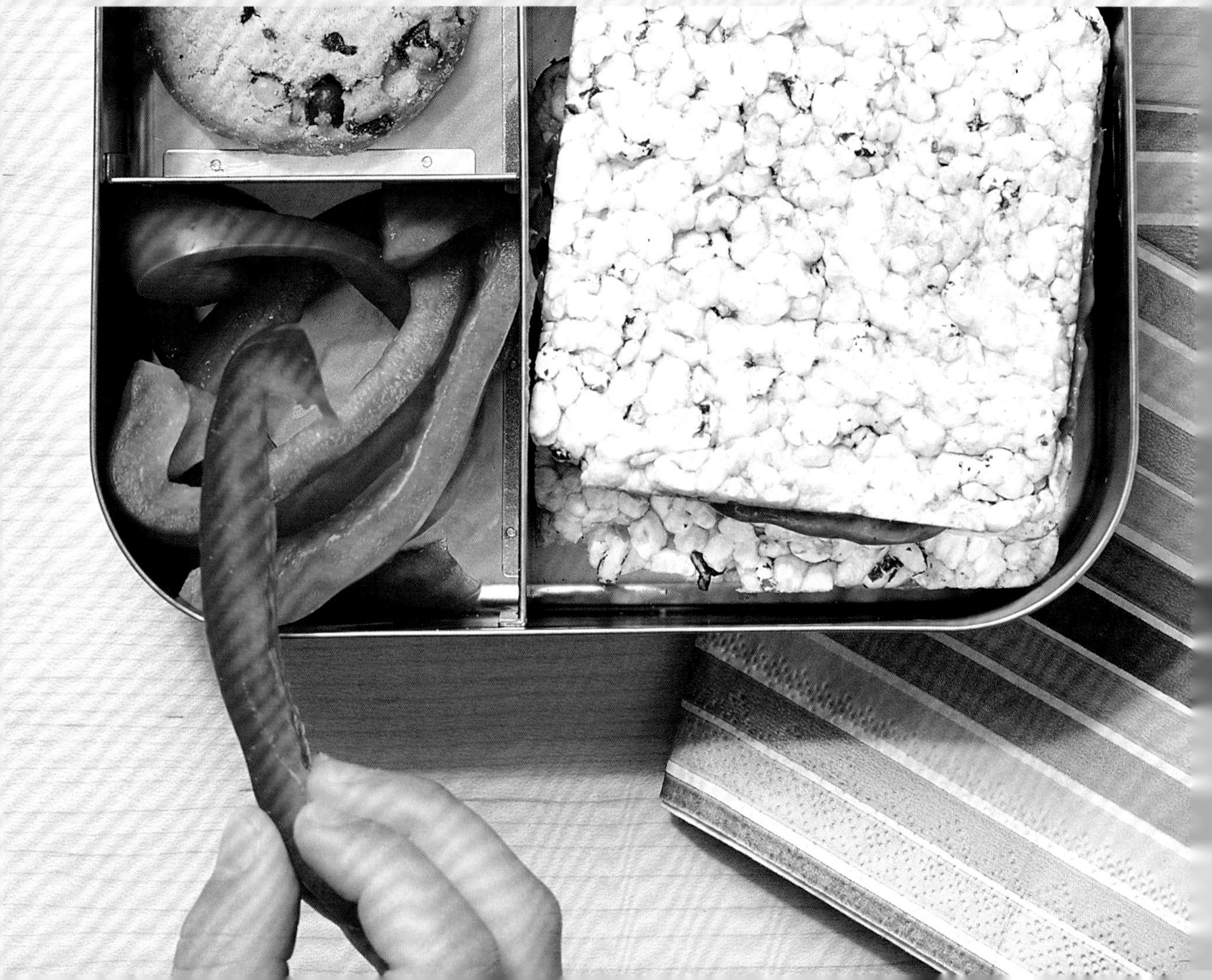

Here are a few quick tips to help your child love veggies eventually:

1. **Put vegetables in their lunch, even if you don't think they'll eat them.** (Psst, this is why our School Lunch Formula contains vegetables—it's a reminder to serve them for exposure!)
2. **Serve a favorite dip.** Cold, raw veggies are often better with hummus, tzatziki, or ranch.
3. **Keep portions very small.** You might assume that your child won't eat the bell pepper strips, but send one thin piece anyway. It's funny how much more likely kids are to try things when they're not overwhelmed by a big pile of them.
4. **Check out the picky eating tip** that accompanies each lunch idea—we have included many fun and simple ideas for making veggies more appetizing.
5. **Use vegetables as part of your cooking and food prep.** No, this doesn't mean we need to "hide" veggies in everything—that usually backfires. Instead, serve veggie-based soups, casseroles, or pasta dishes with vegetables, or cook your entrées with veggies to help your child eat them more often.

Cucumbers

Carrots

Bell pepper and mini bell peppers
(yellow, red, orange, green)

Snap peas

Snow peas

Green peas
(fresh, from frozen, freeze-dried)

Celery

Lettuce
(on sandwiches, as part of salads)

Tomatoes

Cherry/grape/plum tomatoes

Zucchini

Jicama

Corn
(fresh, canned, from frozen, freeze-dried)

Broccoli
(fresh, from frozen)

Green beans
(fresh, canned, from frozen)

Frozen veggie tots

Seaweed

Veggie soup

Sweet potato

Squash

Olives

Beets

Cabbage

Eggplant

Dips

Do you have a kid who loves to dip? Awesome—that can help them love new flavors! Judy uses dips as a "bridge" to less familiar foods; if they love the dip, they might be more inclined to try the dipper.

Usually we find that ketchup and ranch are kid favorites, but there are so many dips and condiments that can add flavor, nutrition, and interest to your child's lunch! Note these can be store-bought or homemade. Some brands even make allergy-friendly sauces and dips.

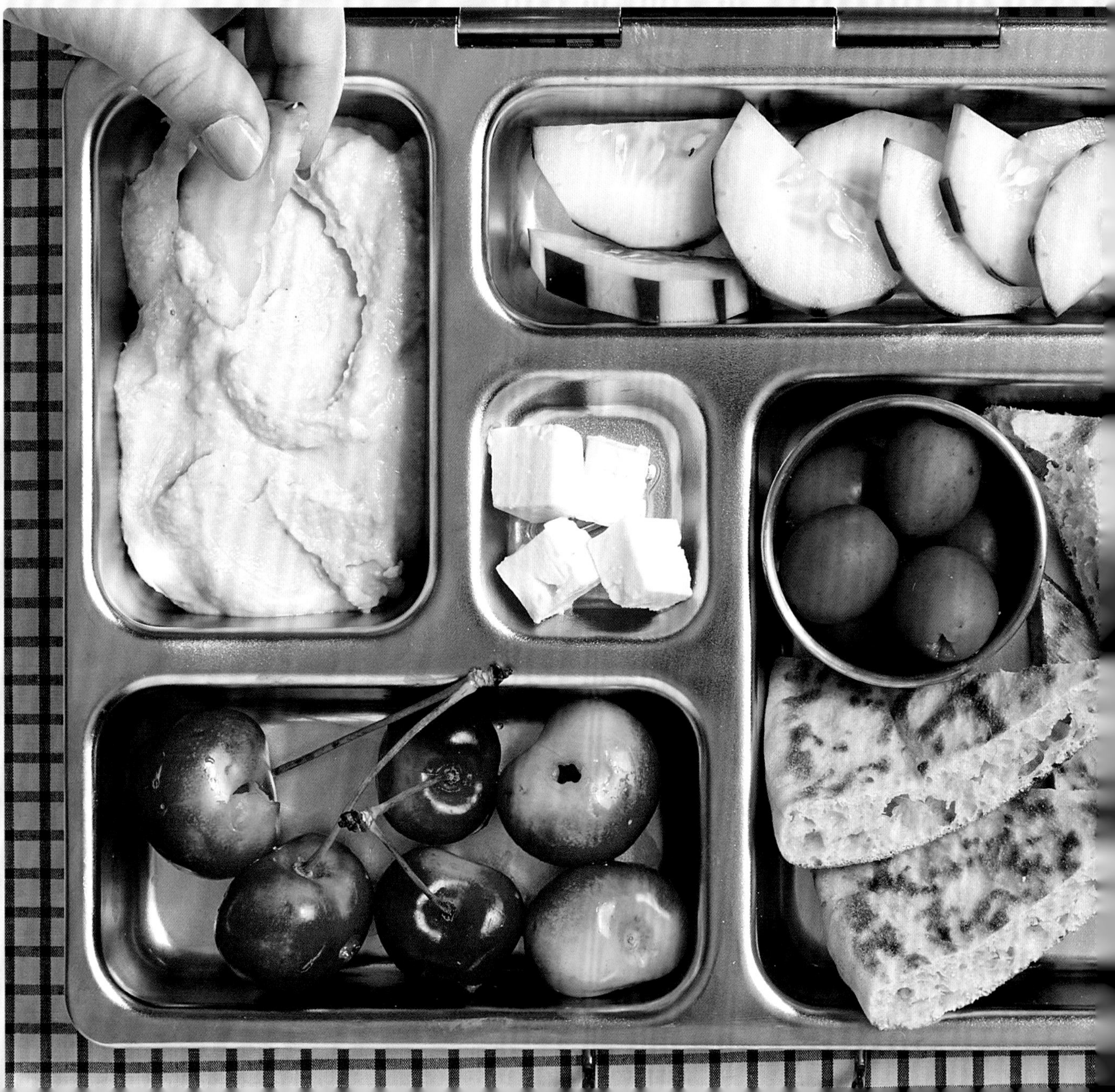

"What if my kid doesn't like dips or sauces?"
This is actually really common, and while kids don't *need* dips or sauces nutritionally, dining out or eating at a friend's house can be tough if they don't enjoy them. Here are a few tips from Judy that might help:

1. **Don't force it.** Some kids and adults just don't like dips or condiments, and that's OK. You can still offer them regularly—sometimes it takes time for kids to warm up to them. Serve them on the side so your child has the choice to use them or not.

2. **Ask if they want to dip** their food in water, then squeeze out the water before eating. It sounds kind of silly, but it can work to get kids used to the idea of dipping.

3. **Make a familiar food a dip.** If your child loves applesauce or yogurt, ask them to dip other favorite foods in them to become accustomed to dipping.

4. **Try a familiar or preferred dipper with a new dip.** For example, when introducing hummus or tzatziki, offer pita bread or cucumber if they already enjoy them.

Ranch

Hummus

Tzatziki

Guacamole

Yogurt-based ranch

Bean dip

Salsa

Ketchup

BBQ sauce

Marinara sauce

Pesto

Yogurt

Baba ghanoush

Mustard

Sour cream

Fruit dip
(can be yogurt-based)

Soy sauce

Balsamic vinaigrette

Teriyaki sauce

Curry sauce

Applesauce

Sandwich Ideas

Sandwiches might be the quintessential American lunch food, but it's super easy to send the same ones over and over again, and that can get boring. Below are a few ideas that your child might like.

Easy Sandwich Options

- Peanut butter,* almond butter,* or sunflower seed butter with jelly or honey
- Peanut butter,* almond butter,* or sunflower seed butter with smashed fruit
- Cream cheese and sliced strawberries
- Turkey and cheese
- Chicken salad, egg salad, or tuna salad
- Chicken pesto*
- BBQ chicken or BBQ tofu
- Caprese sandwich: tomato, mozzarella, and basil with balsamic glaze
- Hummus and veggie or hummus and cheese
- Smashed avocado and bacon, cheese, or veggies (make the morning of, not the night before, to keep the avocado from browning)
- Cold cuts on a sub roll or focaccia

Add condiments and toppings (tomato, lettuce) as desired.

*Contains peanuts or tree nuts

Tips for Preventing Soggy Sandwiches

Soggy sandwiches are the absolute worst, especially for a kid who might be struggling with lunch anyway. Megan hasn't had an issue with this when using hearty, whole-grain bread, but sometimes it happens, depending on what bread you use. Here are tips to prevent it:

1. **Add a spread** to both pieces of bread before making your sandwich. It sounds a little counterintuitive, but a layer of mayo, mustard, or sunflower seed butter helps prevent moisture in the sandwich ingredients (like a tomato slice) from getting to the bread. This is key when doing a smashed raspberry and nut/seed butter sandwich—put the nut or seed butter on both pieces of bread first, then smash the raspberries onto the nut or seed butter.

2. **Use a hearty bread or wrap.** French bread or thicker whole-grain bread can help. Toasting sandwich bread can also prevent sogginess, but sometimes it's not appetizing to kids.

3. If sogginess is a chronic issue with your sandwiches, **pack them the morning of school** instead of the night before.

4. If needed, **send wet ingredients separately** to be added to the sandwich later.

Psssst. It's me showing up in your day with an I LOVE YOU.

Lunch Box Notes

If you're the kind of person who would *never* send a lunch box note, skip right on past this page. This is not a guilt trip or a must-do. Move along, friend.

If you *do* like writing lunch box notes to your reading-aged kids, we wanted to include a little inspiration from our favorite children's book author, Marianne Richmond. She wrote Megan's all-time favorite tear-inducing book, *If I Could Keep You Little*, and including her words in this book is a huge honor for us. We hope you enjoy them as well.

- Thinking of you! Hope you're having a great day!
- I know you're trying your best today, and I'm so proud of you!
- Make your teachers smile today—they are working hard too!
- What kindness can you share today?
- Share your smile today with someone who needs one.
- Hi sweetie! Just a little note to let you know I'm thinking about you!
- Here's your happy reminder that you're loved by me!
- Guess what? I love you big today and always!
- This is a little note from home to remind you how BIG you're loved.
- I believe in you and all the good work you're doing!
- I'm here and you're there but our hearts are always together!
- Just remember—I think you're amazing!
- Just remember—you make a big difference wherever you are!
- I'm looking forward to hearing all about your day!

A FEW FUNNY ONES . . .

- What kind of key opens a banana? A monKEY!
- How can you tell the ocean is friendly? It waves!
- What do you call a bear with no teeth? A gummy bear!
- Why did the math book need to see a counselor? Because he was full of problems!
- Why shouldn't you write with a broken pencil? Because it's pointless!

Take a moment today to breathe and remind yourself that your best is enough!

"How Can My Toddler Eat a Sandwich?"

Big, assembled sandwiches can be difficult for the one- to three-year-old crowd. Not only are they hard to hold, but they can also fall apart easily. Below are some ways to make sandwiches doable for your little one.

Use a sandwich cutter and sealer to keep sandwich fillings contained. (You can buy these sandwiches premade in the freezer aisle, but they'll cost a lot more.) →

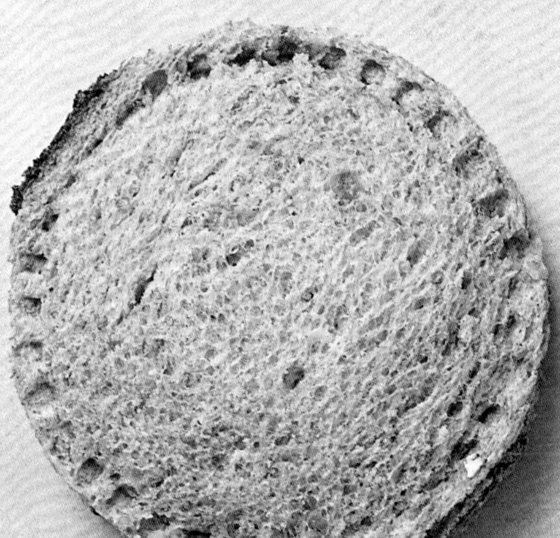

Deconstruct a sandwich so your toddler eats the components separately. →

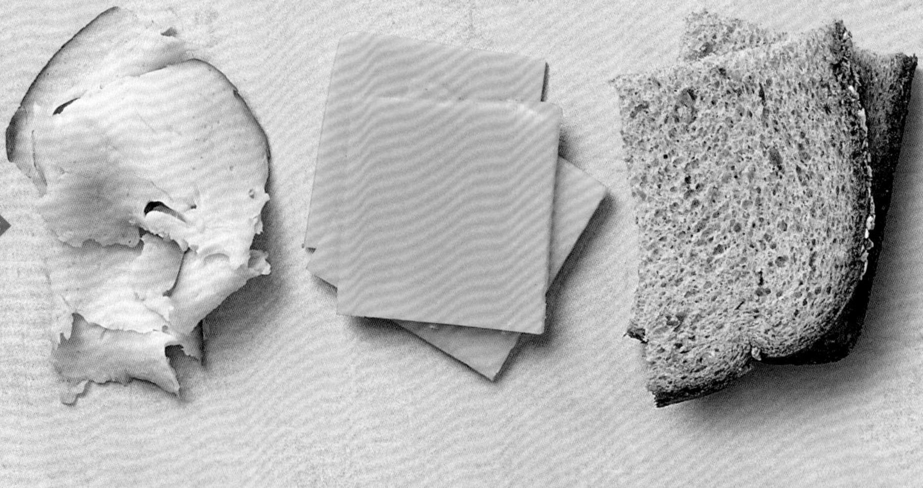

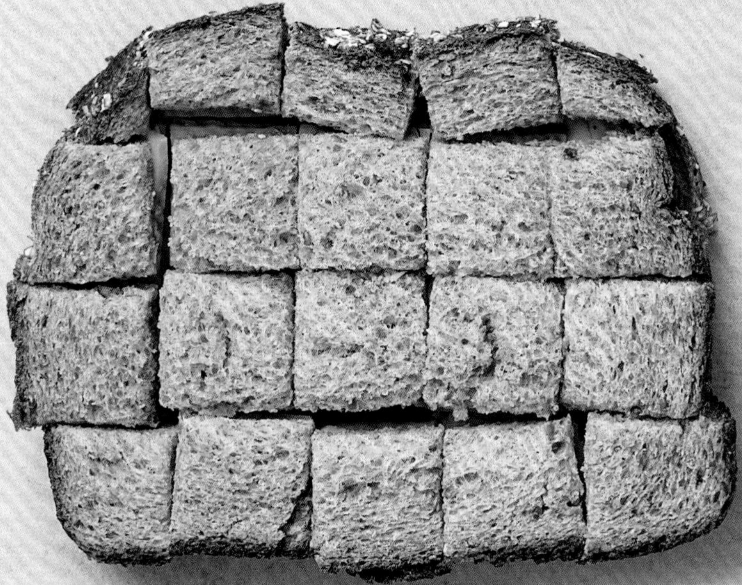

Cut into smaller pieces. A spread like nut or seed butter, mayo, or hummus inside both pieces of bread can help keep these pieces together after you cut them.

Cut into strips. A big sammie might be hard for little hands, but strips are more manageable and easier for them to bite into.

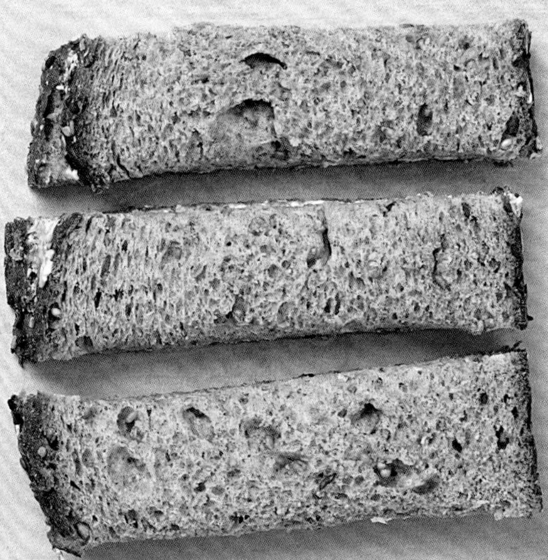

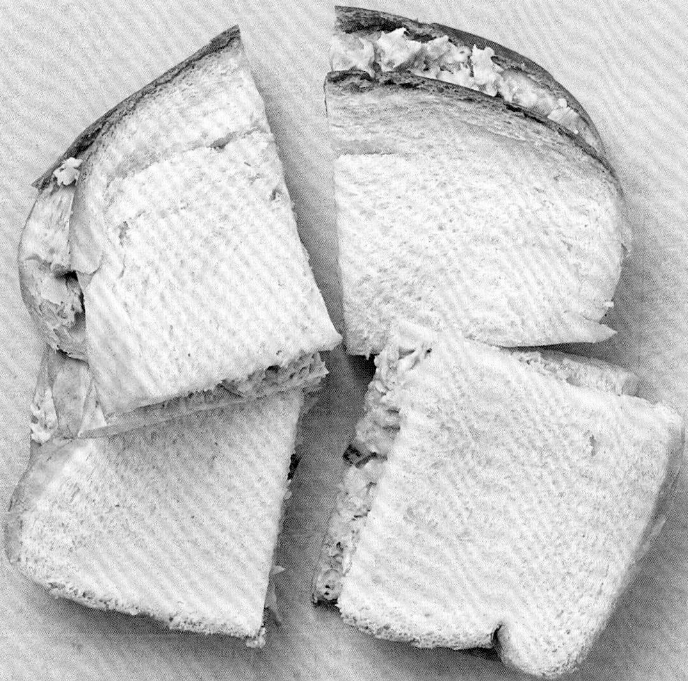

Quarter the sandwich instead of just cutting it in half. It will be much easier to hold.

Add Variety in Small Ways

We know that seeing a bunch of different lunch ideas can be overwhelming when your child wants one and only one specific lunch every single day. If you're ready to introduce more variety but not sure where to start, try these tips:

1. **CHANGE UP THE SIDES:** Use different fruits, veggies, or desserts. Start with things they really enjoy, as this process will be more successful.
2. **USE A DIFFERENT SPREAD:** Instead of cream cheese, as shown here, try a nut or seed butter or a different flavor of cream cheese.
3. **CHANGE HOW IT LOOKS:** Two mini bagels instead of one big bagel might not seem profound, but for a child used to seeing the same lunch, it's a small stepping stone.

Say this is your child's favorite lunch. Let's look at small ways to add a little more variety. →

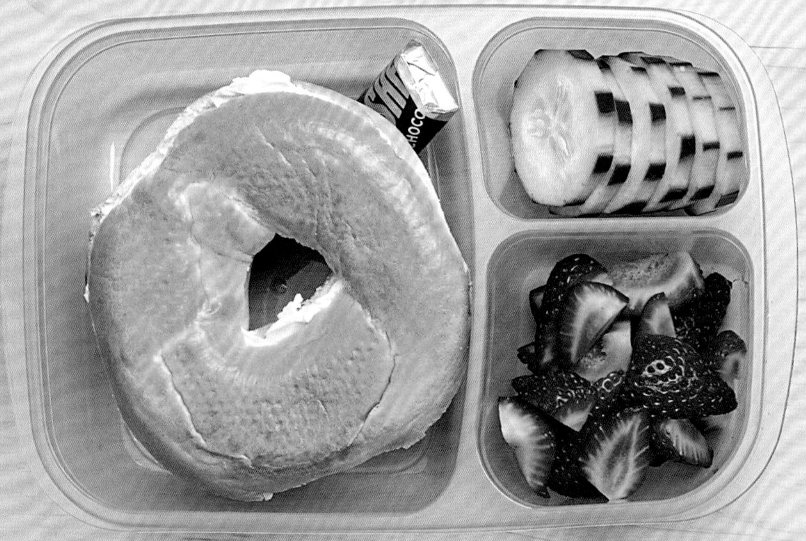

Serve sunflower seed butter or another nut/seed butter instead of cream cheese. →

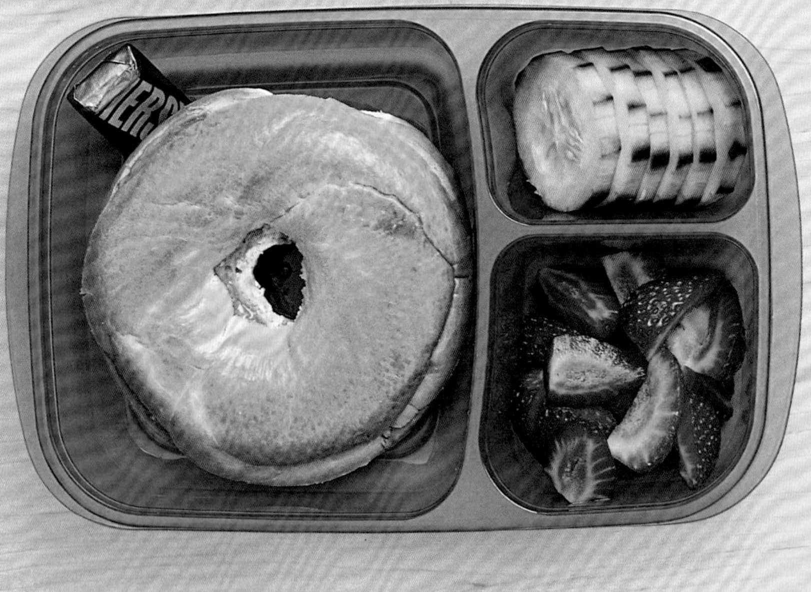

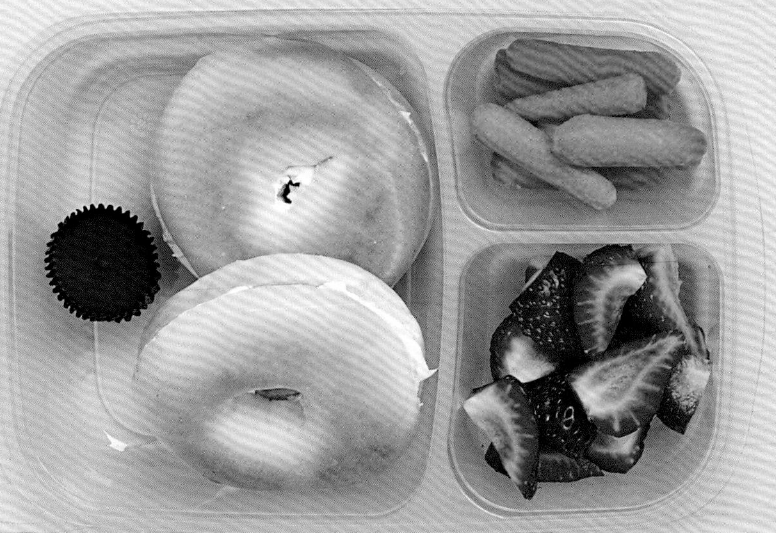

← Use mini bagels instead of full-size bagels and swap cucumbers for carrots. You can also mix up the type or brand of chocolate.

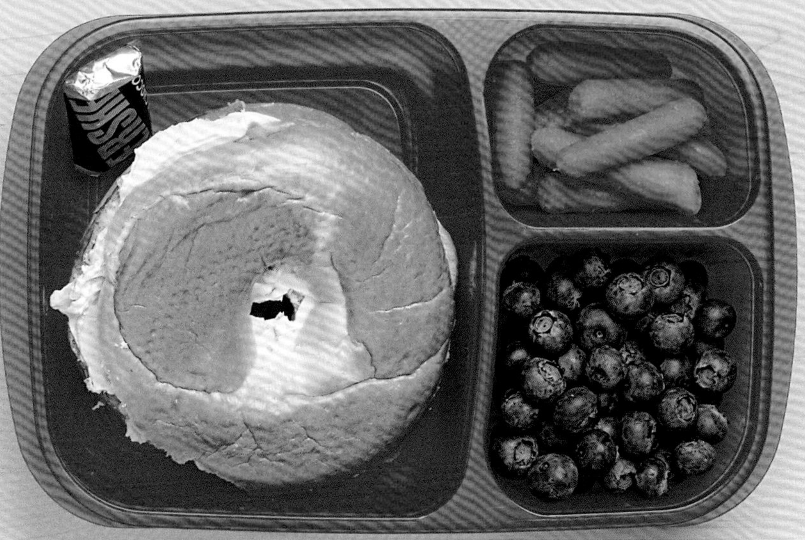

← Offer blueberries instead of strawberries.

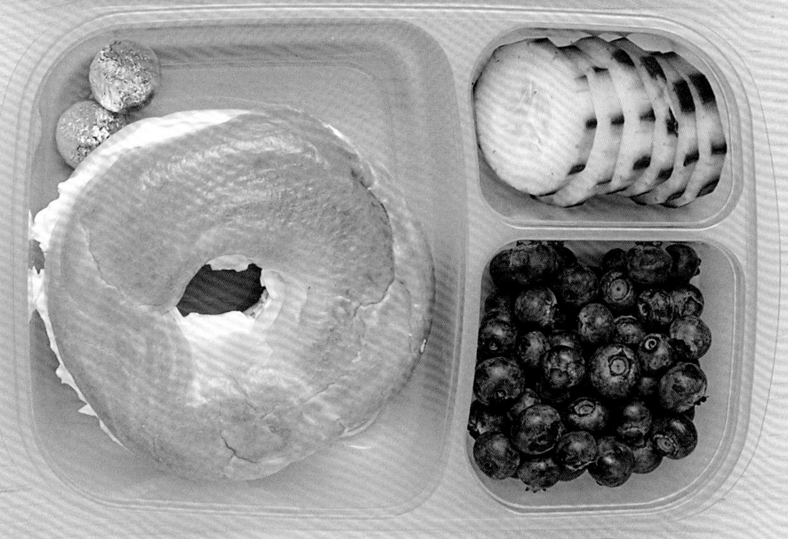

← Change up the chocolate again. Notice that every lunch shown has been a little different without adding a ton of effort—that's the goal!

Non-Perishable Lunch Ideas

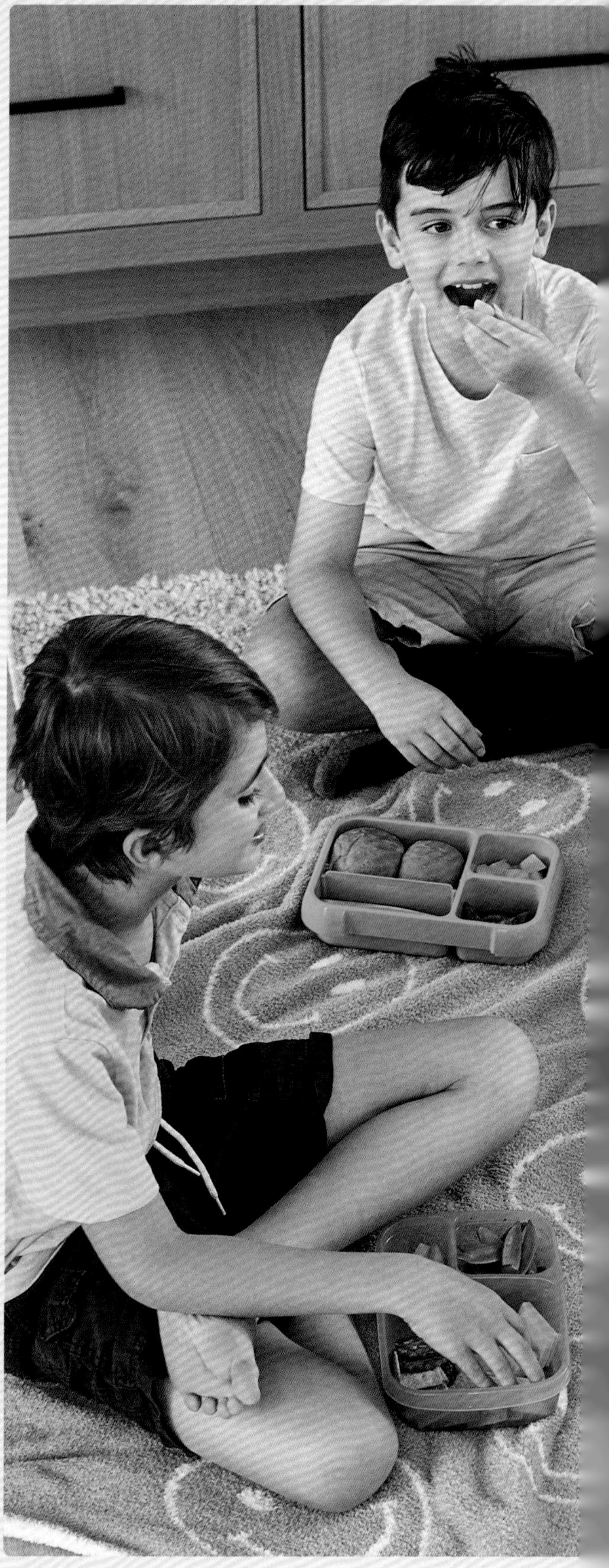

If your child is heading on a field trip or needs a non-perishable lunch for camp, it's important to know what you can and can't send. As mentioned in the Food Safety section on page 34, lunches with any perishable ingredients need two ice sources to keep them safe until lunchtime.

Did you eat warm bologna sandwiches at school when you were younger? Maybe. And were you OK? Likely, yes. Generations before us didn't necessarily know or abide by food safety guidelines for school lunch (nor did they necessarily have the gear to keep food cold). However, it's important to err on the side of safety when it comes to foods, as foodborne illness is a real concern.

Which foods need to be refrigerated or sent with ice? According to the USDA, "Items that don't require refrigeration include whole fruits and vegetables, hard cheese, canned meat and fish, chips, breads, crackers, peanut butter, jelly, mustard, and pickles."*

Some parents send frozen drinks like a frozen water bottle to help keep food cold, although that as the only cold source might not be sufficient for perishable items.

On the next page are a few ideas for lunches you can send that don't need refrigeration.

* "Keeping 'Bag' Lunches Safe," FSIS, USDA, www.fsis.usda.gov/food-safety/safe-food-handling-and-preparation/food-safety-basics/keeping-bag-lunches-safe.

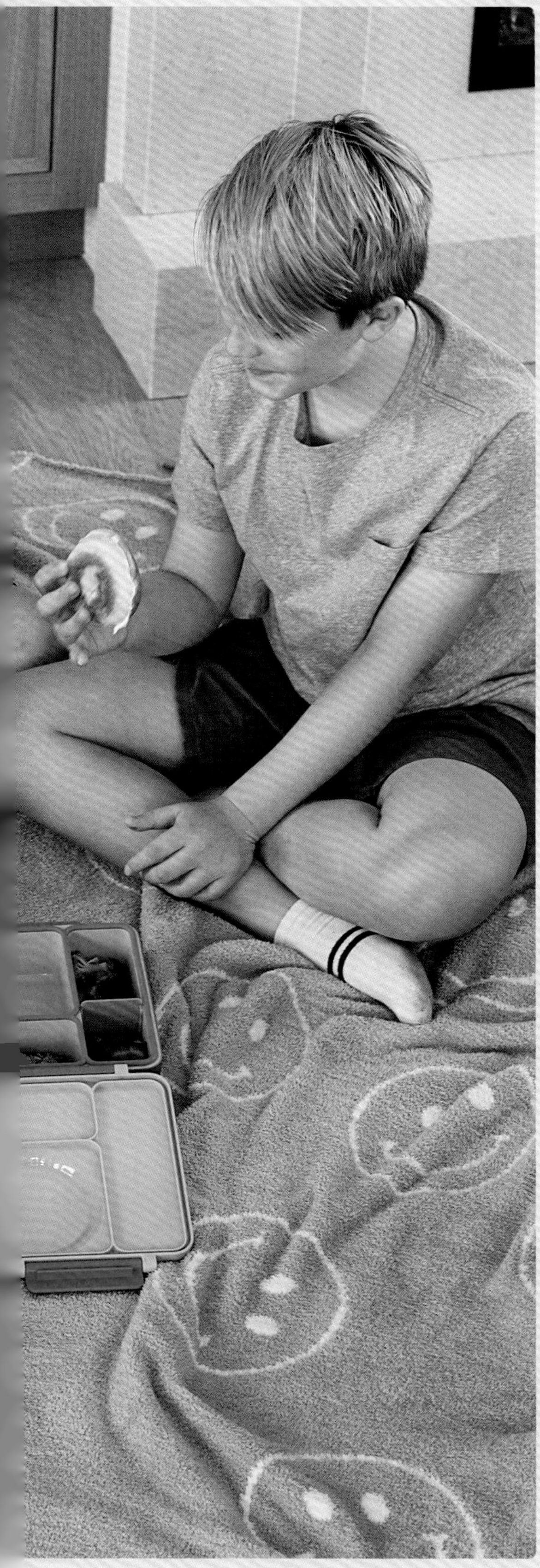

Starches/ Proteins

- Peanut butter or sunflower seed butter and jelly or honey sandwich
- Pita bread or pita chips and dried chickpeas
- Peanut butter or sunflower seed butter and banana rolled up in a tortilla
- Muffin and beef jerky
- Bagel with nut or seed butter
- Hearty whole-grain crackers, frozen string cheese (will thaw by lunch), and turkey jerky
- Kids' protein bar and pretzels
- Trail mix (made with sunflower seeds if nut-free) and crackers or chips
- Chicken salad or tuna salad kit

Fruits

- Whole fruits: apple, orange, pear, banana, peach, nectarine, plum
- Freeze-dried fruits
- Dried fruits
- Individually packed canned/jarred fruits

Veggies

- Grape tomatoes
- Snap peas
- Snow peas
- Freeze-dried veggies
- Crunchy broccoli
- Snap pea crisps

Dips

Ranch cups are shelf-stable.

Chips

Most store-bought chips are shelf-stable.

Desserts

Most chocolates, candies, cookies, brownies, etc. do not require refrigeration.

Sample Lunch Meal Plan

The entire point of this book is to help you simplify packing lunches for your kids (and yourself). In this section we feature a few weeks' worth of lunches to show how you can pack variety without putting in a ton of effort.

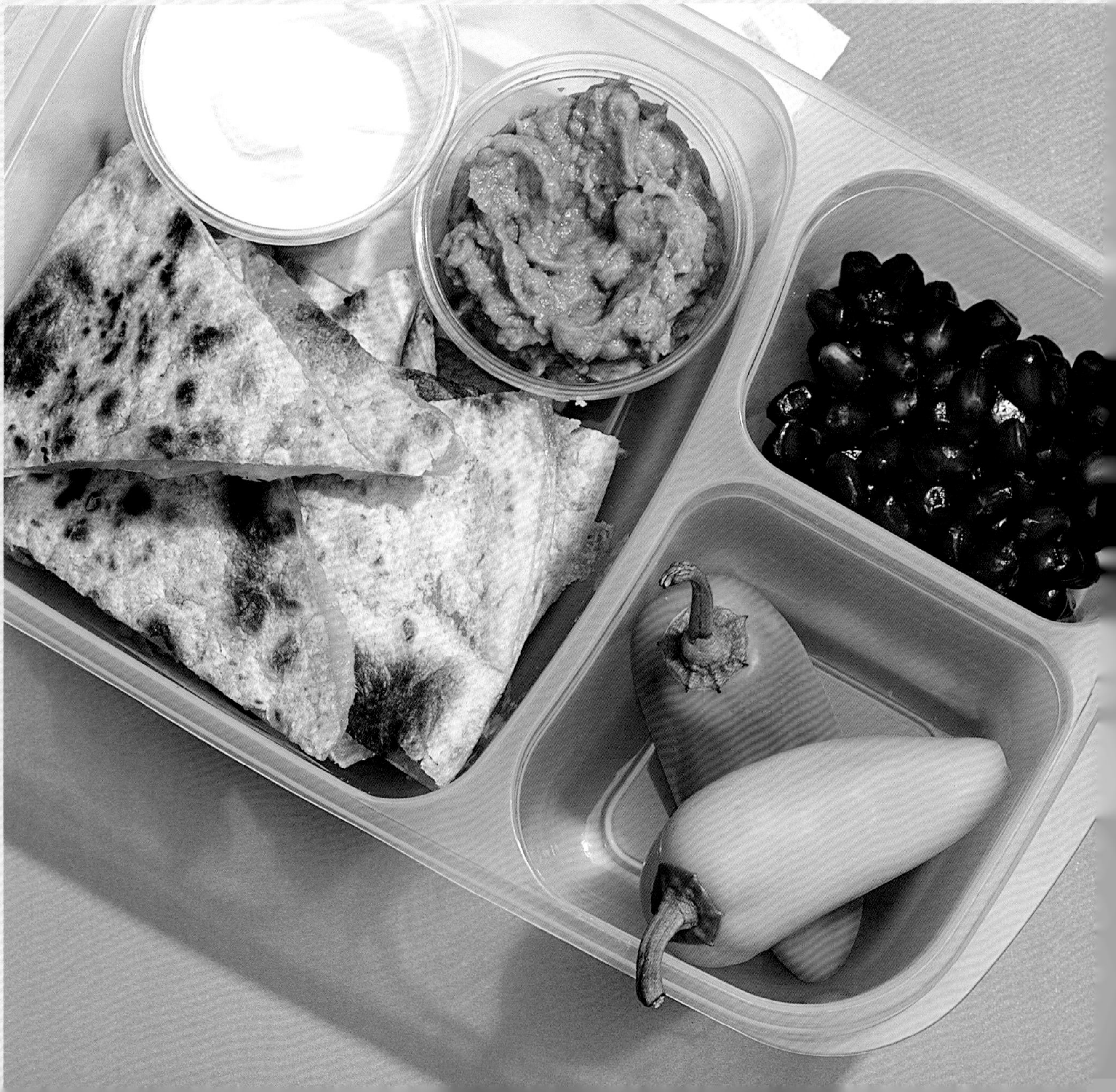

Week 1

These lunches offer a lot of variety without having entirely different ingredients each day.

MONDAY
(Shown on page 83)

- Quesadillas with guac and/or sour cream for dipping
- Pomegranate seeds
- Mini bell peppers

TUESDAY

- Chicken salad
- Crackers
- Strawberries
- Cucumber slices
- Chocolate chunks

WEDNESDAY

- Sunflower seed butter and jelly sandwich
- Dried crunchy broccoli
- Blueberries
- Chocolate chunks and white chocolate chips

THURSDAY

- Chicken salad wraps
- Pomegranate seeds
- Mini bell peppers
- Shredded cheese

FRIDAY
(Shown on page 111)

- Strawberry cream cheese sandwich
- Dried crunchy broccoli
- Trail mix (homemade or store-bought)

SHOPPING LIST

- Tortillas
- Whole-grain crackers
- Whole-grain bread
- Shredded cheese
- Cream cheese
- Chicken salad (homemade or store-bought)
- Sunflower seed butter
- Jelly
- Guacamole or sour cream
- Pomegranate seeds
- Strawberries
- Blueberries
- Mini bell peppers
- Cucumbers
- Dried crunchy broccoli
- Trail mix
- Chocolate chunks
- White chocolate chips

Week 2

This week has a little less variety but shows that you can still mix things up while minimizing how many foods you buy.

MONDAY

- Whole-grain crackers
- Sliced turkey
- Sliced cheese
- Carrot chips
- Grapes, quartered lengthwise

TUESDAY

- Turkey and cheese sandwich
- Raspberries
- Snow peas with hummus
- Small cookies

WEDNESDAY

- Whole-grain crackers and sunflower seed butter sandwich
- Carrot chips
- Raspberries
- Chocolate chips

THURSDAY

- Turkey and hummus sandwich
- Grapes, quartered lengthwise
- Snow peas
- Small cookies

FRIDAY

- Sunflower seed butter sandwich
- Carrot chips
- Raspberries
- Cut-up cheese

SHOPPING LIST

- Whole-grain crackers
- Whole-grain bread
- Turkey
- Cheese
- Sunflower seed butter
- Hummus
- Grapes
- Raspberries
- Carrot chips
- Snow peas
- Cookies
- Chocolate chips

Snacks

Even though this is a lunch book, like most of our clients you're still probably in need of some snack inspo. Snacks are important for kids (and adults) for so many reasons. Kids are growing and need a regular source of energy, so a snack helps tide them over between meals. Snacks also ensure that kids get enough food when they're going through a picky stage.

Sure, "snack foods" are often crunchy beige foods—think chips, crackers, veggie straws, and cheese crackers—but they can be made from veggies, fruits, and protein foods too. Adding some protein and fat makes snacks more filling and wards off the "hangry."

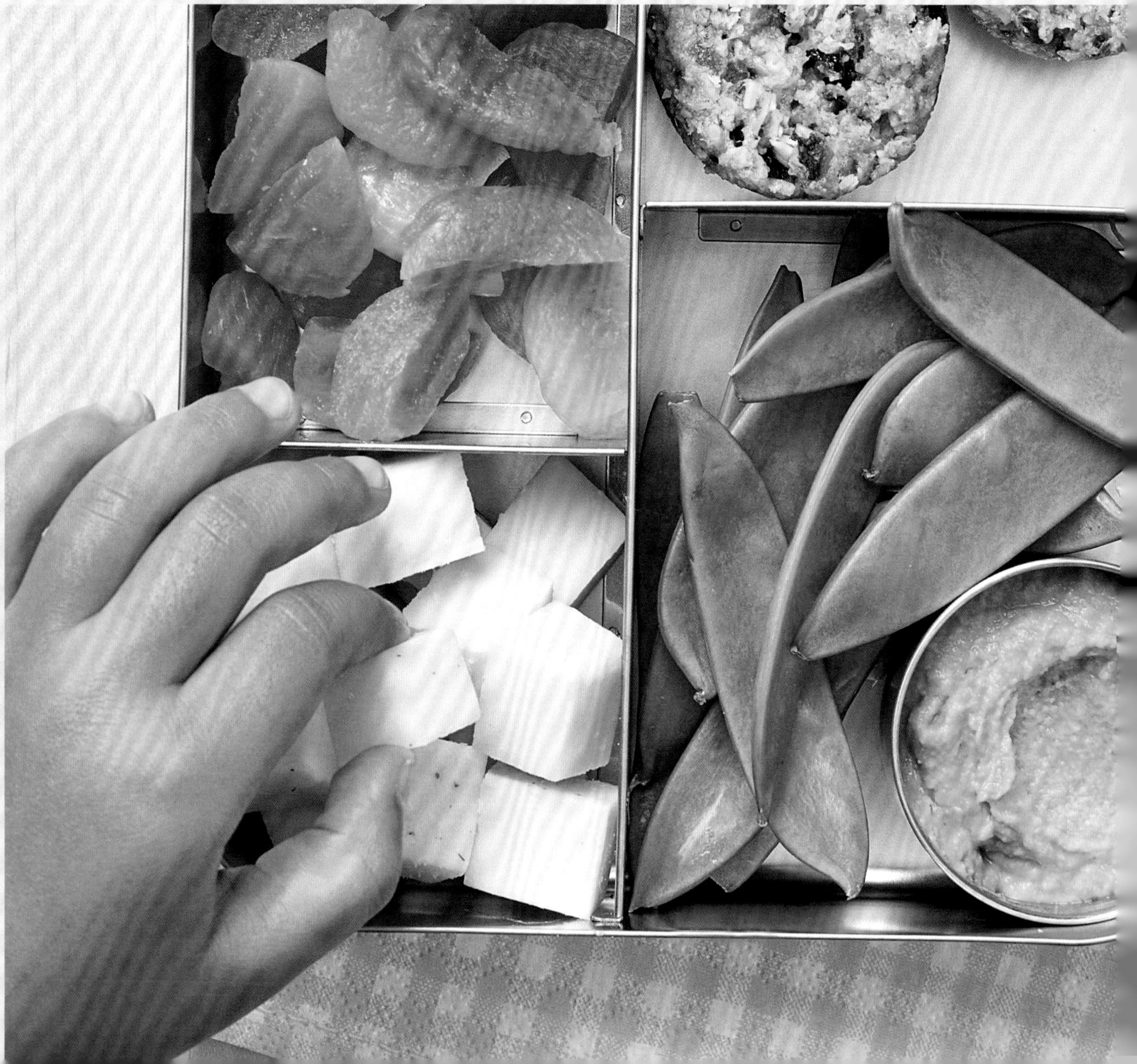

Here are some snack tips:

1. **Offer three meals and two to three snacks to kids ages one and over.** If a young toddler is still breastfeeding or drinking formula, milk feeds might replace their snacks for now.

2. **Cheese, nut butter, energy bites, a protein bar, yogurt, roasted garbanzo beans, or a hard-boiled egg** gives snacks more staying power, due to their protein and fat content. Add a veggie or fruit to their snack if you can!

3. **Make sure to keep snacks safe for toddlers.** The snacks listed here are not necessarily modified for choking hazards. Remember to serve apples thinly sliced, quarter grapes lengthwise, and avoid whole nuts.

Oh, and here's a *super* important reminder: **No matter what time you pick up your kids from school, they most definitely *will* be hungry. Yes, even if they just ate a meal or a snack. It's a thing.** We recommend having a snack ready right away or when you get home to minimize hangry meltdowns.

Snack Ideas

REQUIRES REFRIGERATION OR ICE PACKS

- Whole-grain crackers, cheese cubes, and sliced pears
- Matchstick apples (cut thinly into matchstick pieces) and yogurt dip
- Trail mix and peach slices
- Crackers, cubed chicken, and cucumber slices
- Mini bagels with cream cheese and freeze-dried mango
- Hard-boiled egg and pretzel sticks
- Pita or pita chips and hummus (can also add carrot sticks)
- Cereal and milk of your choice
- Chips, guac, and bell peppers
- Apple and string cheese
- Mini pizza bagels and watermelon
- Cottage cheese and peaches
- Pretzel rods, hard-boiled egg, and blueberries
- Goldfish crackers, rolled turkey slices, and orange segments
- Smashed avocado on toast
- Waffle or pancake (from frozen) and sunflower seed butter

DOESN'T REQUIRE REFRIGERATION/ ICE PACKS

- Cheerios, whole banana or freeze-dried banana, and sunflower seed butter
- Hippeas (dairy-free cheese snack) and freeze-dried strawberries
- Lärabar or other fruit and nut bar
- Pretzels, turkey jerky, and whole apple
- Granola bar or oat bar and frozen string cheese (freeze to keep cold a few hours)
- Pretzel rods and crunchy baked cheese
- Banana and frozen yogurt tube (freeze to keep cold a few hours)
- Aussie Bites and unpeeled mandarin orange
- Roasted garbanzo beans and fruit cup
- Beef stick and snap pea crisps
- Rice cakes, peanut or sunflower seed butter, and sliced banana
- Graham crackers, almond butter, and whole pear

Snack Ideas

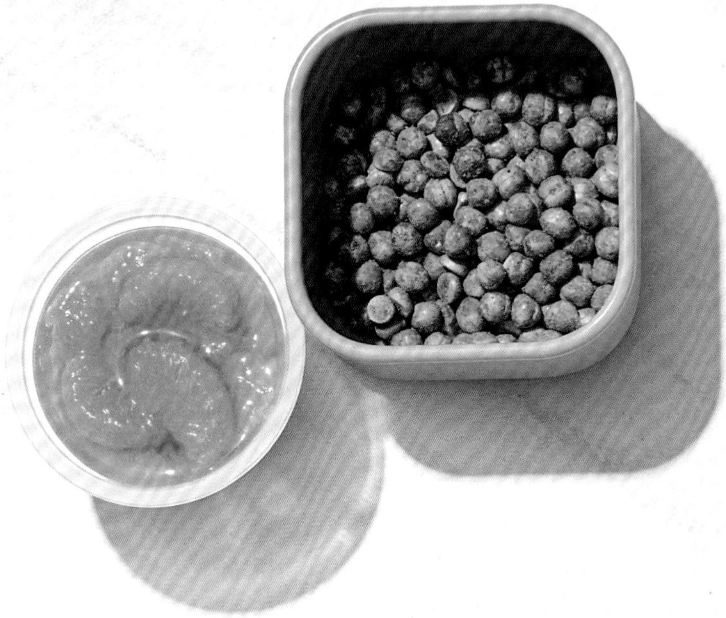

Garbanzo beans and fruit cup →

OMIELIFE OMIESNACK

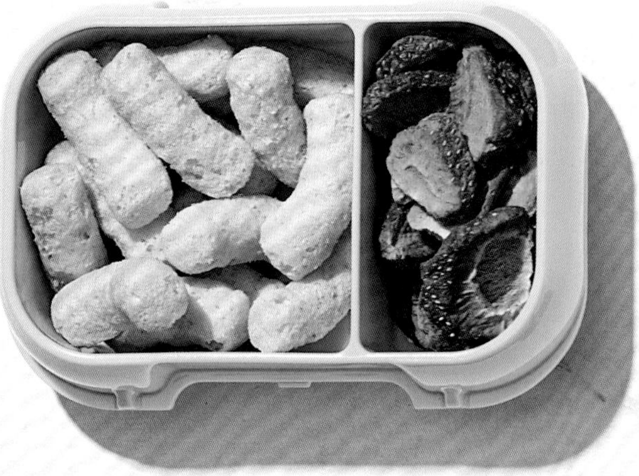

← Hippeas and freeze-dried strawberries

BENTGO KIDS SNACK

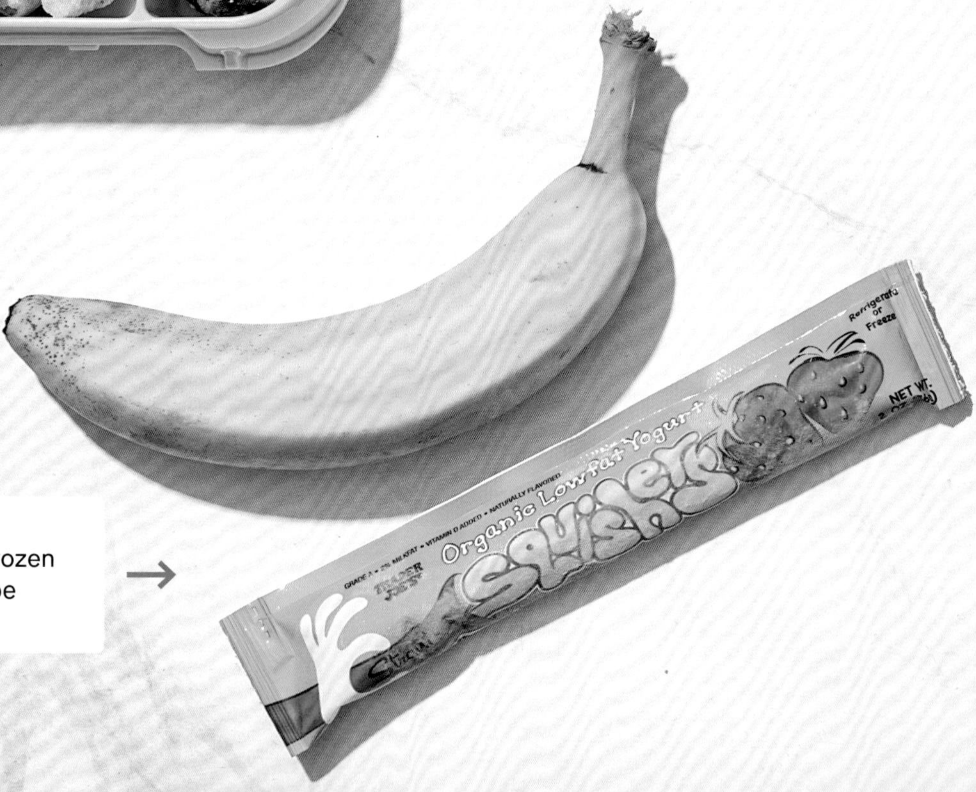

Banana and frozen yogurt tube →

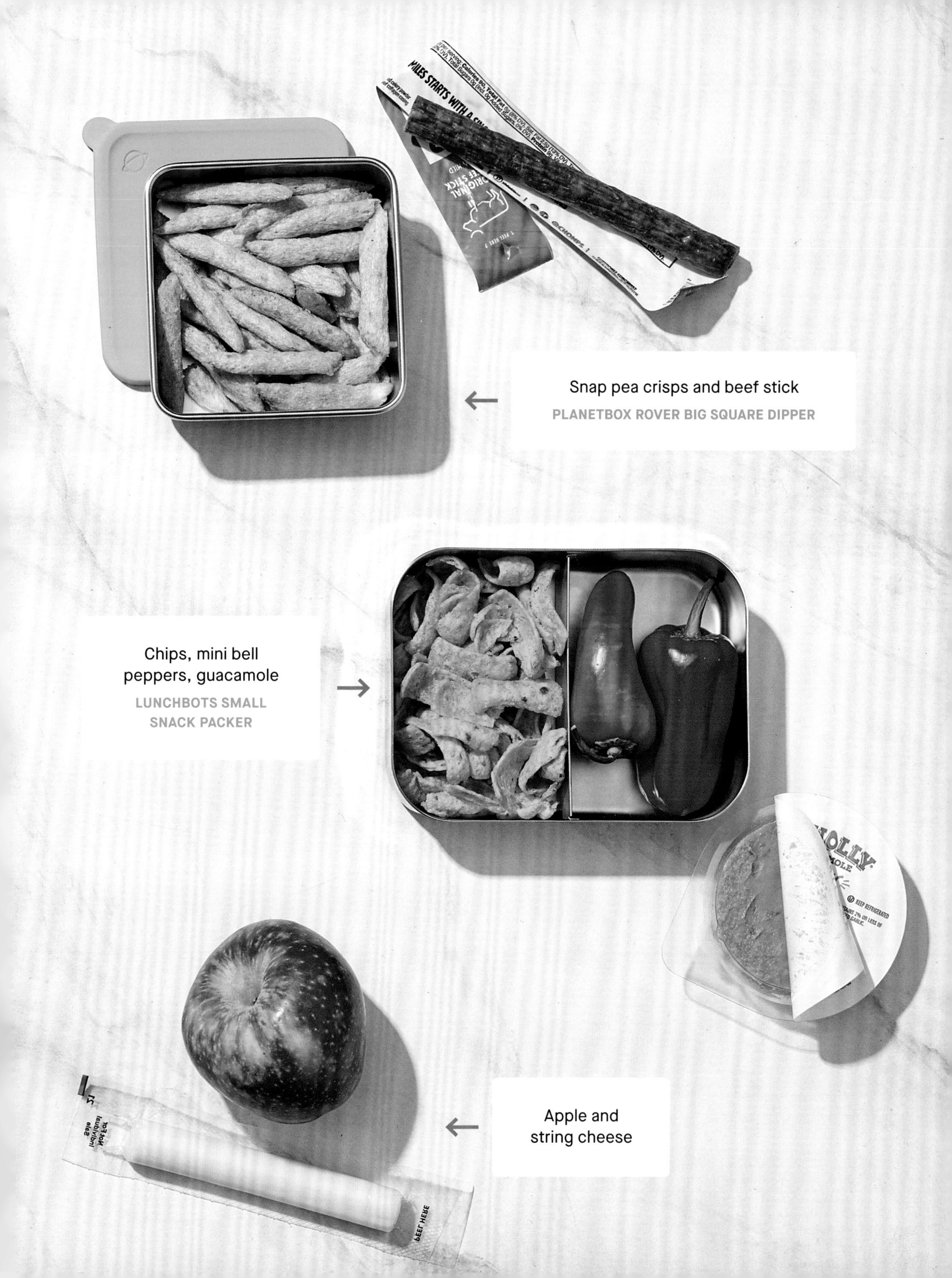

Snap pea crisps and beef stick

PLANETBOX ROVER BIG SQUARE DIPPER

Chips, mini bell peppers, guacamole

LUNCHBOTS SMALL SNACK PACKER

Apple and string cheese

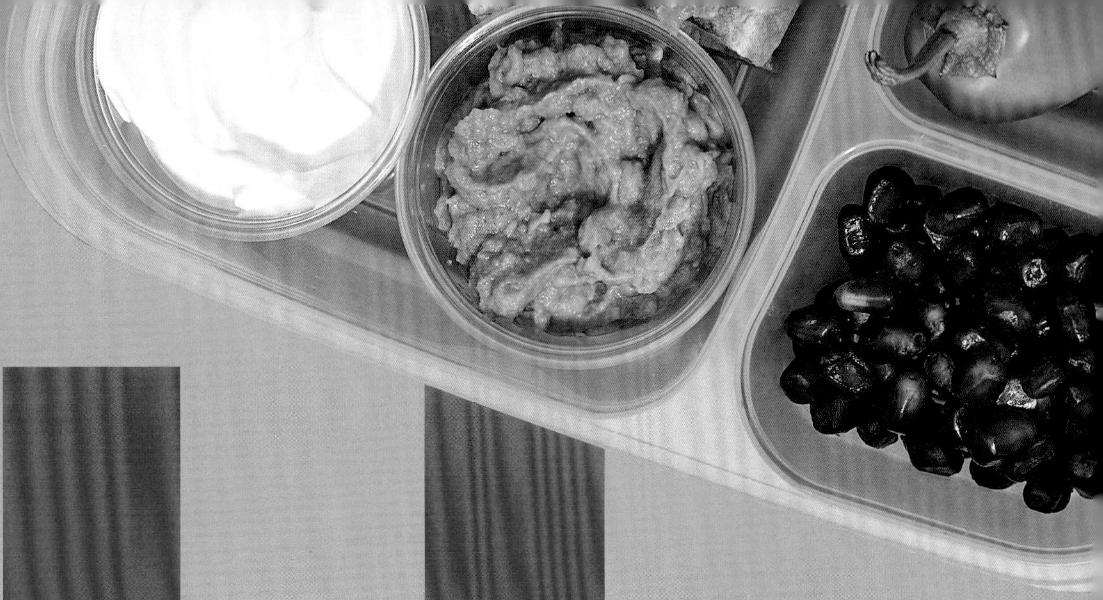

THE LUN

The rest of this book contains lunch inspo for you (and your child) to look through. Not everything will be a "yes" for your family, but we hope that you discover something delicious and doable for you. In each lunch idea you'll find a list of components, which are the foods that make up that lunch, plus allergy tips for those who have to be free from certain top nine allergens. You'll also find our thoughts for making these lunches safer and easier for kids ages one to three to eat, as well as picky eating tips. Some lunches will also have prep advice or "I Can't Even" tips to make assembly of that lunch even easier, as well as vegetarian swaps if the lunch contains meat, poultry, or fish. We hope you enjoy these ideas!

CE

HS

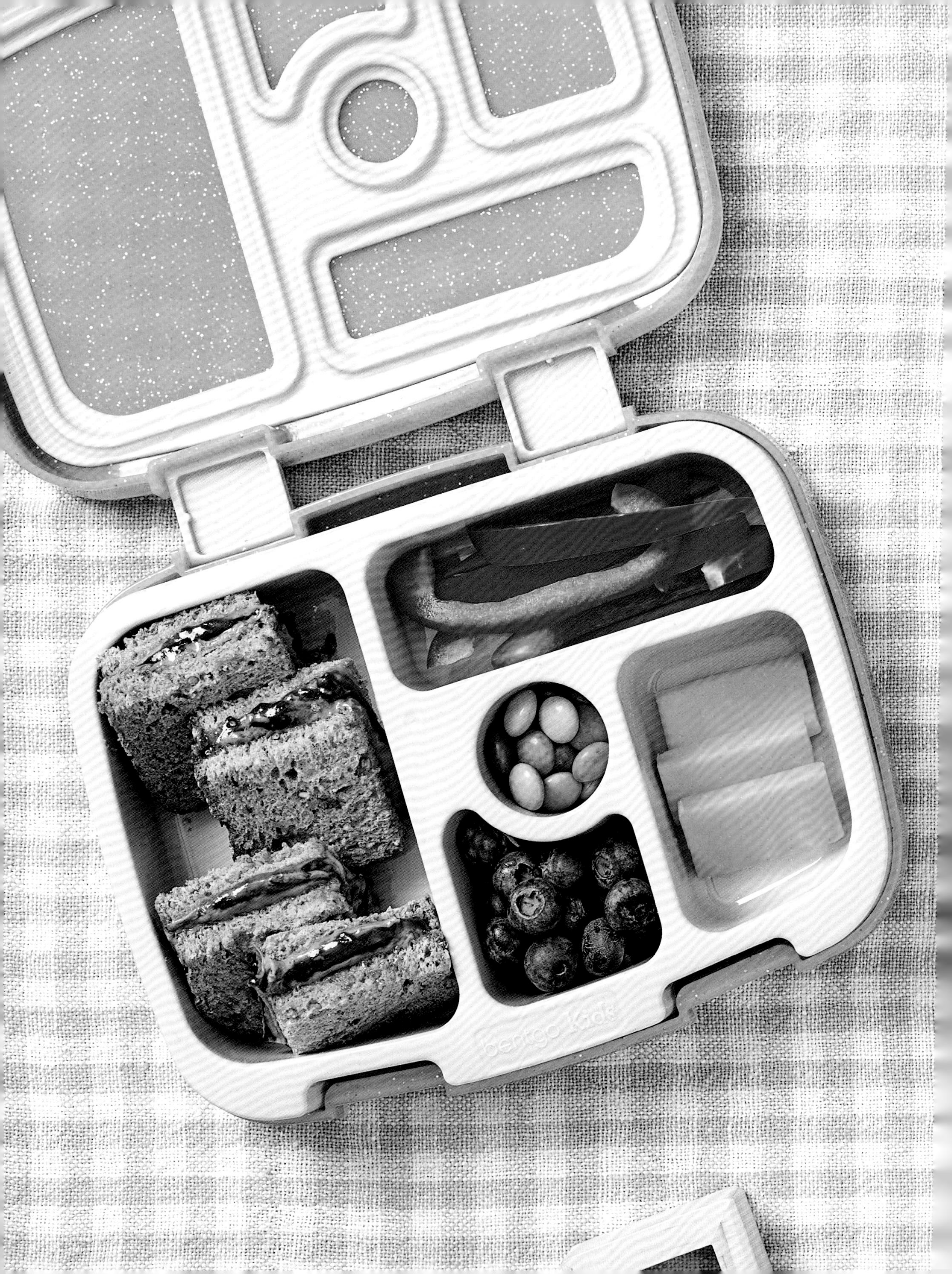
bentgo kids

Traditional PB&J

Peanut butter and jelly is a classic kid favorite, something many students eat every day at school. The protein, fat, and fiber from the sandwich offer nice staying power for a day of play and learning. Of course, many schools are nut-free, so use the substitutes listed below to make this allergy-friendly.

Peanut butter and jelly sandwich on whole-grain bread,
cut into quarters

Blueberries

Thinly sliced red bell pepper

Cheddar cheese

Candy-coated milk chocolate
(Trader Joe's brand shown)

ALLERGY TIPS

PEANUTS: Use sunflower seed butter, almond butter, granola butter, soy butter, or cream cheese instead of peanut butter.

WHEAT: Use gluten-free bread or a rice cake instead of whole-wheat bread.

DAIRY: Use dairy-free chocolate chips or another dessert option. Swap the cheddar cheese for a dairy-free cheese your child enjoys.

TODDLER TIP

Make sure your bread doesn't have large seeds, as they can be a choking hazard for kids under four.

PICKY EATING TIP

If bell peppers are a non-preferred food for your child, serve just a few thin slices of peppers and consider adding a favorite dip in a separate container on the side.

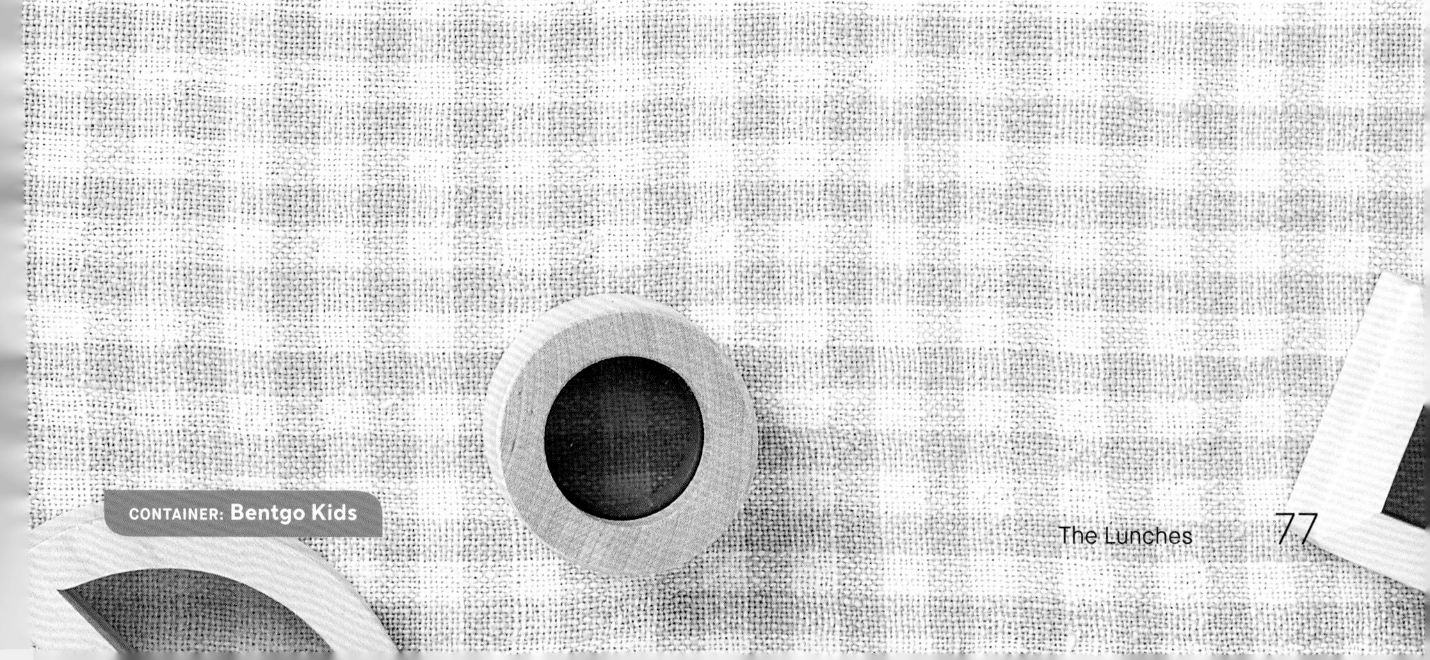

CONTAINER: Bentgo Kids

Mix Up Your PB&J

We get it—PB&J is delicious (and easy)! We love it too. But for many kids, seeing the exact same PB&J every day can start to limit their willingness to try other foods. Adding a little variety to how you serve their beloved sandwich can slowly help them become used to different foods (and can offer some different nutrients too). Here are our favorite ways to mix up PB&J.

Change up the jelly (try grape instead of strawberry). →

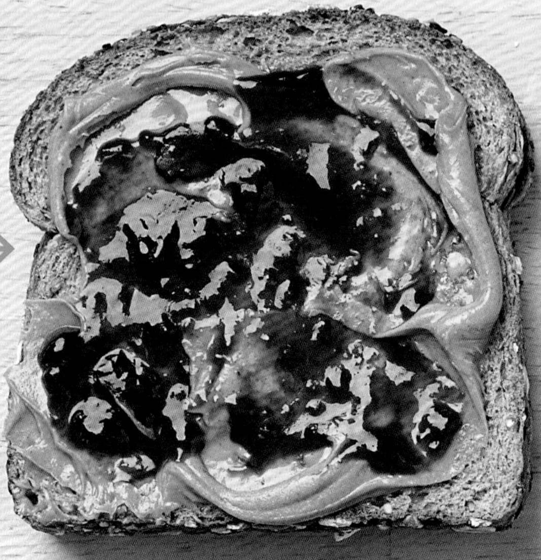

Swap a toasted waffle for the bread. →

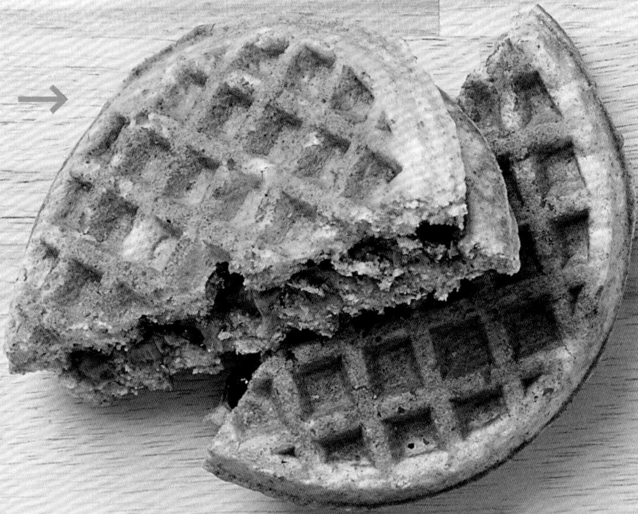

Use fresh sliced or smashed fruit instead of jelly (we love smashed raspberries, sliced strawberries, and sliced banana). →

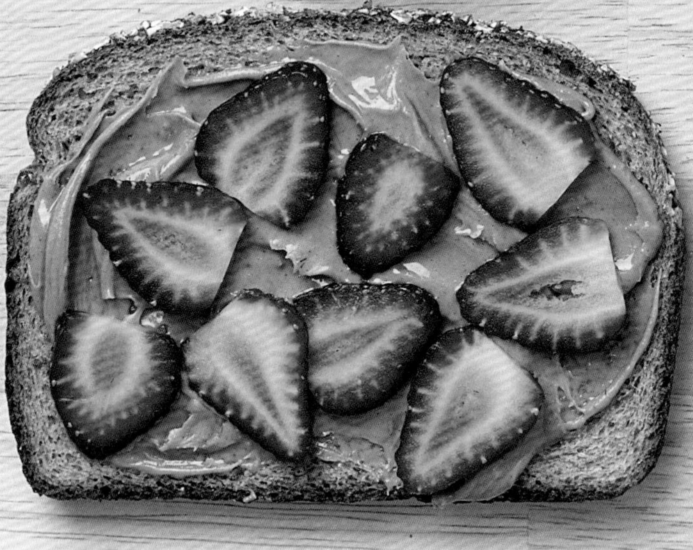

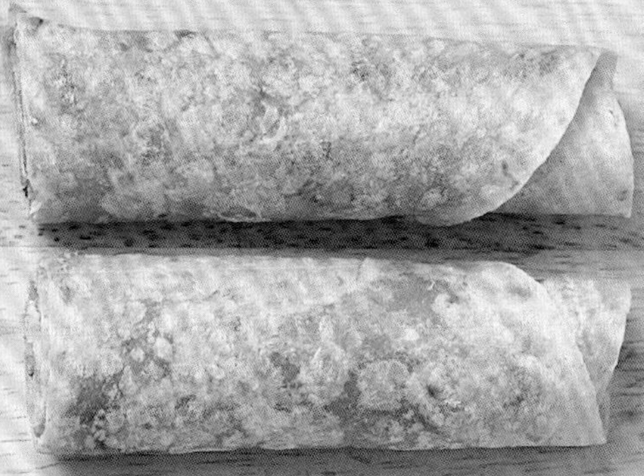

Serve it rolled up in a tortilla.

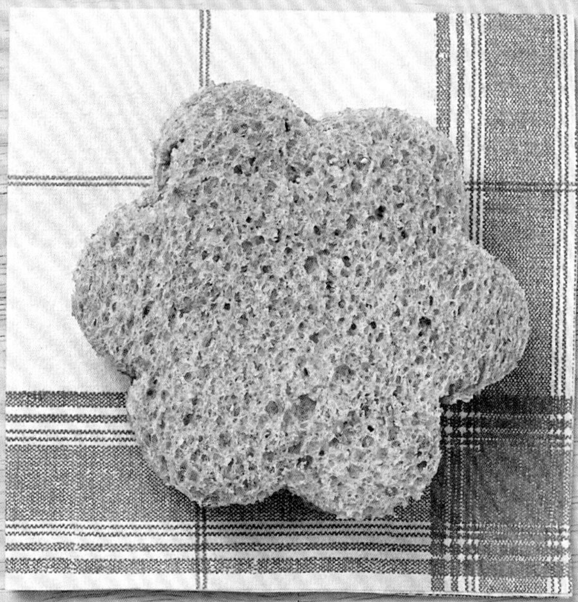

Use a cookie cutter (this is a great first step for kids who really struggle with any changes to their lunch).

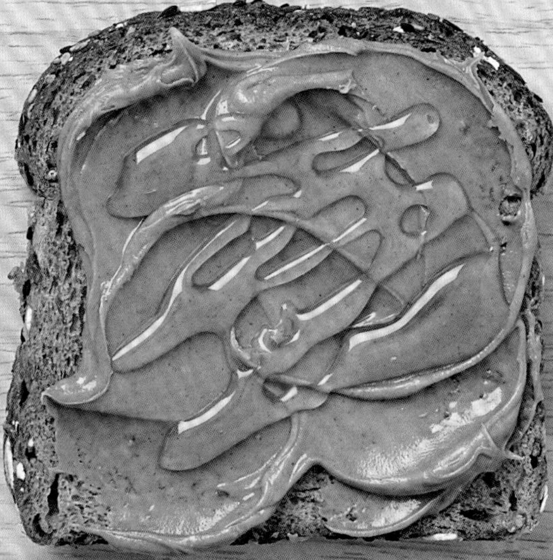

Try honey instead of jelly (not appropriate for babies under twelve months).

No Crust Raspberry and Nut Butter Sandwich

Does your kid love those frozen premade PB&Js, but you're sick of paying a fortune for them? Enter this amazing sandwich cutter, which can be found at the QR code below. It seals the sandwich edges so the filling is less likely to pop out. Try smashed raspberries instead of jelly to add a nice tart flavor and some extra vitamins and fiber. (It's also a great way to use up any squishy raspberries your kid doesn't want to eat!)

Nut butter or sunflower seed butter and smashed raspberries on whole-grain bread, cut with a sandwich cutter/sealer

Freeze-dried bananas

Rainbow baby carrots

Sun chips

White and dark chocolate chips

https://sites.prh.com/feedinglittleslunches

PREP TIP

Spread nut or seed butter on both pieces of bread first. This will help keep the bread from getting soggy from the raspberries. Wash and fully dry raspberries before using a fork to smash them atop the layer of nut/seed butter, then assemble the sandwich.

ALLERGY TIPS

PEANUTS: Use sunflower seed butter, almond butter, granola butter, soy butter, or cream cheese instead of nut butter.

WHEAT: Most gluten-free breads don't work well with these sandwich cutters because the bread doesn't seal well. If you want to use something fun, try a cookie cutter instead with your gluten-free bread.

DAIRY: Use dairy-free chocolate chips.

TODDLER TIPS

This lunch contains multiple crunchy foods that kids love, but they might pose an increased choking risk for toddlers under four.

- Some freeze-dried bananas are very hard and crunchy. If this is all you can find, serve a whole banana or another fresh fruit instead.
- Cut carrots thinly, lengthwise.
- Sub pretzel sticks or a puffed snack for chips.

PICKY EATING TIP

It's amazing how effective a sandwich cutter and sealer can be with kids when they are reluctant to eat sandwiches. Give it a try!

CONTAINER: Yumbox Presto

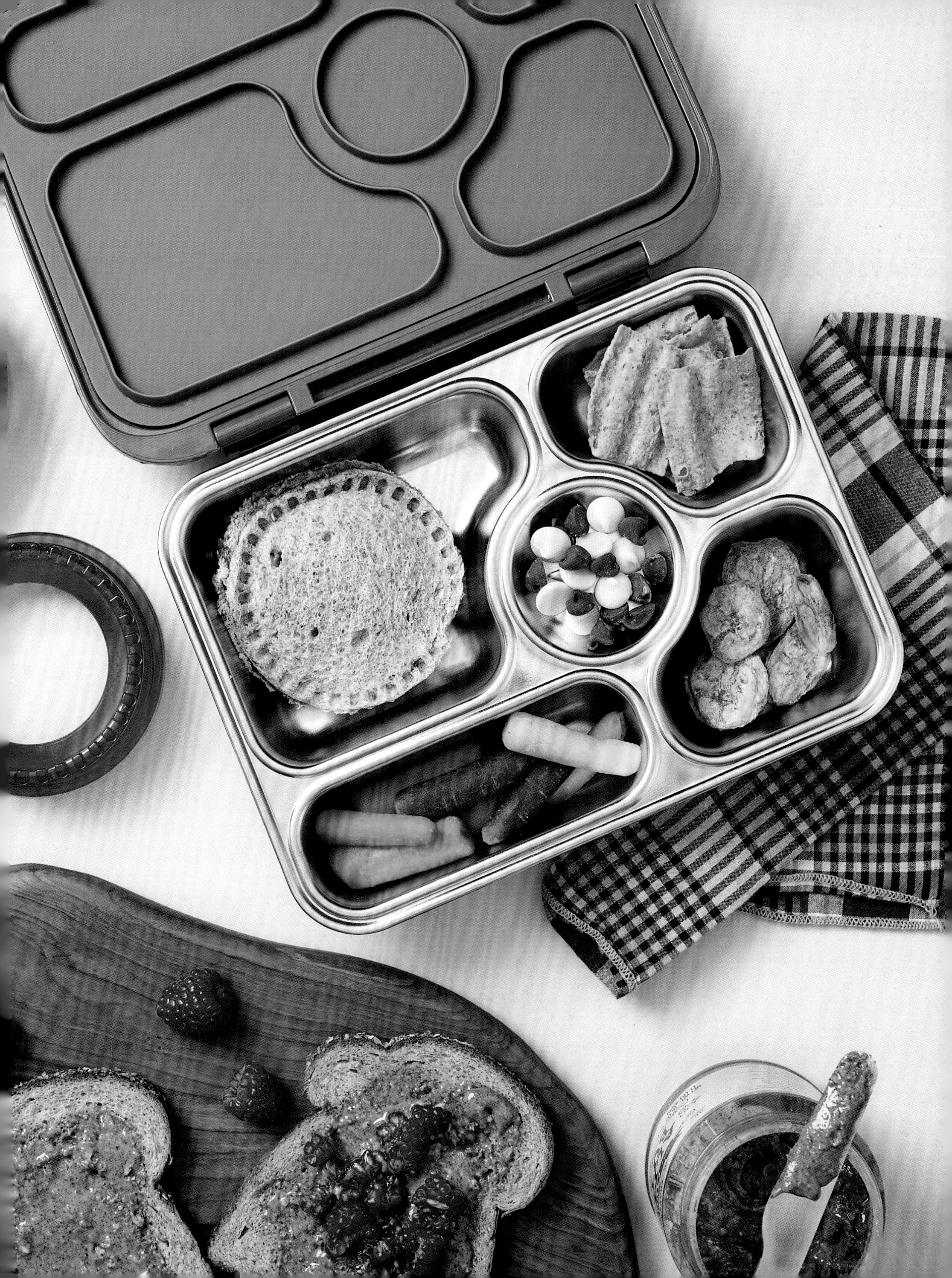

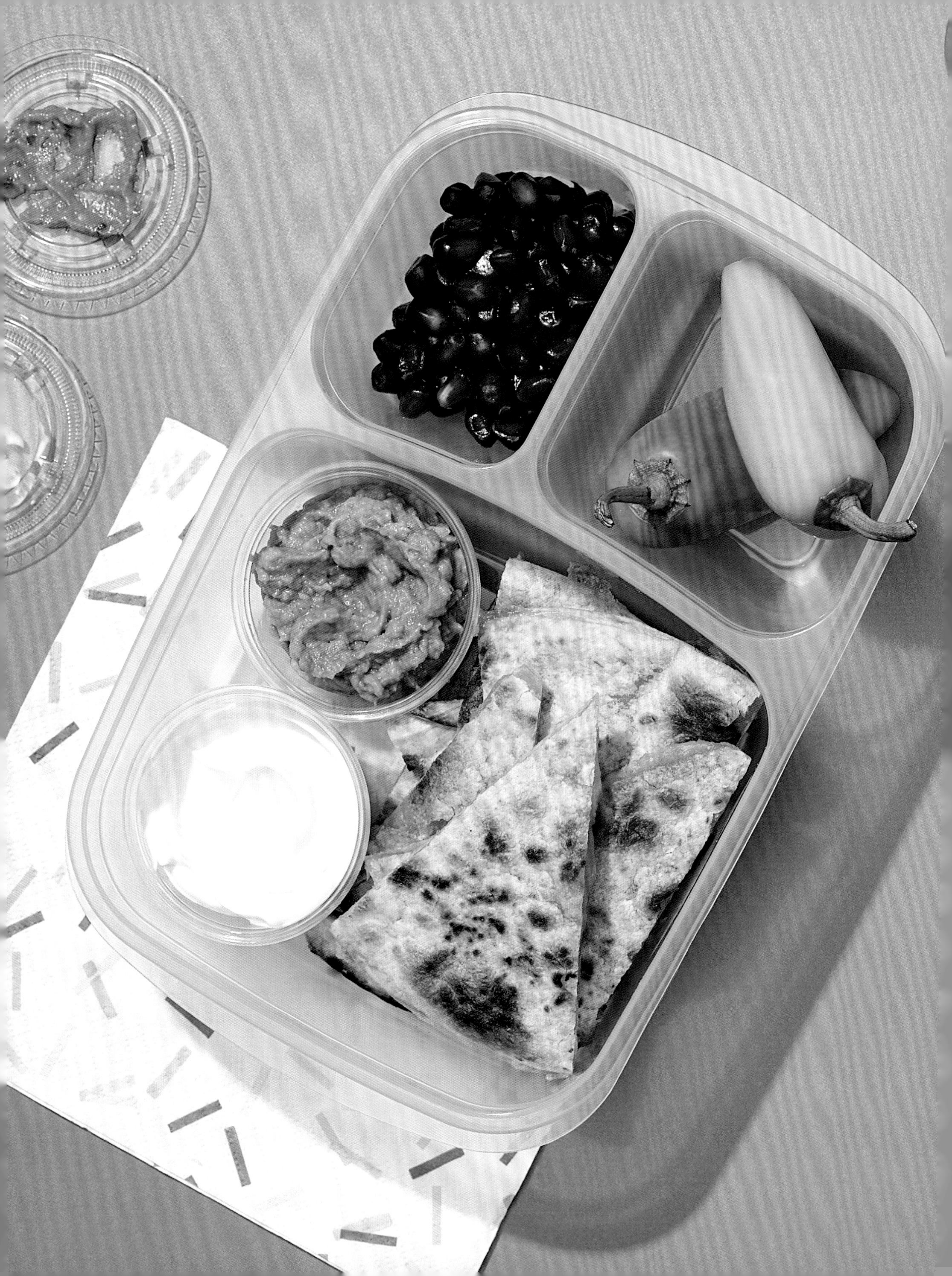

Quesadilla

Many parents don't think of sending quesadillas in a cold lunch box, but quesadillas are kind of like pizza—they're delicious at any temperature! Make your quesadilla with cheese only, or add shredded veggies, black beans, or chicken for a little extra nutrition and flavor. Kids love to dip, so sour cream, guacamole, or salsa can be a delicious addition to this lunch.

Cheese quesadilla

Guacamole and sour cream
(in separate containers)

Pomegranate seeds

Mini bell peppers

PREP TIP

Use a leftover quesadilla from dinner the night before, or make it easily in the microwave with tortillas and shredded cheese.

ALLERGY TIPS

WHEAT: Use a gluten-free tortilla instead of a wheat tortilla.

DAIRY: For best results with dairy-free cheese, heat one tortilla in a pan. In a separate small pan, add your dairy-free cheese on medium heat so it melts properly. Slide the melted cheese onto the heating tortilla, then add the second tortilla and flip right away. You'll also want to use a dairy-free sour cream of your choice.

TODDLER TIPS

Pomegranate seeds are really hard, so they might constitute a choking hazard for kids under four. Serve cut-up oranges or strawberries instead.

Cut a bell pepper into thin strips.

PICKY EATING TIP

Mini bell peppers are novel and fun—they look like regular bell peppers, just shrunken, and can be an appealing option for a reluctant eater who might normally not go for them.

CONTAINER: Bentgo Easyboxes 3-Compartment Meal Container (formerly EasyLunchboxes brand)

Pasta Salad

Boiling water is a no-go on busy mornings, but if you have leftover plain pasta from dinner the night before, toss it with some tomatoes, garbanzo beans, and (optional) Italian dressing for a delicious and colorful pasta salad entrée.

Tricolor rotini pasta salad

with plum tomatoes quartered lengthwise, canned garbanzo beans, and (optional) Italian dressing

Quartered mozzarella cheese

Applesauce

Chocolate chip cookie

ALLERGY TIPS

WHEAT: Use gluten-free or legume-based pasta instead of wheat pasta. Just know that many gluten-free pastas do not make great leftovers. This lunch might be best eaten at home using freshly made gluten-free pasta. Use a gluten-free cookie instead of a regular chocolate chip cookie.

DAIRY: Use dairy-free cheese of your choice. Make sure the cookie you send is dairy-free as well.

TODDLER TIP

This lunch is already modified for choking hazards, but if you're not ready to send desserts to school, add fresh or freeze-dried fruit.

PICKY EATING TIPS

Sometimes a little note is a nice surprise for a reluctant eater. We're not saying that you have to do this all the time—or ever—but if your kiddo is struggling with food, a sweet reminder from you can be encouraging. (Plus, it's a nice way to "fill up" a space in the lunch box that isn't used.)

Also, if your child isn't familiar with a new color pasta, try a familiar pasta instead.

CONTAINER: Bentgo Easyboxes 5-Compartment Meal Container (formerly EasyLunchboxes brand)

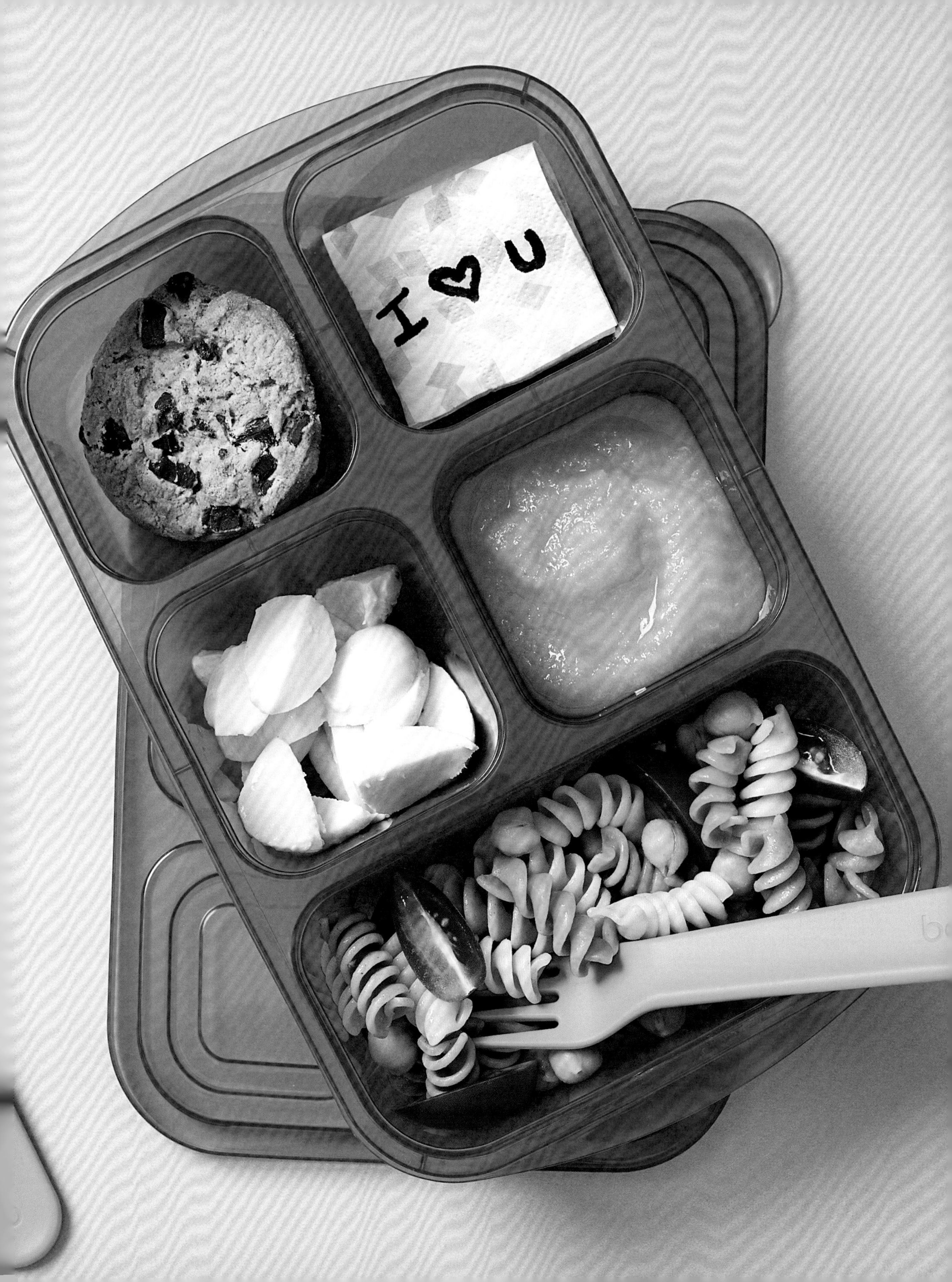
I ♥ U

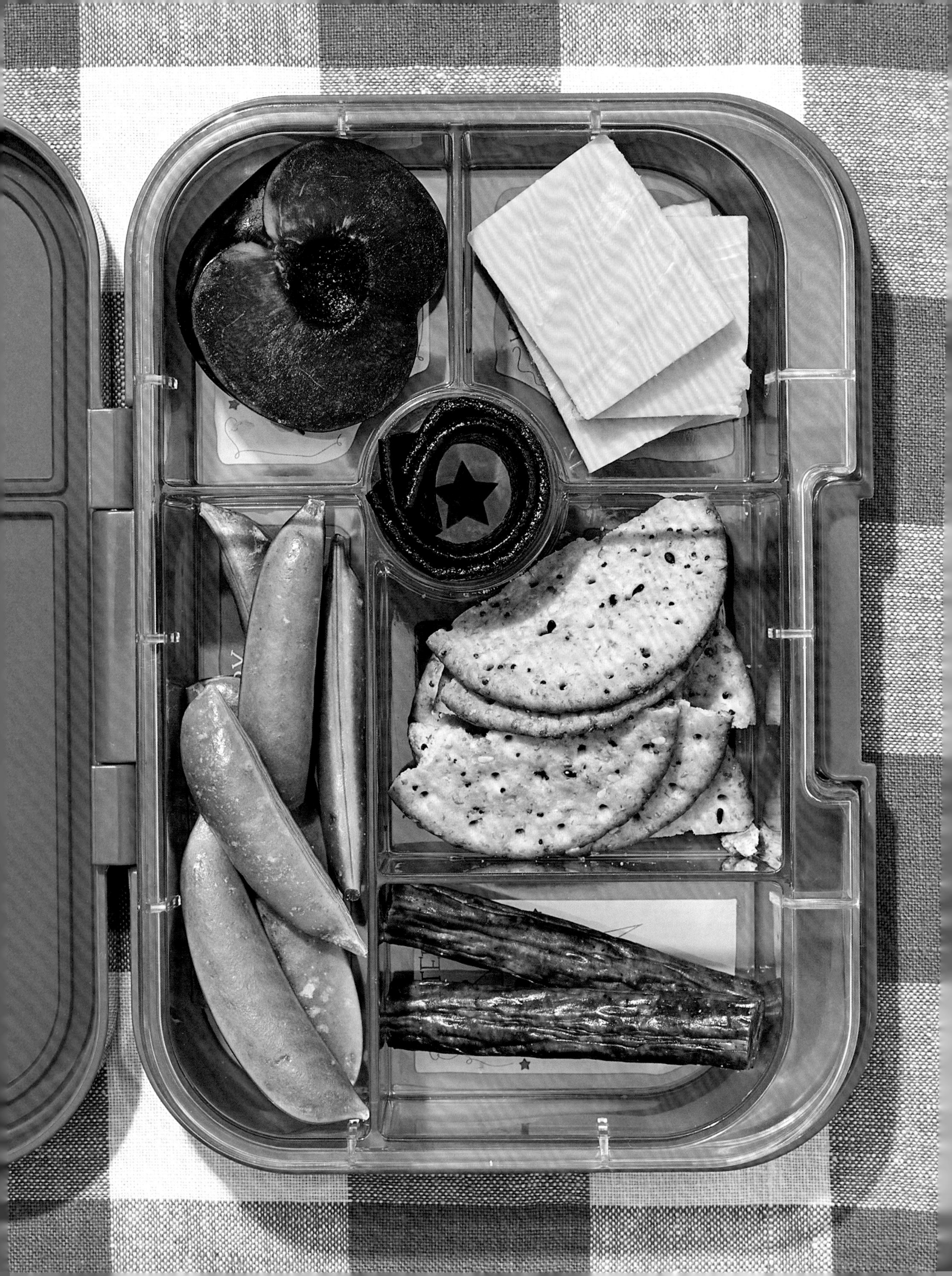

Cheese, Crackers, and Beef Stick

Do your kids like "snack" lunches? Yup, ours do too. This is an especially awesome one because it's so easy to make and can be a big hit in the cafeteria. Use whole-grain crackers for a little extra fiber and staying power.

Sliced cheddar cheese

Whole-grain crackers

Beef stick

Halved plum

Snap peas

Fruit leather

ALLERGY TIPS

WHEAT: Use gluten-free crackers instead of wheat crackers.

DAIRY: Use dairy-free cheese or replace with kidney beans or garbanzo beans.

TODDLER TIPS

To minimize choking risk, dice the beef stick into small pieces (not rounds) or serve roast beef slices instead.

If your fruit leather is sticky or hard to chew, try chocolate chips or a piece of fruit.

PICKY EATING TIP

If your child has never seen a plum before, it might help to serve it at home first. However, don't be surprised if they try something unexpected at school—remember, the environment is wildly different than it is at home, and kids can really surprise us by what they eat there!

VEGETARIAN SWAP

Sub a hard-boiled egg or kidney beans for the beef stick.

CONTAINER: Yumbox Original

Chicken Salad with Mini Brioche Toasts

These little brioche toasts, found at many grocery stores in the cheese or cracker section, are fun and interesting starch options that make perfect dippers for chicken salad. They also happen to fit in the Bentgo Kids compartment perfectly!

Premade chicken salad
(you can make it at home too)

Cheese stick

Brioche toasts

Grapes,
quartered lengthwise

Thinly sliced celery

Sunflower seed butter cup

PREP TIP

We served this in a unique way, using a silicone insert to separate the chicken salad from the cheese, but you could also just serve the cheese stick on the side.

ALLERGY TIPS

WHEAT: Serve gluten-free bread (cut into small squares) or crackers instead of mini brioche toasts.

DAIRY: Omit string cheese; use dairy-free chocolate or a dairy-free filled chocolate cup instead of the sunflower seed butter cup.

TREE NUTS: Watch for whole nuts in premade chicken salad (pecans and walnuts are often used).

EGG: Make chicken salad at home using vegan mayo instead of store-bought chicken salad, which might contain egg.

TODDLER TIPS

If your brioche toasts seem too crunchy for your toddler to eat, send soft crackers instead.

Make sure that your premade chicken salad doesn't contain whole nuts, whole grapes, or whole celery pieces, which can be a choking hazard for kids under four.

PICKY EATING TIP

Some selective eaters love mayo-based salads; others won't touch them. If this is a really tough option for your child, try sending shredded chicken first. Consider sending the mayo separately so they can add it as a spread at school (depending on their age).

VEGETARIAN SWAP

Try a chickpea "chicken" salad (many recipes can be found online) or egg salad.

CONTAINER: Bentgo Kids

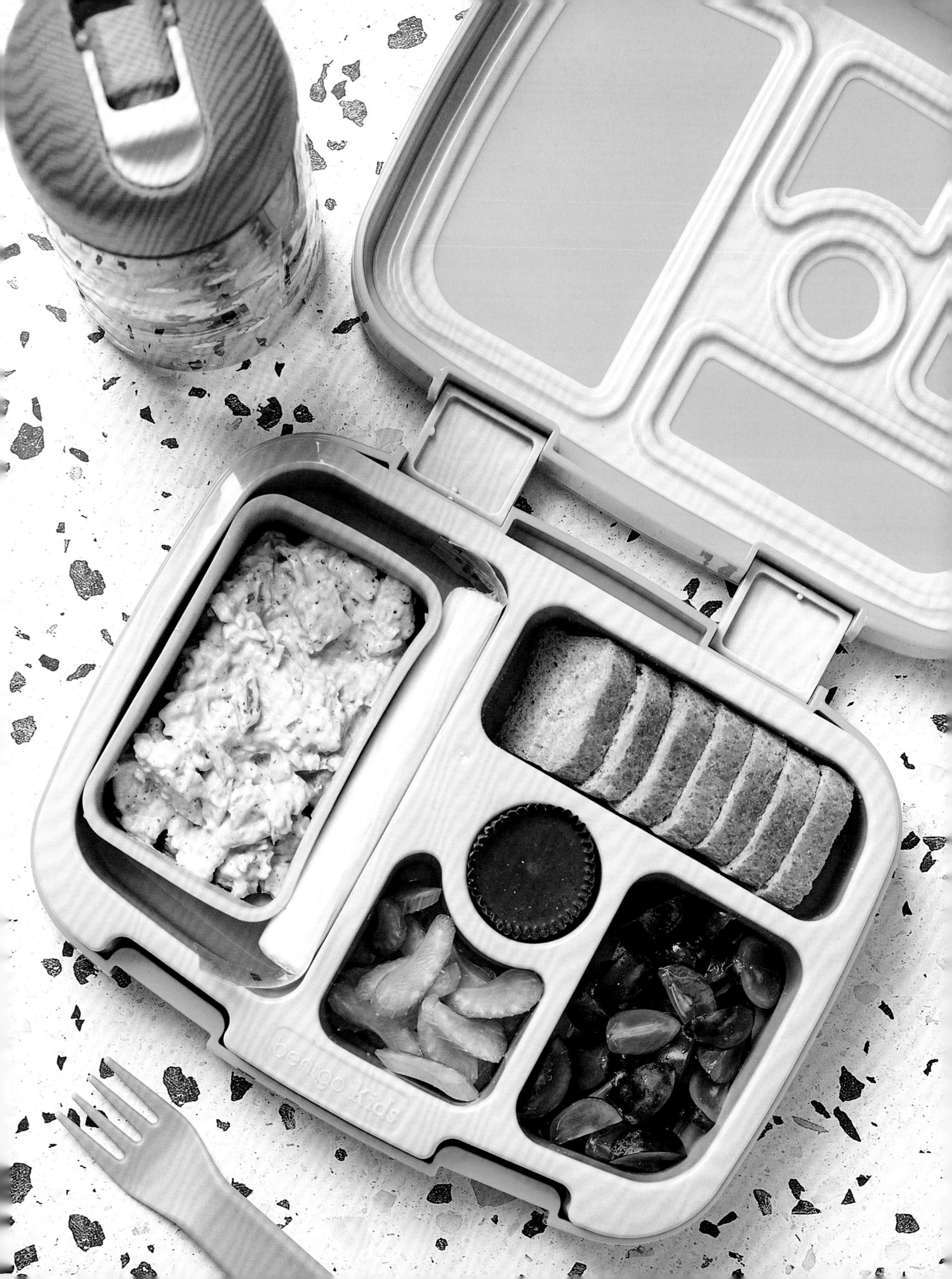
bentgo Kids

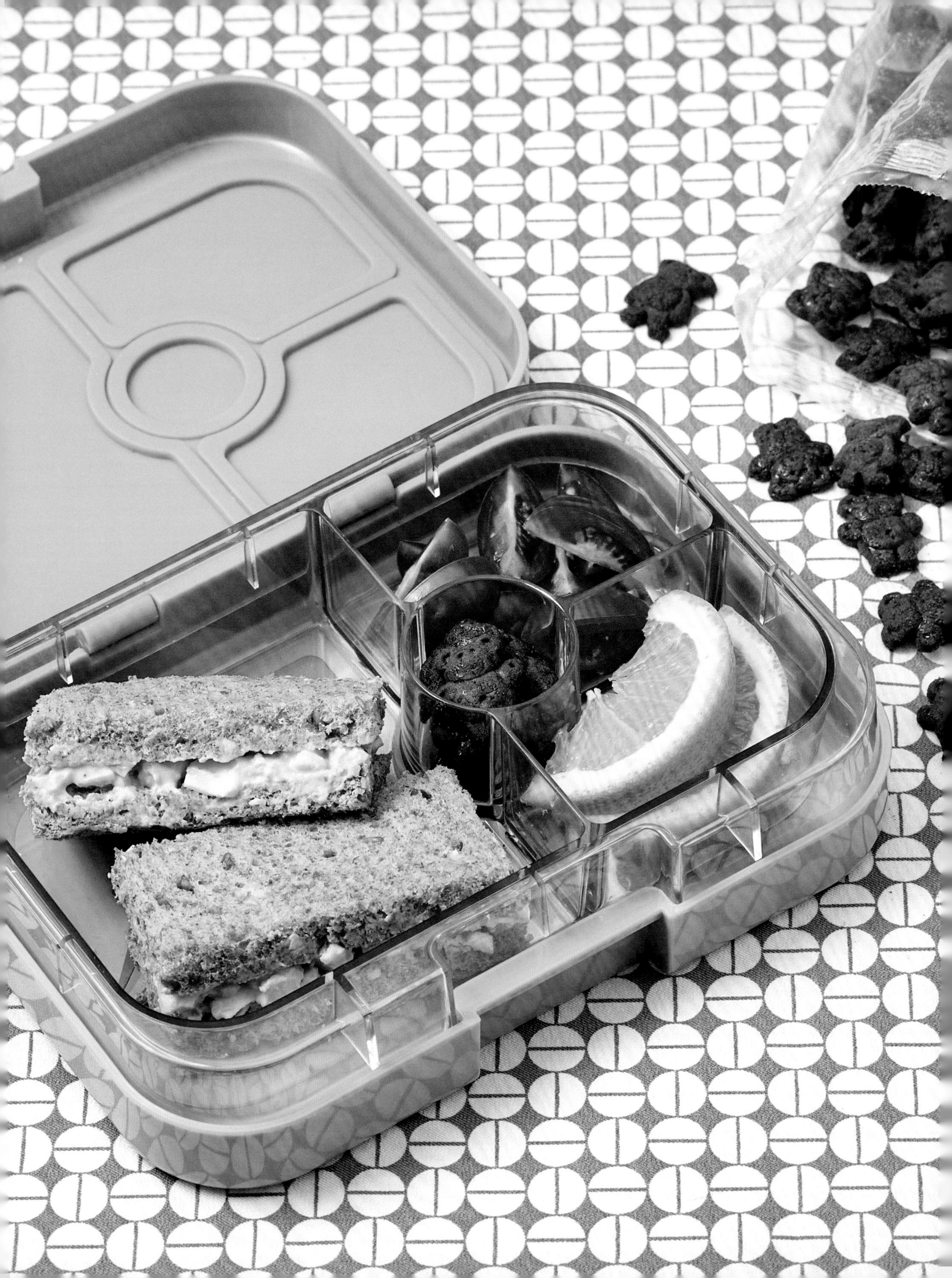

Egg Salad Sandwich

Egg salad is quite the underrated lunch option for kids who enjoy scrambled or hard-boiled eggs. It's easy to whip up in a big batch or to buy premade, and it makes for a very satisfying lunch!

Egg salad sandwich on whole-grain bread
(store-bought or homemade; shown without crust and cut in half)

Orange wedges

Plum tomatoes,
quartered lengthwise

Chocolate bear cookies

PREP TIP

Scared of a soggy sandwich? Pack this the morning of school—not the night before—to keep the bread intact. Counterintuitively, a thin layer of mayo (or mustard) on both pieces of bread can help prevent the bread from getting soggy.

ALLERGY TIPS

WHEAT: Use gluten-free bread instead of whole-grain bread and a wheat-free alternative to the chocolate bear cookies.

DAIRY: Use a dairy-free alternative to the chocolate bear cookies.

EGG: Serve chicken or tuna salad (made with vegan mayo) instead of egg salad; you can also find vegan egg salad recipes (usually made with tofu) online.

TODDLER TIP

This lunch is already modified for choking hazards, but if your child struggles to eat orange wedges with the peel, remove it before sending.

PICKY EATING TIP

Reluctant eaters can be sensitive to a strong "egg" smell when they open their lunch box. To help minimize that smell if you're making egg salad from scratch, make sure you don't overboil your eggs. Practice having the little ones peel eggs at home to get more comfortable with the smell before sending it to school. This is one of those foods that are an automatic turnoff to many people's noses, so if your child is especially sensitive, talk to them about it first.

CONTAINER: Yumbox Panino

Tuna Salad with Crackers

Your kid might shy away from a tuna salad sandwich, but pairing tuna salad with crackers might be a big *yes* for them because the tuna salad becomes a dip. Fresh cucumbers and sweet strawberries offer interesting flavors and textures to round out the meal.

Tuna salad
(premade or homemade)

Crackers

Strawberries,
quartered lengthwise

Sliced cucumber

Chocolate chunks

PREP TIP

If your child's lunch box doesn't have enough compartments, use a silicone cupcake liner to "create" another space for things like chocolate chunks, shown here. To keep it in place on the way to the lunchroom, make sure there is plenty of food in that compartment—in this case, notice how the strawberries are closely packed together.

ALLERGY TIPS

WHEAT: Use gluten-free crackers instead of wheat crackers.

DAIRY: Serve dairy-free chocolate chunks.

EGG: Use vegan mayo to make the tuna salad.

FISH: Use egg salad, chicken salad, or shredded beef/chicken instead of tuna salad.

TODDLER TIP

Make sure that your premade tuna salad doesn't contain large pieces of raw celery, fresh apple, or sliced almonds, which can be choking hazards.

PICKY EATING TIP

We serve desserts not just because they're delicious—they can also be a selective eater strategy. When kids see something familiar and preferred, they're more likely to start eating . . . and if they start eating, they're more likely to continue eating. Chocolate chunks (or a cookie or some graham crackers) might be just the food that "gets them going" on the meal. Yes, they might eat it before anything else, and that's OK.

VEGETARIAN SWAP

Sub vegetarian chickpea salad (many recipes can be found online) or roasted chickpeas for the tuna salad.

CONTAINER: Bentgo Kids Stainless Steel

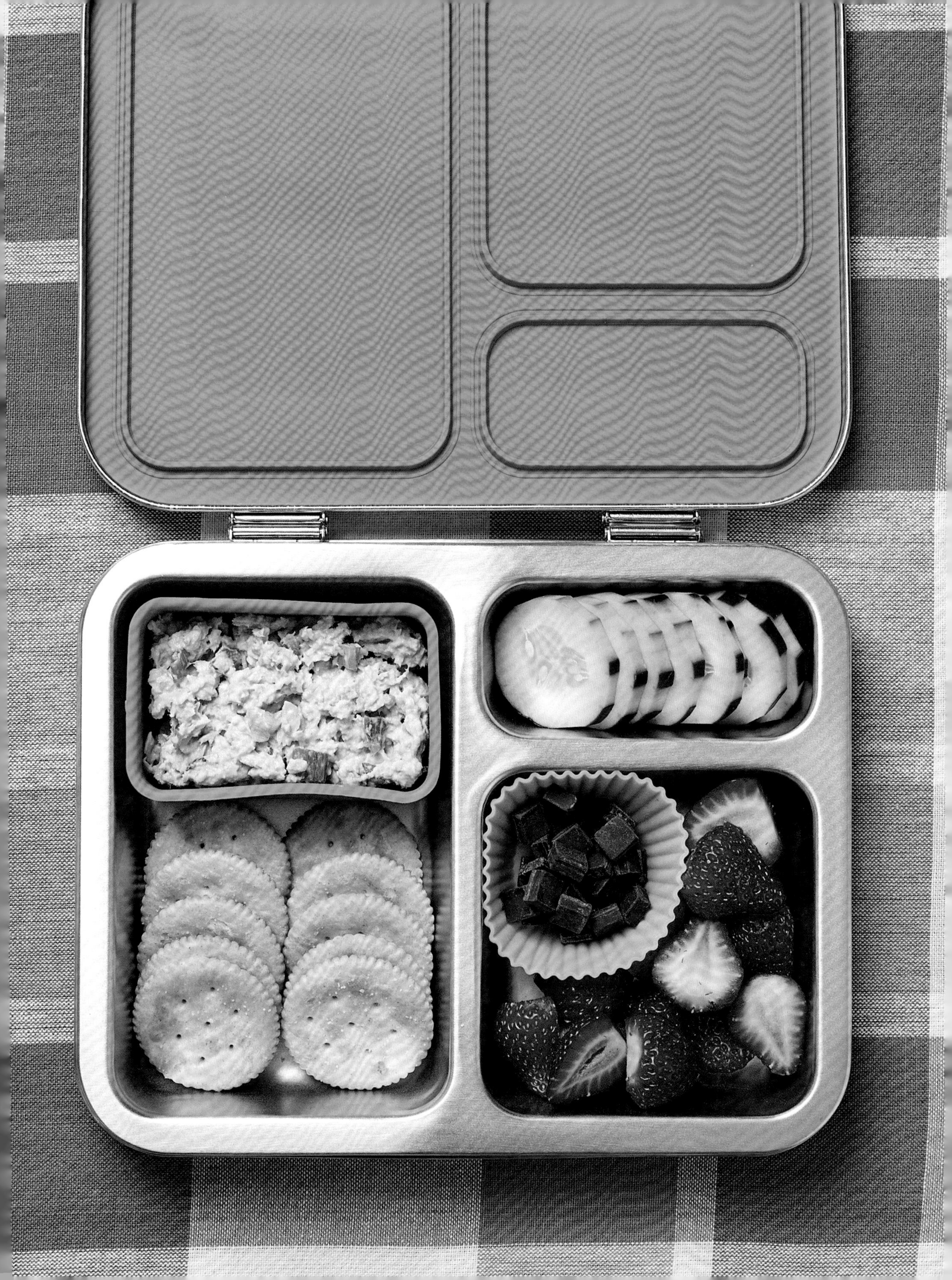

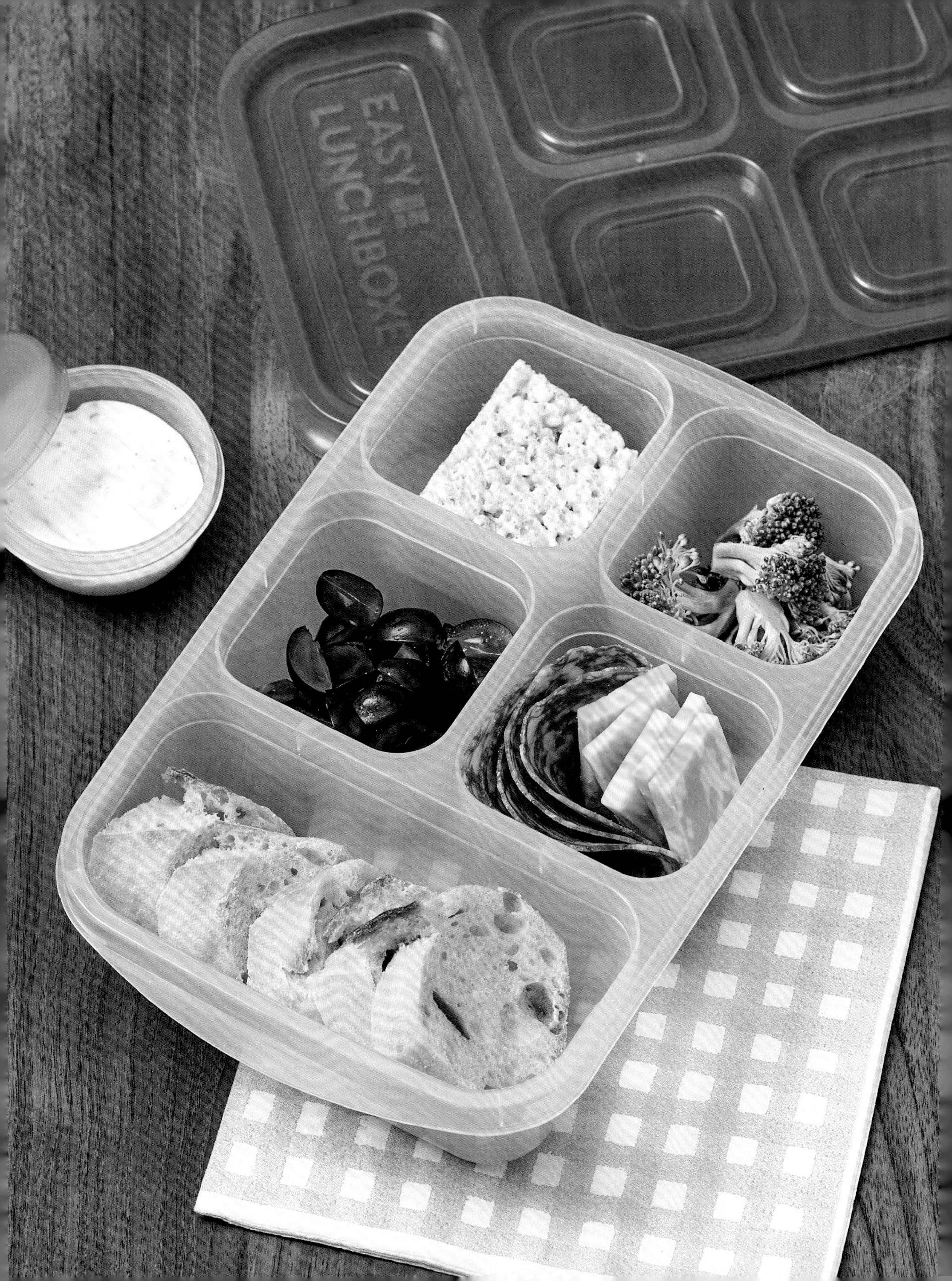
EASY
LUNCHBOXE

Sliced Baguette with Cheese and Salami

When Megan visited Europe after college, almost every lunch consisted of a baguette with meat and cheese—and it was *delicious*. This lunch is a kid-friendly, build-your-own option that bread lovers will enjoy.

Sliced baguette

Sliced cheese

Thinly sliced salami

Red grapes, quartered lengthwise

Small raw broccoli pieces

Crispy rice treat

Ranch dressing

PREP TIP

Place baguette slices in a separate compartment from other foods to keep the bread as fresh as possible.

ALLERGY TIPS

WHEAT: Use gluten-free bread or gluten-free crackers.

DAIRY: Use dairy-free cheese or hummus, olive tapenade, or another spread instead of cheese. Offer an allergy-friendly crispy rice treat. Salami may contain dairy—sub with pepperoni. Use dairy-free ranch dressing.

EGG: Use egg-free ranch dressing.

SOY: Use soy-free ranch dressing.

TODDLER TIP

This lunch is already modified for choking hazards. If your child struggles to bite into crusty bread, consider cutting it into smaller pieces.

PICKY EATING TIP

If your kid doesn't like cooked broccoli, they might still like raw broccoli—the flavors and textures are very different. Small pieces of raw broccoli served with ranch dressing helped Megan's oldest daughter enjoy broccoli again after boycotting it for years.

VEGE-TARIAN SWAP

Sub a plant-based meat alternative for the salami.

CONTAINER: **Bentgo Easyboxes 5-Compartment Meal Container (formerly EasyLunchboxes brand) with Bentgo Easyboxes Salad-to-Go dressing container**

Thin Rice Cake Sandwiches

You might associate rice cakes with diet food from the '90s, but they're actually a delicious and crunchy vehicle for various toppings like sunflower seed butter, cream cheese, Nutella, or avocado. These toppings add fat and protein, which transform rice cakes from a lower-calorie food to a deliciously crunchy lunch option. Megan's kids *love* these rice cake sammies—just be sure to send a few of them because one on its own isn't super filling.

Thin Stackers rice cakes with nut or seed butter

Fresh mango slices

Orange and red bell pepper,
cut into strips

Babybel cheese

M&M cookie

ALLERGY TIPS

DAIRY: Swap cubed chicken or turkey, or edamame or other beans, for the cheese. Alternatively, Babybel sells a coconut-based, dairy-free cheese option now. You can also purchase blocks of dairy-free cheese and cube it at home.

TREE NUTS: Use sunflower seed butter, granola butter, cream cheese, or smashed avocado instead of nut butter.

TODDLER TIP

Cut the bell pepper into thin slices, especially for very young toddlers still learning how to chew.

PICKY EATING TIP

Many reluctant eaters love crunchy food, and that's why this rice cake sandwich can be such a hit. Help them learn to love new foods by offering crunchy versions first: think freeze-dried fruits and veggies, crunchy baked cheese, and store-bought (or homemade) roasted garbanzo beans.

CONTAINER: LunchBots Large Cinco

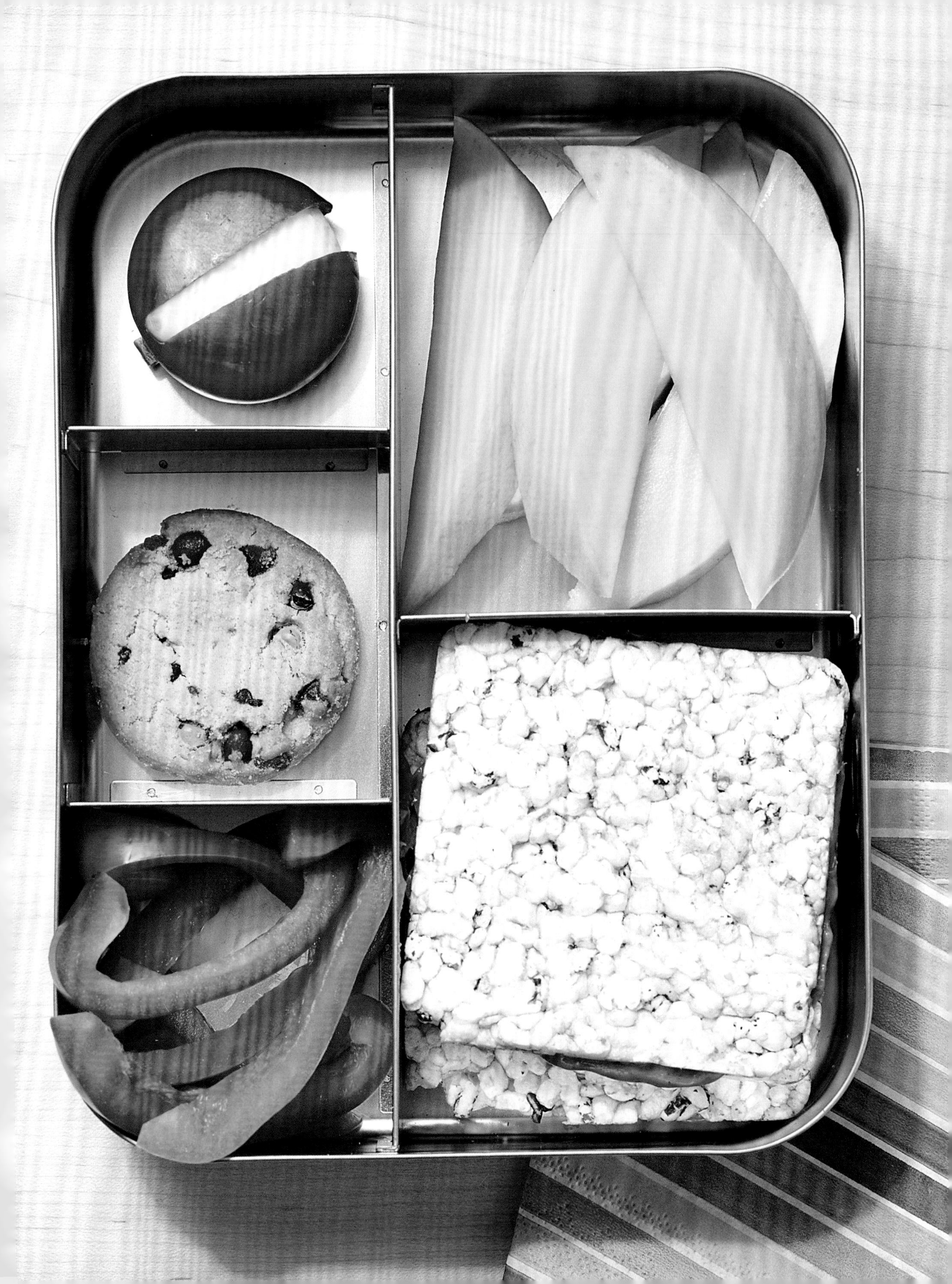

Hard-Boiled Egg and Pretzel Thins Snack Box

Don't fall for the lie that you have to send a formal "entrée" to school. Snack-style lunches can be just as filling and nutritious if they have a balance of nutrients. This one contains chocolate hummus, which is a somewhat sweet version of hummus that pairs well with graham crackers. Many of our clients love it, so we've included it as a unique idea for dessert!

Hard-boiled egg and pretzel thins

Blackberries

Cooked peas

Graham cracker strips

Chocolate hummus

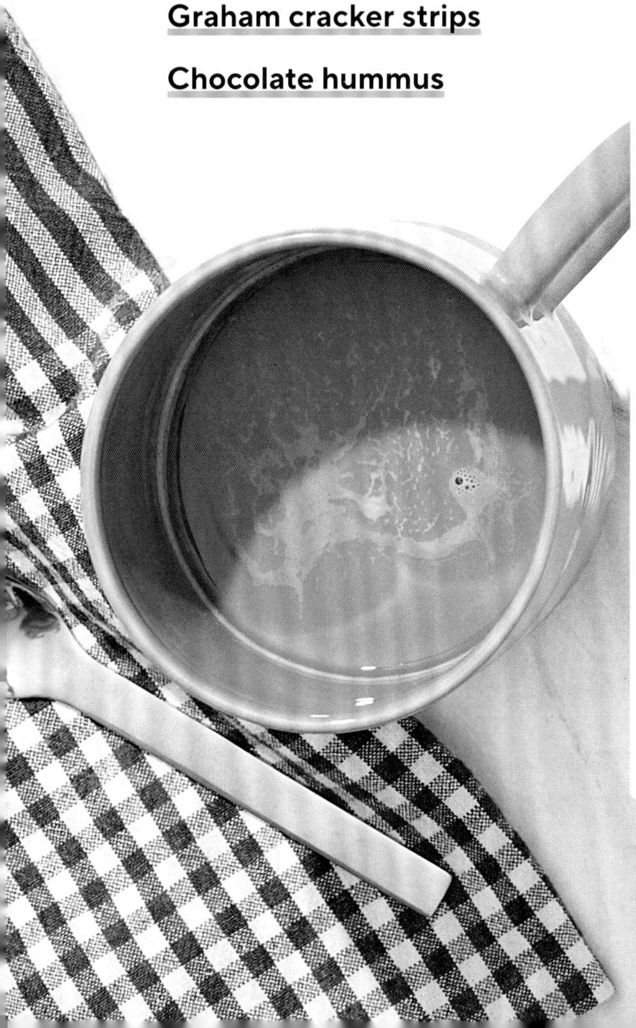

PREP TIP

Add a little salt to your cooked-from-frozen peas; it will bring out their flavor and make them more appealing to your kid.

ALLERGY TIPS

WHEAT: Use gluten-free pretzels and gluten-free graham crackers instead of wheat-based versions.

EGG: Sub shredded chicken, cubed ham, or tofu slices for the hard-boiled egg.

SESAME: Most store-bought hummus contains tahini, a sesame product. However, chocolate hummus usually does not—as always, make sure to check the label. You can also purchase chocolate chickpea butter as an alternative.

TODDLER TIP

Quarter the blackberries lengthwise for kids under four to make them less of a choking risk.

PICKY EATING TIP

Dips can be a powerful tool for reluctant eaters—Judy uses them in her practice all the time! Pair a familiar dip (like ranch) with a less familiar food (like broccoli) to help your selective eater try something new. Similarly, pairing a familiar dipper (graham cracker strips) with a less familiar dip (chocolate hummus) can help them branch out.

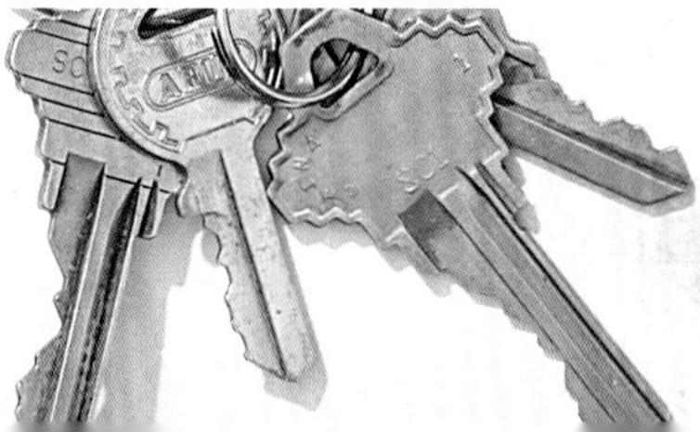

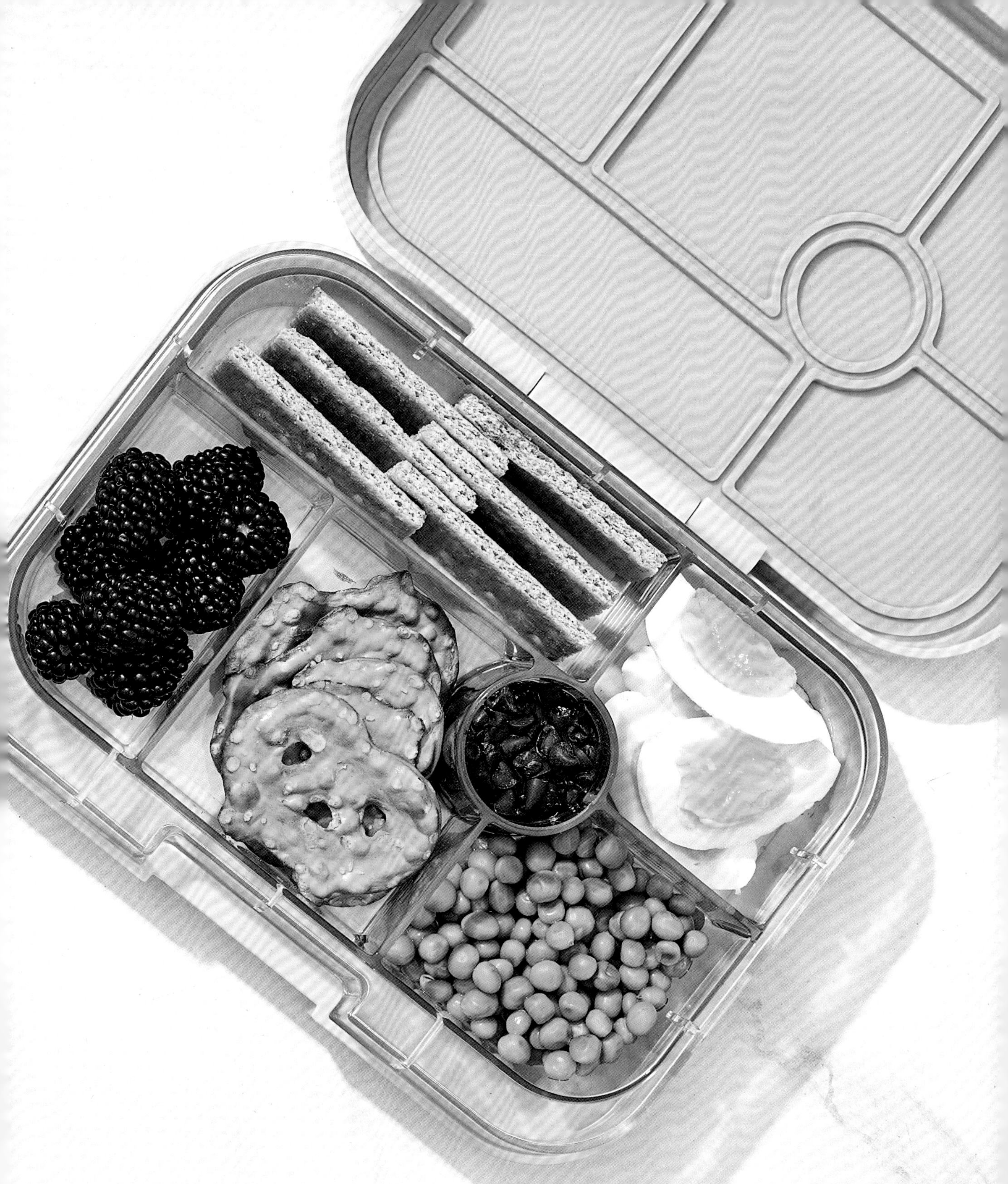

CONTAINER: **Yumbox Original**

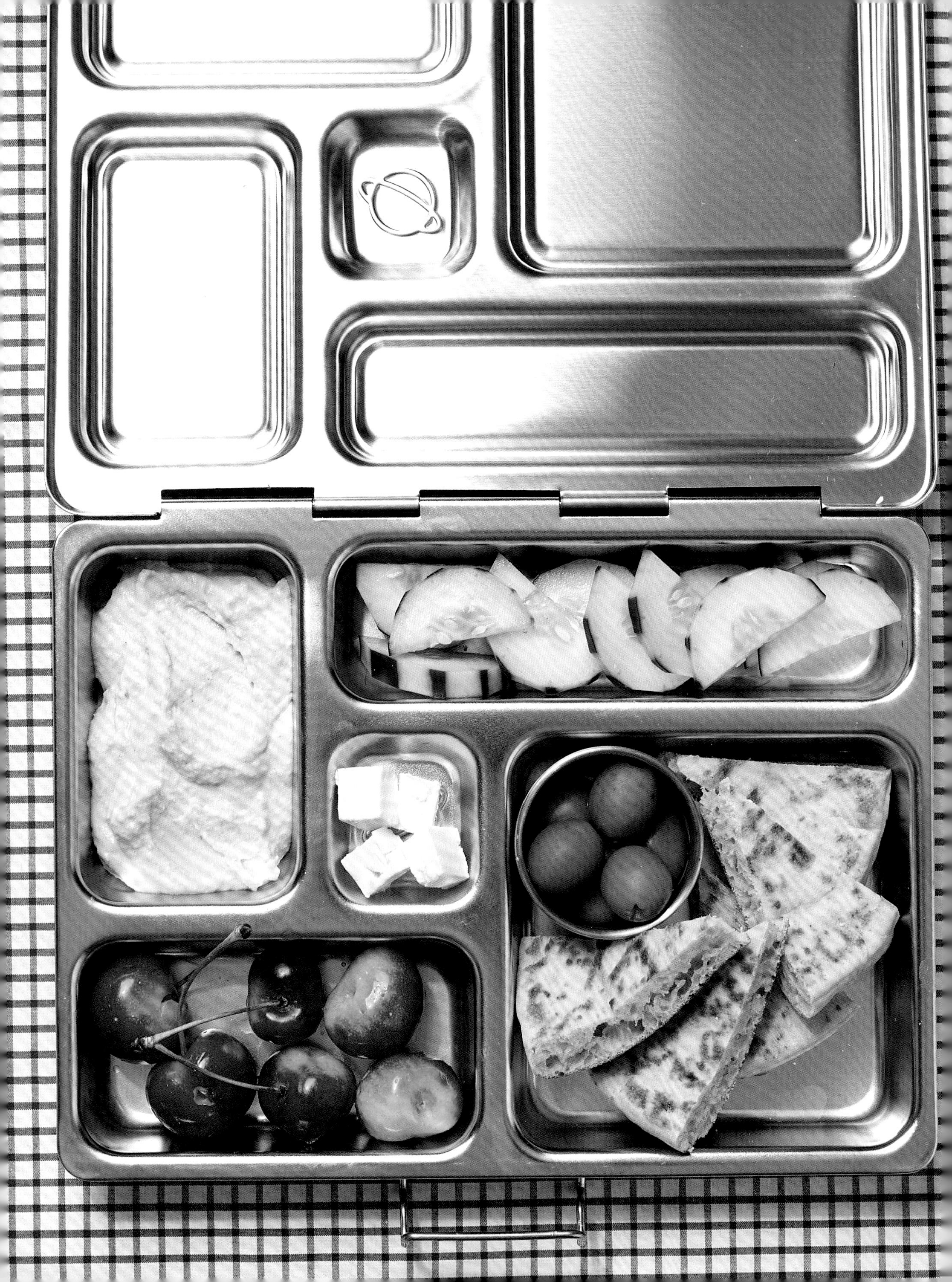

Hummus, Pita, and Feta Box

Hummus is a kid favorite across the globe, and it's also a decent source of protein. When paired with soft pita, some tangy feta, and salty olives, it's a simple but elevated lunch that eaters of all ages can enjoy.

Soft pita
(white or whole wheat)

Traditional hummus

Cubed feta

Pitted cherries

Cucumber slices

Whole olives

PREP TIP For kids four years and older who can safely eat whole cherries, pit the cherries but keep the stems on. This is an idea from our food stylist Hadas—her daughter loves to eat cherries this way! It's a more novel presentation, which means she's more likely to eat them.

ALLERGY TIPS

WHEAT: Use a gluten-free pita instead of a wheat pita.

DAIRY: Use dairy-free feta or omit feta, or sub with whole garbanzo beans.

SESAME: Use homemade tahini-free hummus or sub with tzatziki.

TODDLER TIP Quarter the pitted cherries and olives lengthwise to make them safer for kids under four to eat.

PICKY EATING TIPS Olives and feta both have very strong flavors and might be new foods for your selective eater. Consider trying one at a time or subbing with something more familiar (like mozzarella cheese for the feta, pickles for the olives) as your child gets used to seeing new foods in their lunch box.

CONTAINER: PlanetBox Rover

Leftover Pizza

Megan's all-time favorite lunch to pack is leftover pizza. Her kids love it, it uses up cold pizza leftovers, and it's super easy. Pair it with a fruit and a veggie (consider throwing a dessert in there) and you have a yummy leftover lunch that's filling, balanced, and kid-approved.

Leftover pizza,
cut into small pieces

Watermelon chunks

Baby carrots,
thinly sliced lengthwise

Hershey's kisses

PREP TIP Use a pizza cutter to slice leftover pizza into smaller triangle shapes. They look like mini pizza pieces and are easy to pick up.

ALLERGY TIPS

WHEAT: Serve gluten-free pizza.

DAIRY: Offer dairy-free pizza and use dairy-free chocolate.

TODDLER TIP Remove any black seeds from the watermelon, as they can be a choking hazard.

PICKY EATING TIP If your child is old enough, ask them to help you cut the pizza into smaller pieces, using a pizza cutter. Their involvement in the process might be enough to encourage them to eat it at lunchtime . . . fingers crossed!

CONTAINER: Bentgo Pop

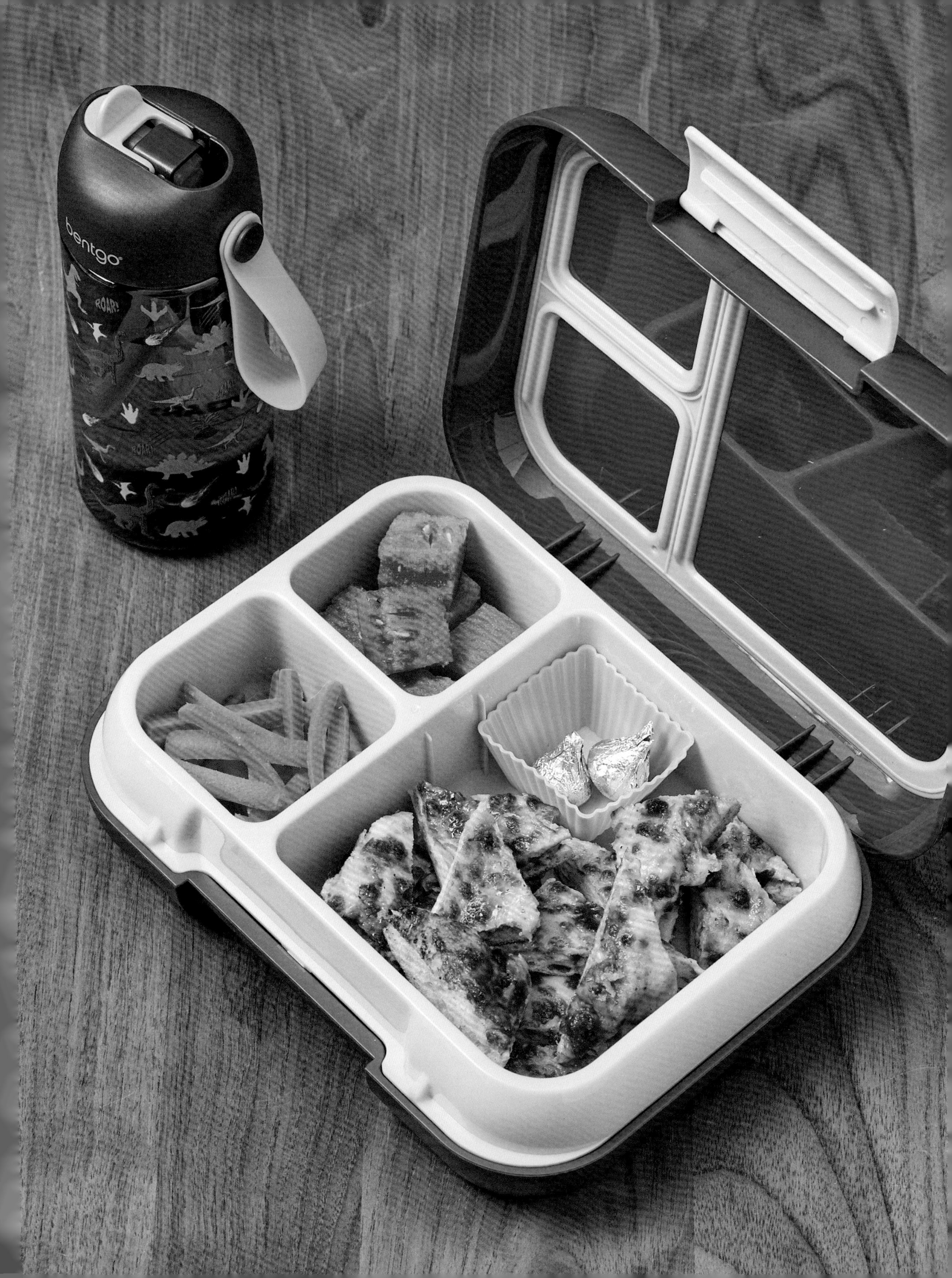
bentgo

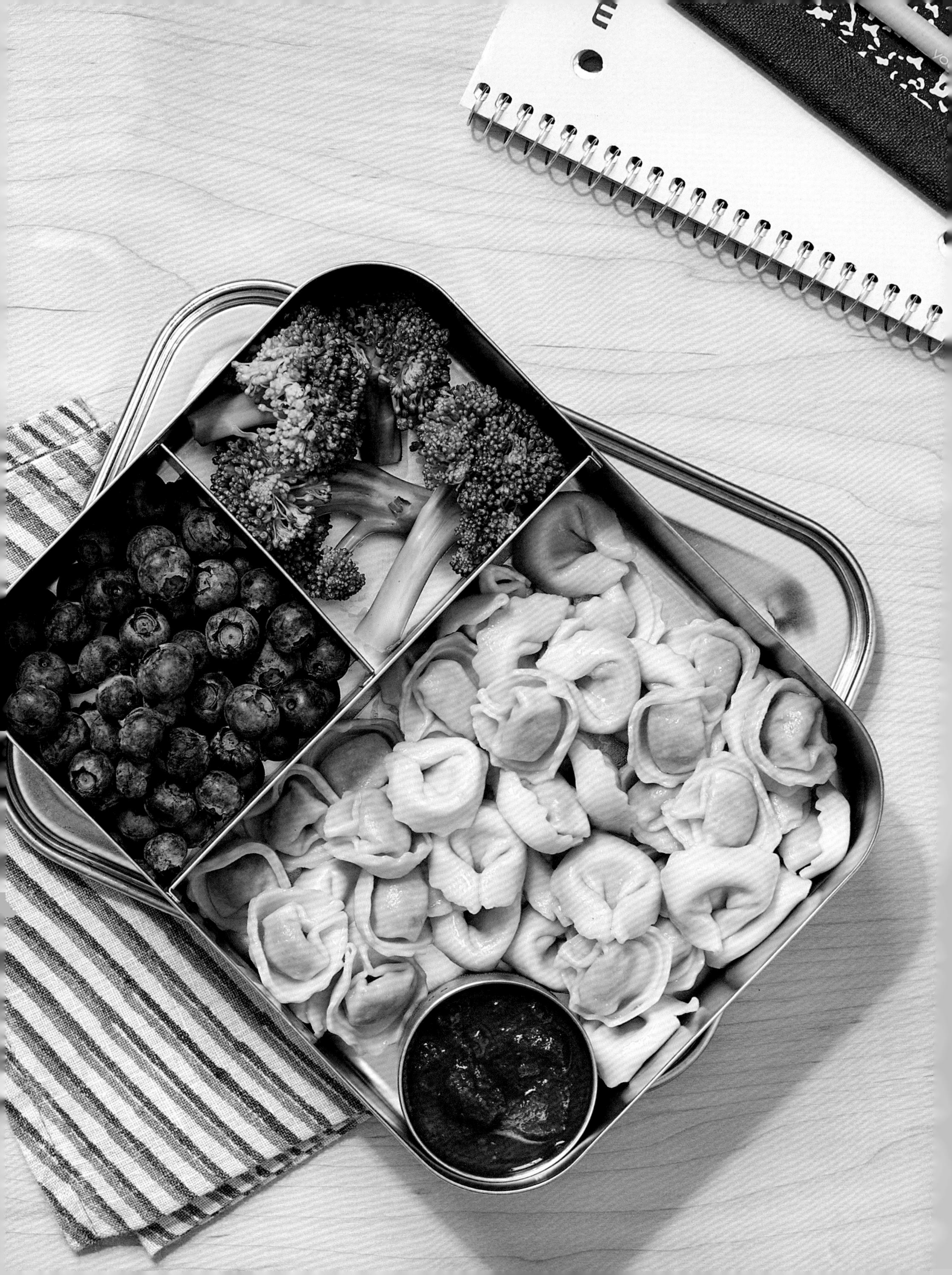

Leftover Tortellini

This is one of our favorite leftover lunches. Tortellini is *amazing* served cold, and it's a satisfying option for busy mornings when you need to throw leftovers in a box and get your little one to school quickly.

Leftover spinach and cheese tortellini
(or just cheese tortellini)

Blueberries

Steamed broccoli

Marinara sauce "dip"

PREP TIP Add a little garlic powder, salt, and pepper to the steamed broccoli for enhanced flavor.

ALLERGY TIPS

WHEAT: Try gluten-free tortellini.

DAIRY: Serve plant-based tortellini or spiral pasta with dairy-free meatballs.

TODDLER TIP Show your tot how to dip the tortellini in the sauce before they head off to school.

PICKY EATING TIP Deconstructing foods can help reluctant eaters feel more comfortable eating those dishes. This lunch is a very simple example—instead of adding sauce to the tortellini, we served it separately from the pasta as a dip. Try this at home with other pasta dishes that are a struggle for your kid.

CONTAINERS: LunchBots Large Trio and LunchBots 1.5-oz Dip

Leftover Chicken and Rice

Chicken and rice is a beloved meal for many families. It can make for a tasty lunch the next day too, especially when paired with a veggie, a fruit, and a dessert.

Leftover grilled chicken

Leftover buttered rice

Leftover steamed green beans

Mandarin orange segments

Chocolate bar pieces

PREP TIP Make sure to refrigerate all leftovers soon after dinner is done to ensure proper food safety. You can pack them in your child's lunch box right away and store it overnight in the fridge.

ALLERGY TIP **DAIRY:** Offer dairy-free chocolate. Use a cooking fat of your choice (olive oil, dairy-free butter) on the rice, if desired.

TODDLER TIP Cut the mandarin orange segments into smaller pieces for young toddlers.

PICKY EATING TIP If your child loves to peel mandarin oranges, send one whole and unpeeled! Sometimes the process of peeling fruit motivates reluctant eaters to try a new fruit.

VEGETARIAN SWAP Send leftover tofu or tempeh instead of chicken.

CONTAINER: Bentgo Kids Chill

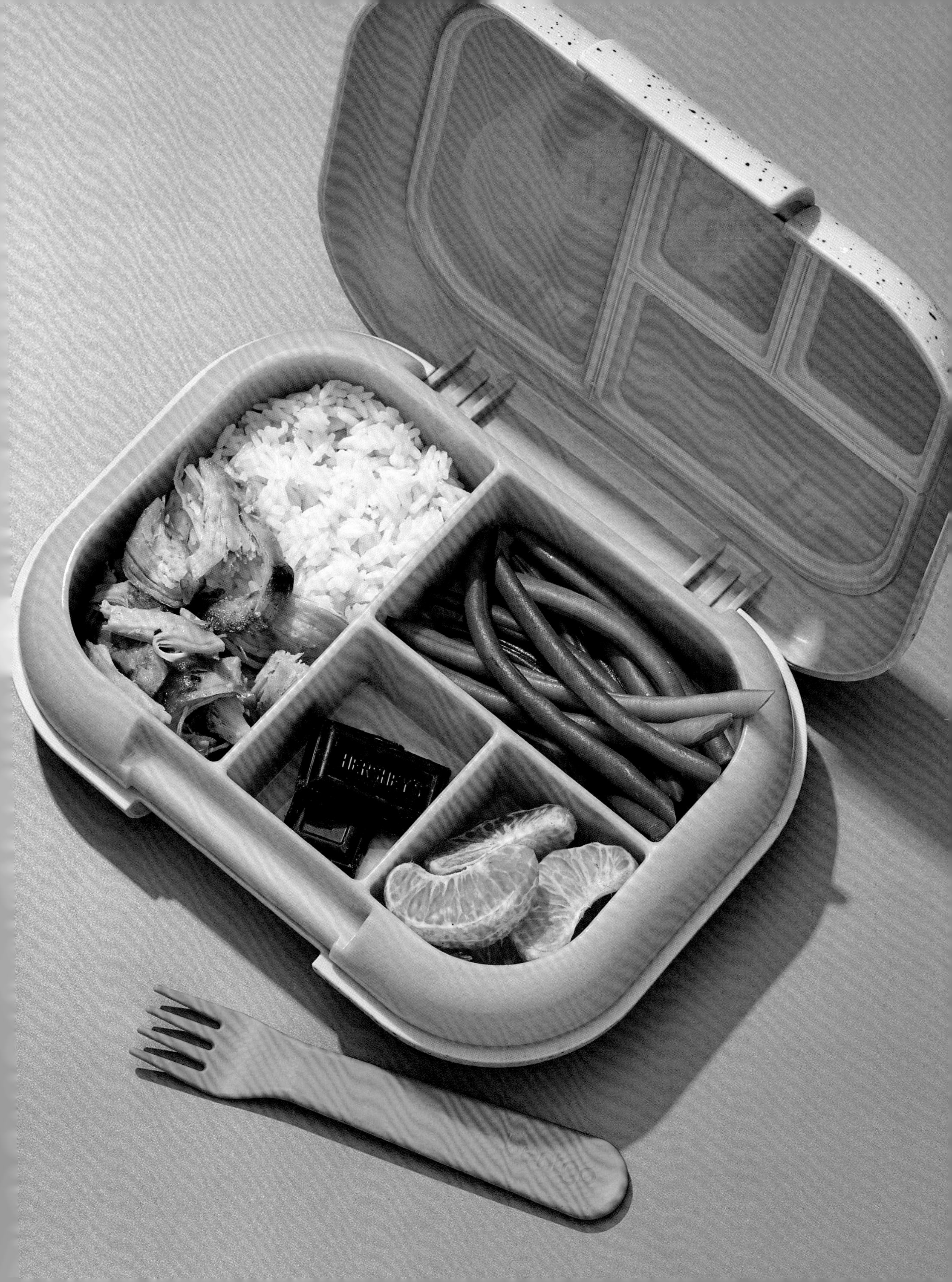
HERSHEY'S

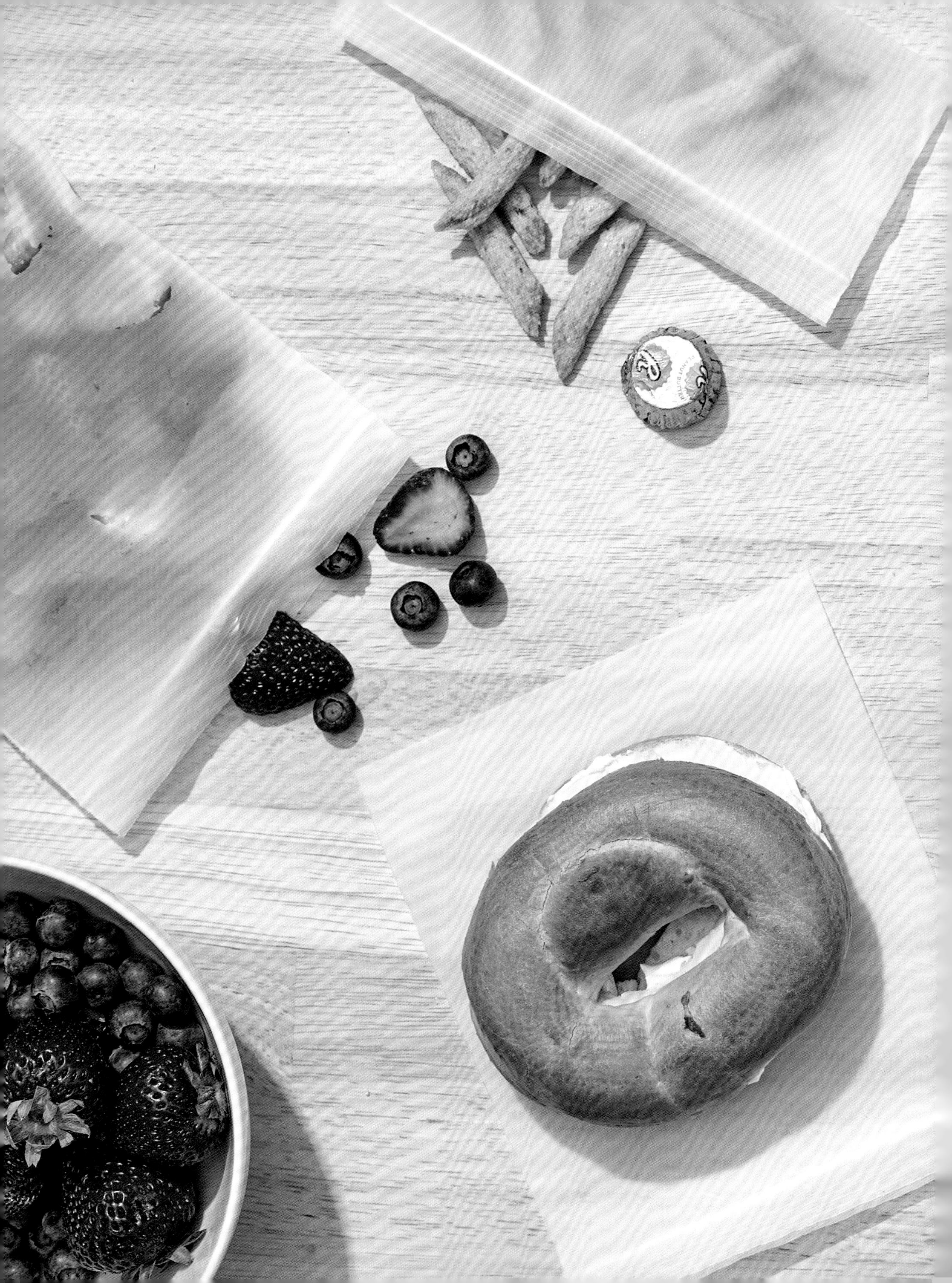

Easy Bagel and Cream Cheese

When in doubt . . . send a bagel. It's a no-brainer option for busy mornings and is dense and satisfying for kids of all ages. Whole-wheat and protein bagels have a little extra nutrition, but get whatever kind sounds good to your family—and don't forget about blueberry or everything bagel flavors!

Bagel and cream cheese

Halved strawberry and blueberry mix

Dried snap pea crisps

Mini peanut butter cup

PREP TIP

This is a great lunch to put in disposable bags, as the components are not as likely to get squished as other foods.

ALLERGY TIPS

WHEAT: See our Allergy Guide QR code (page 42) for gluten- and wheat-free bagel suggestions. Alternatively, spread cream cheese on a safe tortilla and roll it up.

DAIRY: Use dairy-free cream cheese or sunflower seed butter instead of cream cheese.

TREE NUTS: Serve a sunflower seed butter cup or regular chocolate instead of a peanut butter cup.

TODDLER TIP

Cut the bagel into quarters to make it easier for little hands to hold.

PICKY EATING TIP

Snap pea crisps are made with peas but are more like a puff or a cracker. They're a great "gateway food" for kids reluctant to eat vegetables because they have a mild pea flavor but a predictable "snack food" texture. Bonus: They're a great source of protein and fiber.

CONTAINER: EcoSoul Compostable Resealable Bags

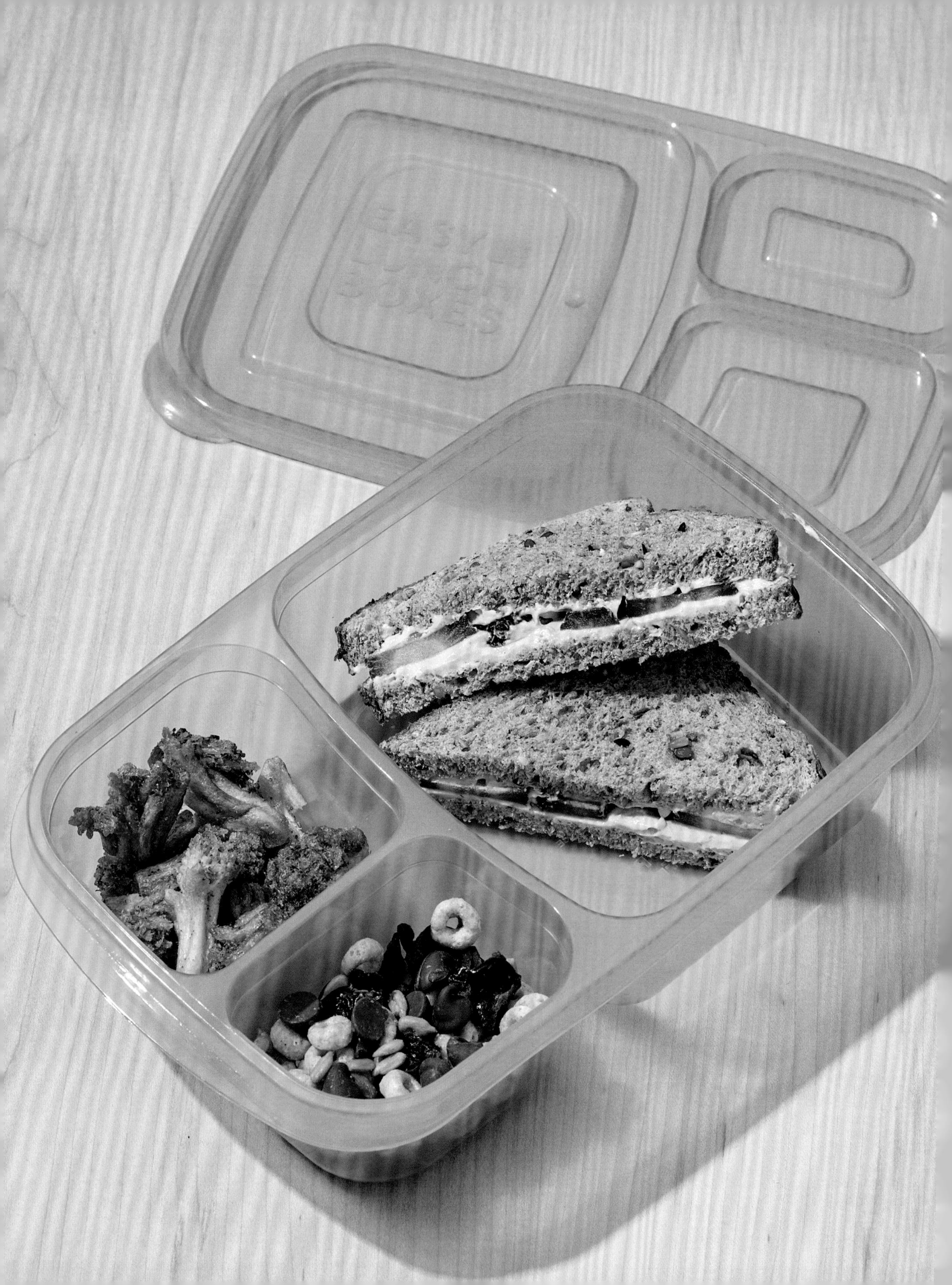

Strawberry Cream Cheese Sandwich

Not everyone loves strawberries in their sandwich, but if you have a fruit lover in your house, this might be just up their alley! Megan's husband, Greg, tried this at the photo shoot for this book and proceeded to eat the whole thing on the spot. The tang of the cream cheese pairs really well with fresh strawberries, and using strawberry cream cheese—while not required—adds an extra boost of flavor.

Strawberry cream cheese sandwich on whole-grain bread with freshly sliced strawberries

Freeze-dried broccoli
(try Trader Joe's crunchy broccoli)

Trail mix
(Cheerios, cranberries, sunflower seeds, chocolate chips)

PREP TIP Spread strawberry cream cheese on both pieces of bread before adding sliced strawberries. This creates a barrier that helps keep the bread from getting soggy.

ALLERGY TIPS

WHEAT: Use gluten-free bread for the sandwich. Use a safe-for-you cereal to make the trail mix.

DAIRY: Use dairy-free plain or strawberry cream cheese. Serve dairy-free chocolate chips in the trail mix.

TODDLER TIP Some toddlers might struggle to eat sunflower seeds in the trail mix—replace them with soft raisins or dried cranberries, if necessary.

PICKY EATING TIP We love freeze-dried broccoli as a unique way to enjoy this often vilified food. Many picky eaters will eat this before they try fresh broccoli, so it's a great first step. If they love crunchy broccoli, try making it for dinner in your air fryer!

CONTAINER: Bentgo Easyboxes 3-Compartment Meal Container (formerly EasyLunchboxes brand)

Leftover Mac and Cheese with Peas

One of our favorite "I Can't Even" dinners is boxed macaroni and cheese, especially since leftovers can be sent cold to school the next day! We love tossing in frozen peas for a little pop of color and flavor, but you can add diced cooked chicken, small pieces of broccoli, or canned beans to amp it up too. Is your kid not ready for anything in their mac and cheese? Totally OK—keep it out.

Prepared boxed mac and cheese, made with frozen peas

Hard-boiled egg slices

Raspberries

PREP TIP Frozen peas are amazing because you just open the bag and pour them into boiling water! Add them during the last few minutes the pasta is boiling. Drain the pasta/pea mixture, then add milk, butter, and the cheese packet, as directed.

ALLERGY TIPS **WHEAT/DAIRY:** Gluten-free and/or dairy-free boxed mac and cheese doesn't taste good left over or cold to many people. Unfortunately, not all free-from families have a safe or palatable mac and cheese option. Instead, send a safe pasta with ragu or meatballs. Gluten-free pasta, immersed in red sauce, usually tastes good the next day.

EGG: Sub with diced chicken or turkey.

TODDLER TIP Send this with a fork or spoon, but don't be surprised if your toddler uses their hands to eat this meal. Their day-care provider or preschool teacher will not be surprised—kids default to their hands when silverware gets tricky, and that's OK! As long as they are practicing with silverware and have the ability to use it, ditching utensils and using their hands instead is developmentally normal and expected.

PICKY EATING TIP Changing up a beloved food like mac and cheese by adding peas can be a *major* no-no for your reluctant eater. Instead, try serving cooked peas on the side for this lunch.

CONTAINER: **Lille Home Kiddiebox**

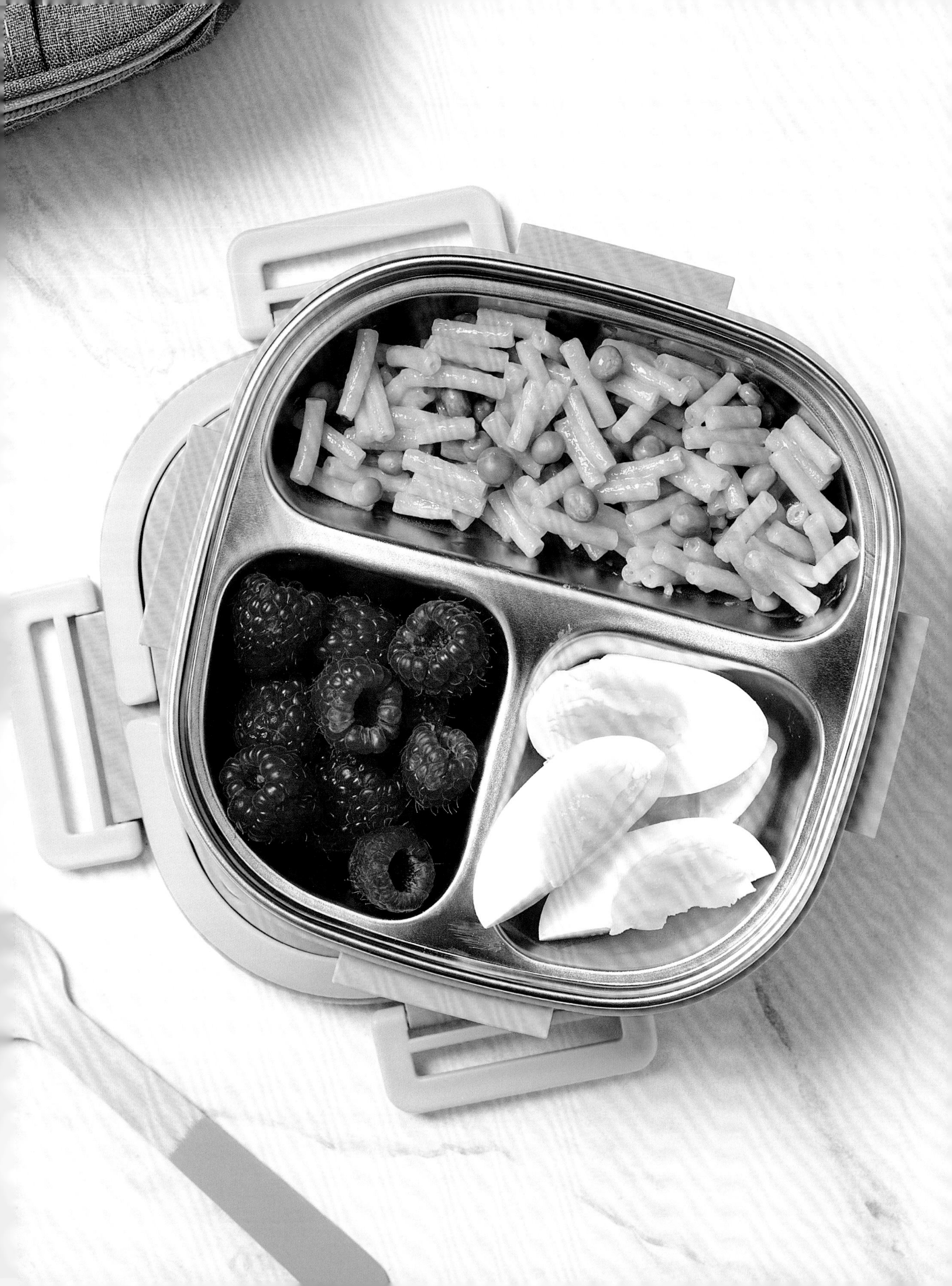

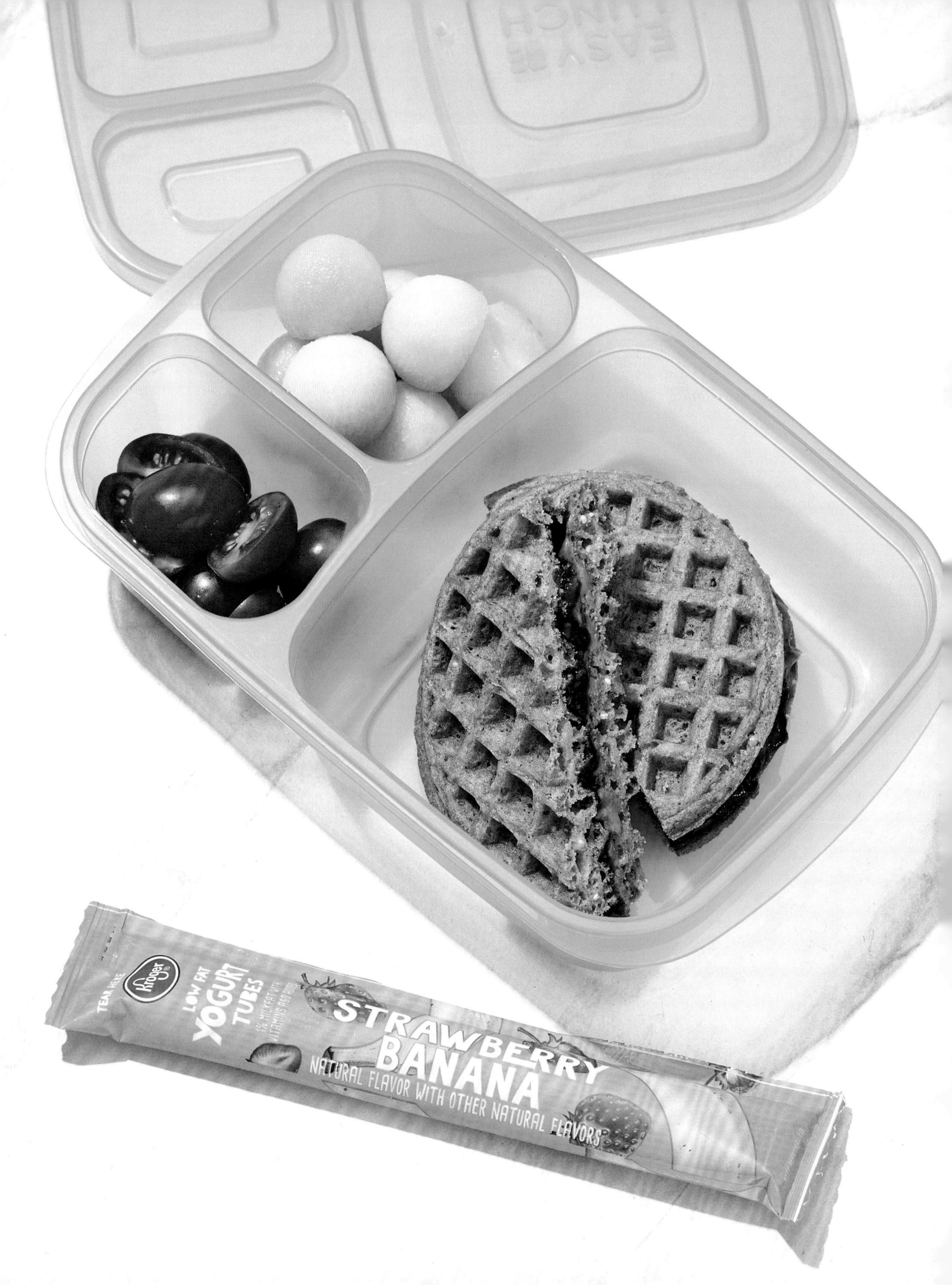
TEAR HERE
Kroger
LOW FAT YOGURT TUBES
STRAWBERRY BANANA
NATURAL FLAVOR WITH OTHER NATURAL FLAVORS

Waffle Sandwich

It's so easy to forget that breakfast for lunch (or dinner) is just as delicious as it is for . . . breakfast! These waffle sandwiches are almost as easy as a bread-based sandwich and might help you break out of your lunch rut. Plus, many frozen waffles on the market are filled with fiber, protein, and whole grains and can be really filling options for school lunch.

Frozen waffles, toasted and made into a sandwich with sunflower seed butter and jelly
(or other fillings as desired)

Honeydew melon balls

Cherry tomatoes

Yogurt tube

PREP TIP Toast the waffle at home before adding the toppings. It takes just a few minutes but makes for a better texture at lunchtime. If your kid's not into sunflower seed butter and jelly, try cream cheese, Nutella (contains tree nuts), smashed fruit, or butter.

ALLERGY TIPS

WHEAT: Use gluten-free frozen waffles instead of wheat-based waffles.

DAIRY: Swap the yogurt tube for a dairy-free yogurt cup from your favorite brand—don't forget a spoon!

EGG: Many frozen waffles contain egg. Substitute with a plant-based toaster waffle or a vegan homemade waffle.

TODDLER TIP To minimize choking risk, cut the tomatoes into quarters lengthwise. Since melon balls are the size and shape of grapes, cut them into quarters lengthwise for kids under four or serve as strips/pieces.

PICKY EATING TIP Never thought to send melon balls? Most people don't, but they're a great technique for selective eaters. Whenever you add a little novelty—like this new shape—you might pique your child's interest. You might be surprised how much they love these, even if they generally don't go for melon when it's cut into wedges. Bonus: Ask your child to use the melon baller to prep their own lunch. When they prep it, they're more likely to eat it!

CONTAINER: **Bentgo Easyboxes 3-Compartment Meal Container (formerly EasyLunchboxes brand)**

Roast Beef on Focaccia

Another fun sandwich base for kids (and adults) is focaccia bread. It's soft and delicious and adds a ton of flavor to a simple sandwich.

Roast beef on focaccia with desired toppings
(mayo, mustard, lettuce, tomato)

Watermelon triangles

Snap peas and baby carrots

Chocolate-covered pretzels

PREP TIP

Spread mayo or mustard on the focaccia to add a protective layer against the tomato and lettuce, which could make the bread soggy.

ALLERGY TIPS

WHEAT: Use gluten-free focaccia or gluten-free bread instead of focaccia. Send gluten-free chocolate-covered pretzels instead of wheat-based chocolate-covered pretzels.

DAIRY: Most focaccia has cheese on top. Use vegan focaccia (store-bought or homemade) or sub with tolerated bread. Send vegan chocolate-covered pretzels or a mix of pretzel pieces and non-dairy chocolate chips instead of chocolate-covered pretzels.

TODDLER TIPS

Select seedless watermelon and cut the baby carrots into quarters lengthwise to minimize choking risk. You can also soften the carrots in boiling water if your toddler struggles to chew them when thinly sliced.

This sandwich might be hard for a toddler to eat, so consider deconstructing it and sending the bread separately from the roast beef. You can cut it into small pieces that are easy to pick up.

PICKY EATING TIP

If your child struggles with new types of bread, it's OK to go slowly and serve this on their favorite bread instead. Serve focaccia (or another type of bread you're trying to expose them to) as a dinner side, and as they get more familiar with the new flavors and textures at home, they might be willing to enjoy focaccia as a sandwich bread at school.

CONTAINER: **OmieLife OmieBox**

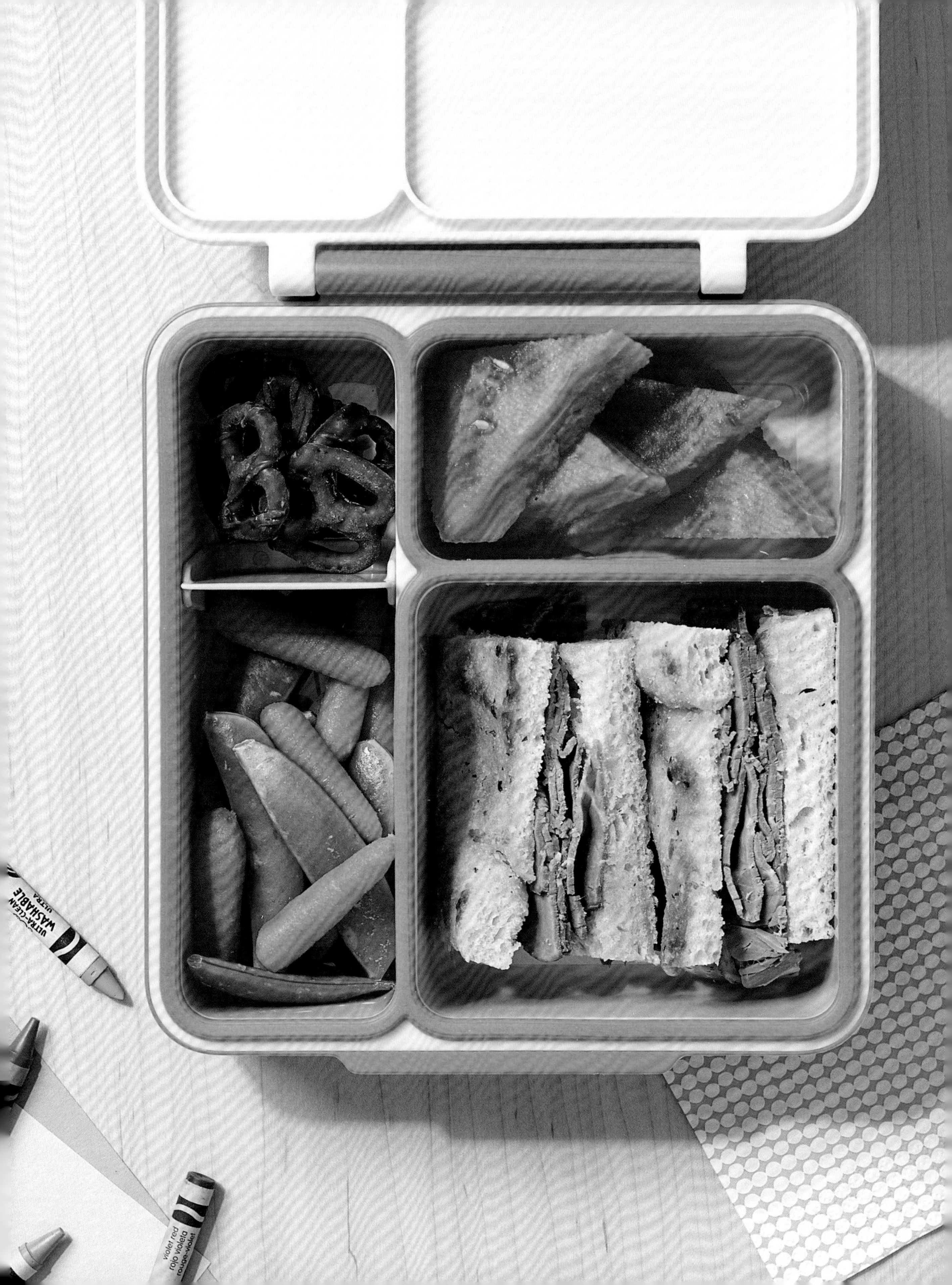
ULTRA-CLEAN WASHABLE
violet red
rojo violeta
rouge-violet

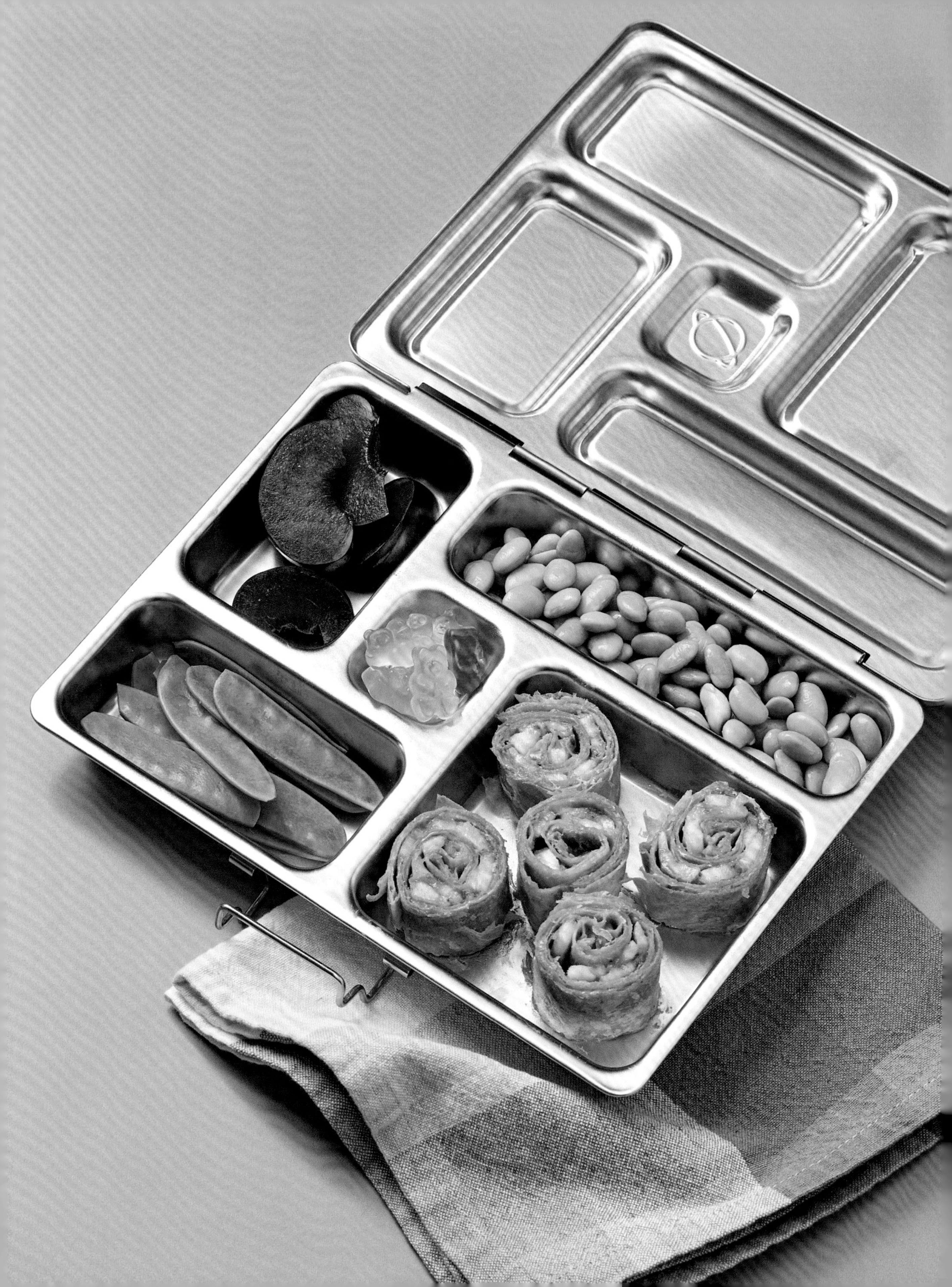

Sunflower Seed Butter Banana Roll-Up "Sushi-Style"

When Megan's kids were younger, she discovered this amazingly tasty snack: Spread sunflower seed butter or peanut butter on a tortilla, then roll it around a banana (or chopped banana). Cut into one-inch-wide pieces to make "sushi-style" rolls. They're nutritionally balanced and delicious, and her kids still love them to this day.

Sunflower seed butter and banana,
rolled in a tortilla and cut "sushi-style"

Edamame

Plum slices

Snow peas

Gummy bears

PREP TIP You can make this a few different ways. Either keep the banana whole as you roll it up, or chop the banana into pieces before rolling up the tortilla, as shown. Then cut it into one-inch-wide rounds. The banana will brown a little bit, but it's usually not a big deal when mixed with sunflower seed butter or another nut/seed butter. This lunch is best prepped the morning of school, not the night before.

ALLERGY TIPS **WHEAT:** Use a gluten-free or grain-free tortilla instead of a wheat tortilla. Store-bought gluten-free tortillas are more pliable when heated. You might want to heat them for twenty to thirty seconds in the microwave in the morning before rolling them up.

SOY: Omit edamame, or send black beans or hummus.

TODDLER TIP Sometimes it's easiest to leave these as long, thin tortilla roll-ups (don't cut them into rounds) when serving this to a young eater. It can be easier for them to pick up and keep together. Cut gummy bears into small pieces or omit for kids under four, as they can be a choking hazard.

PICKY EATING TIP This is another great lunch to deconstruct if your child is hesitant to mix banana and tortilla/sunflower seed butter. Simply serve the tortilla with the sunflower seed butter only, rolled up into a thin, long piece, and serve an unpeeled banana on the side.

CONTAINER: PlanetBox Rover

Build-Your-Own English Muffin Pizza

Who remembers home economics class? Anyone? When Megan was growing up in Minnesota, English muffin pizzas were the first thing she made in middle school home ec. This build-your-own version is a little different because it's served cold, but it remains a delicious, balanced option that kids and adults both love. Opt for whole-wheat or sprouted-wheat English muffins whenever possible, as they offer more fiber and B vitamins.

Sliced English muffin

Marinara sauce

Shredded mozzarella cheese

Pineapple chunks

Carrot shreds and thinly sliced celery sticks

PREP TIP

Making this at home? Throw it in the microwave for thirty seconds or the toaster oven (on the convection setting) for a few minutes to melt the cheese.

ALLERGY TIPS

WHEAT: Use a gluten-free English muffin.

DAIRY: Use dairy-free shredded cheese. If your cheese tastes best melted, microwave or broil the pizzas before packing.

TODDLER TIP

This can be a messy yet fun lunch for toddlers. If you're sending this to preschool or day care, you might want to practice assembling the pizzas at home first so your toddler understands how to do it. Conversely, you can heat the English muffin pizzas at home to melt the cheese and send them in their lunch box cold, cut into wedges. Note: The carrots and celery are thinly cut in this lunch to reduce choking risk, as whole raw carrots and celery can be a hazard for kids under four.

PICKY EATING TIP

Notice how we sent pineapple chunks on the side? Yup, they technically can be a topping for this pizza, although many kids will choose to eat them separately. That's OK—we're all allowed to have preferences about food, and some people just *really* don't like pineapple and pizza together (including Judy and Megan!). If you're dealing with picky eating, it can help to remember that all of us have foods we don't enjoy. Your kid doesn't need to love *everything* either.

CONTAINER: Yumbox Presto

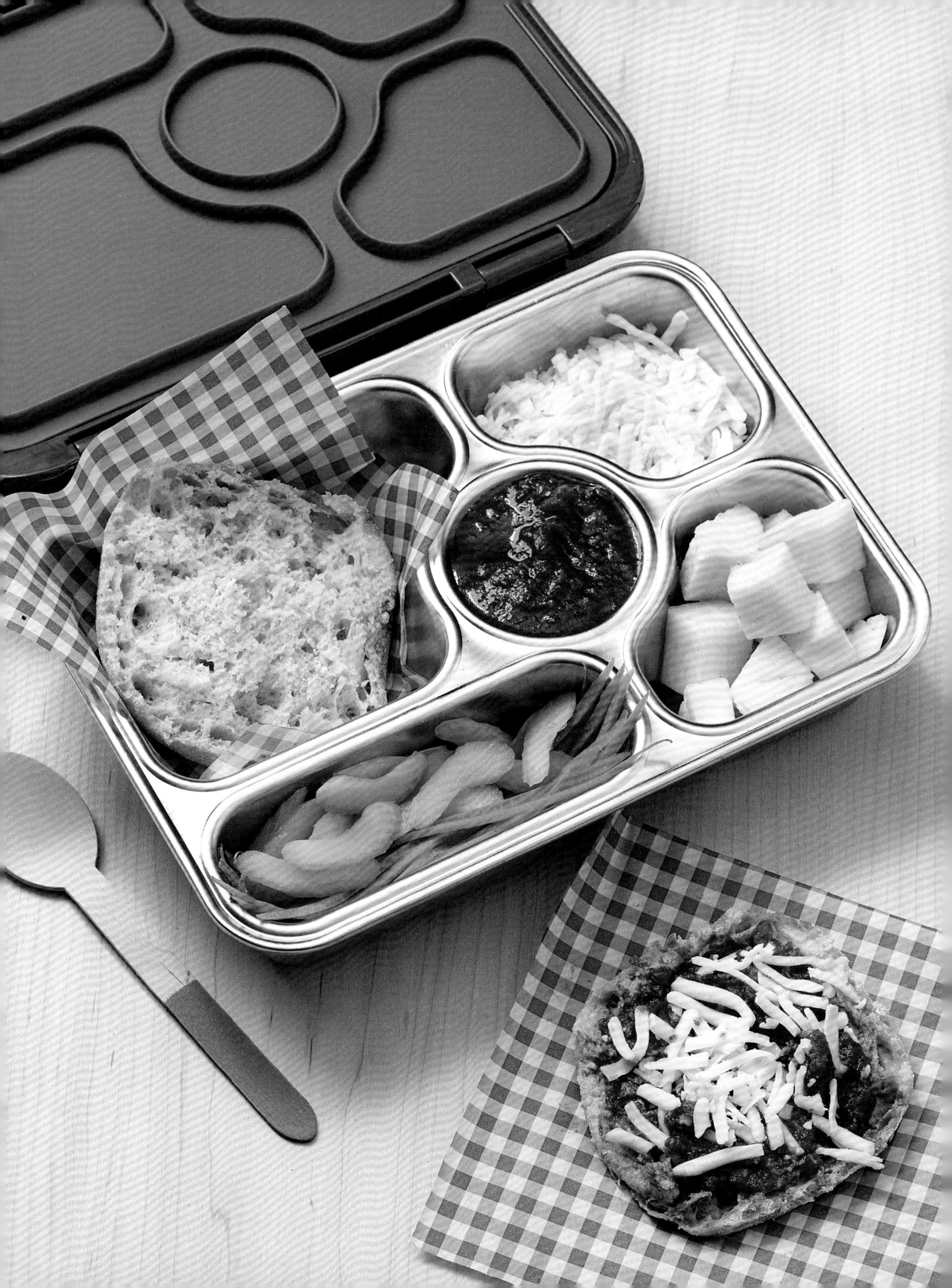

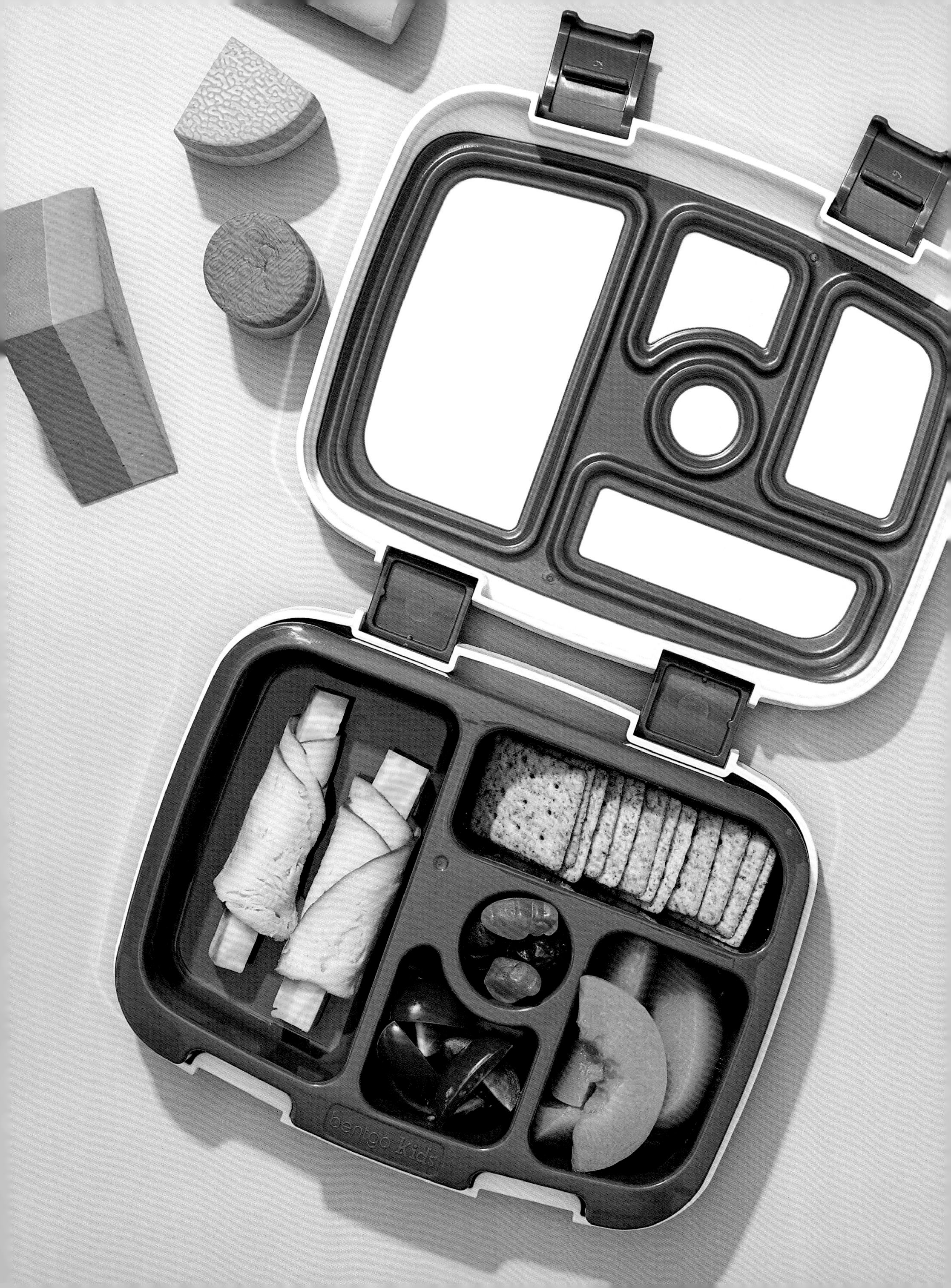
bentgo kids

Turkey and Colby Jack Cheese Stick Roll-Ups

Sometimes simple ideas can become our kids' favorite foods. These roll-ups are just that: simple *and* delicious. We love them because they're high in protein for growing kids (and hungry adults), they're easy to grab, and they taste amazing.

Turkey and Colby Jack cheese stick roll-ups

Whole-wheat crackers

Canned peaches

Cherry tomatoes, quartered lengthwise

Fruit snacks

PREP TIP These look fancier than they are to make. Simply roll a folded piece of turkey (opt for nitrate/nitrite-free whenever possible) around a Colby Jack cheese stick and place it in their lunch compartment. These would also taste great with mustard or honey mustard as a dip.

ALLERGY TIPS Many fruit snacks contain major allergens. Check out our Allergy Guide QR Code (page 42) for alternatives.

WHEAT: Use gluten-free crackers instead of whole-wheat crackers.

DAIRY: Use a piece of dairy-free cheese you enjoy, or use a dairy-free cheese spread instead. Alternatively, omit the cheese and roll the turkey around a pickle or send it with guacamole.

TODDLER TIP Fruit snacks, like gummies, can be a choking hazard for toddlers. Cut them into small pieces or serve another type of dessert or freeze-dried strawberries.

PICKY EATING TIP This is a simple and fun lunch for your child to help you prep. Let them roll the turkey around the cheese stick or place the crackers in the box. They might want to eat it more if they had a hand in prepping it!

VEGETARIAN SWAP Use a plant-based deli meat alternative instead of turkey, or simply omit the turkey.

CONTAINER: Bentgo Kids

Grilled Cheese Dippers and Tomato Soup

Grilled cheese and tomato soup are a quintessential kid (and adult) pairing. Even when paired with cold grilled cheese, hot tomato soup can add some much-needed comfort to our midday meal. Many of us forget that soups are a great way to enjoy vegetables, and tomato soup is no exception. Cooked tomatoes have a *lot* more lycopene—a heart-healthy compound—than raw tomatoes. One cup of tomato soup has up to six times more lycopene than a medium tomato. Cool, right?

Grilled cheese sandwich,
cut into strips

Hot tomato soup
(in an insulated container)

Whole green grapes

Strawberry granola minis

PREP TIPS

Make this grilled cheese sandwich in your toaster oven or air fryer! Once it's cooked, cool it slightly, then cut into strips to make dippers.

TOASTER OVEN (CONVECTION SETTING): 375°F for about ten minutes, flipping halfway through the cook time.

AIR FRYER: 375°F for four minutes, flipping halfway through the cook time.

ALLERGY TIPS

WHEAT: Use gluten-free bread.

DAIRY: Since dairy-free cheese can be tricky to melt, heat it on a pan all on its own before transferring it to your bread. Many people love mayonnaise instead of butter as the spread for the outside of their grilled cheese. This is a great dairy-free option to try; olive oil or plant-based butter work well too. To omit dairy from soup, try a plant-based tomato soup or another dairy-free premade soup like minestrone (check labels, as some do contain dairy).

CONTAINER: LunchBots Large Trio and LunchBots Thermal Dots 8-oz Insulated Container

TODDLER TIPS

Soup can be tricky for young toddlers, especially if they're still working on their spoon skills. Consider sending these dippers with marinara sauce instead.

Cut grapes into quarters lengthwise, as they're a common choking hazard.

Some granola products are very hard to chew—if you can't find softer options, send additional fresh, dried, or freeze-dried fruit.

PICKY EATING TIP

One novel way to enjoy this soup? Send it with a straw! Kids who don't love eating soup with a spoon (or with grilled cheese dippers) sometimes love to drink it through a straw. Consider a wider straw—kids find these fun and unique, meaning they're more likely to use them.

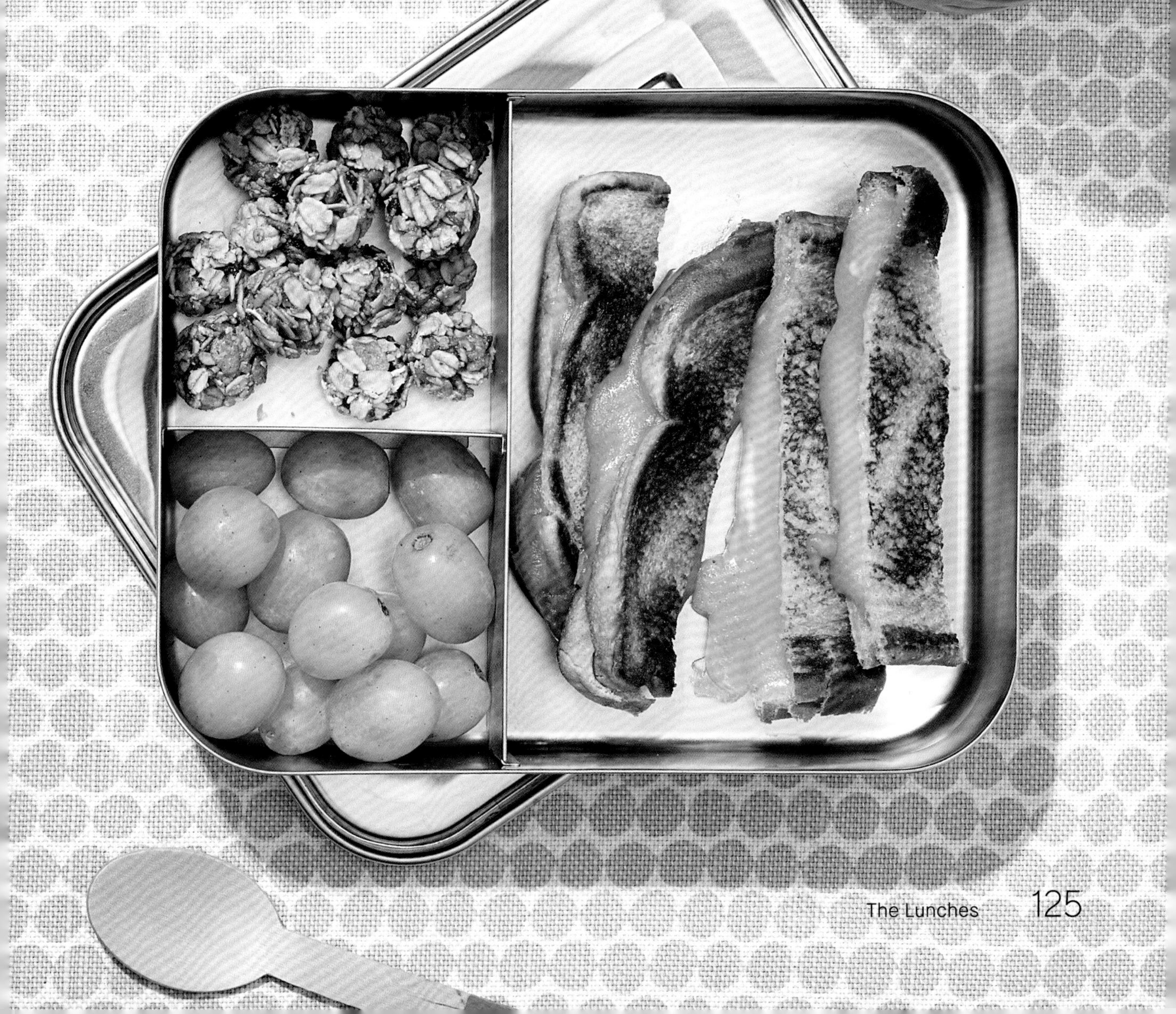

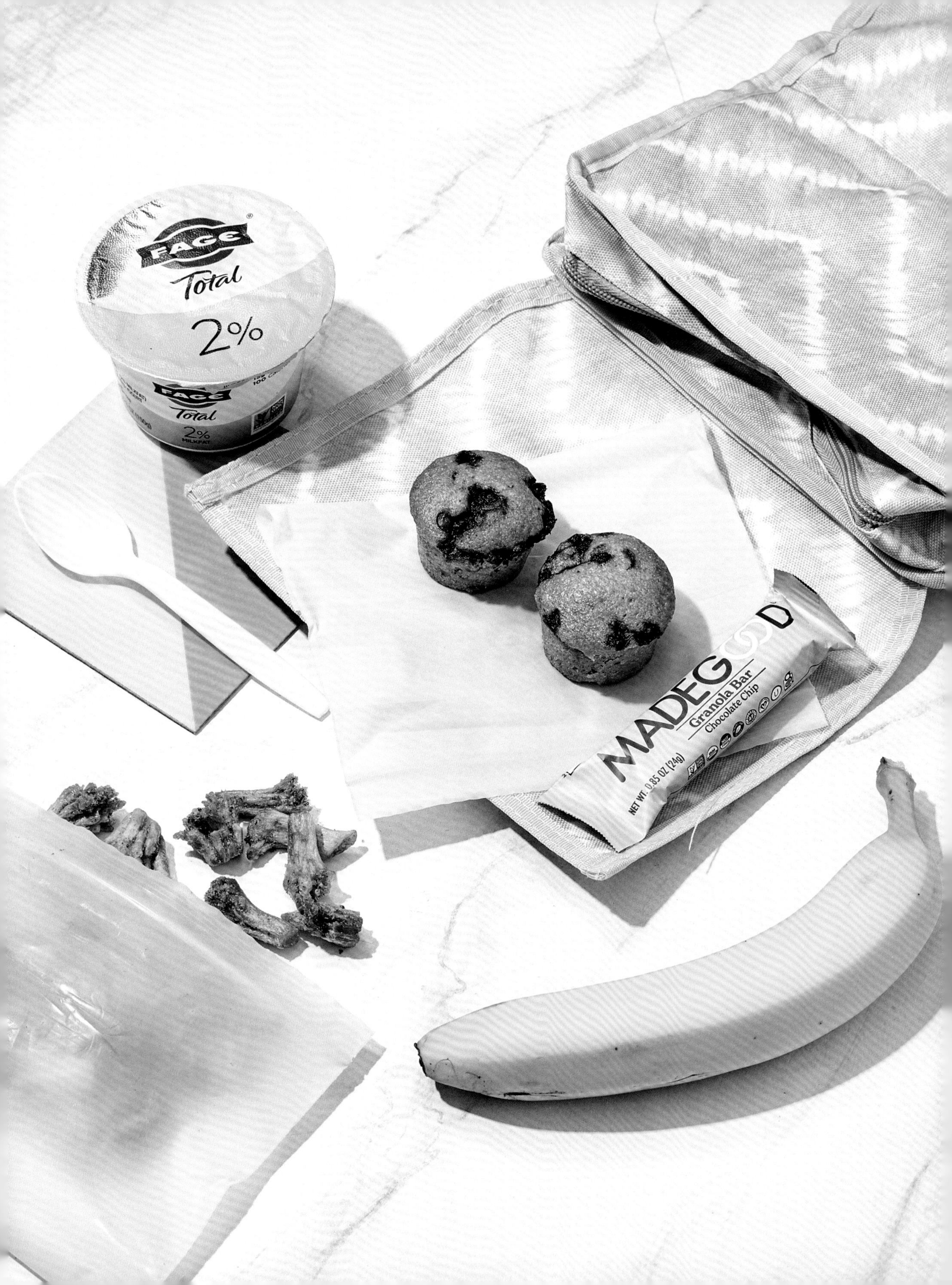
FAGE
Total
2%
FAGE
Total
2%
MILKFAT
MADEGOOD
Granola Bar
Chocolate Chip
NET WT. 0.85 OZ (24g)

Muffin and Yogurt

We're back with another breakfast-for-lunch option: muffins! You can purchase any store-bought muffin or make some at home and send them as leftovers for lunch. By the way, you never have to cook or bake anything just for lunch—that's why we don't have recipes in this book. However, if you're already making muffins at home, they're great to throw in a lunch box.

Blueberry muffin
(or any favorite muffin flavor)

Whole banana

Freeze-dried broccoli

Yogurt

Granola bar

PREP TIP

This entire lunch is shelf-stable except for the yogurt, meaning the other components don't require ice packs or refrigeration. If you'd like, send a frozen yogurt tube without an ice pack—it should be the perfect temperature by the time lunch rolls around.

ALLERGY TIPS

WHEAT: Send a gluten-free or grain-free muffin instead of a wheat-based muffin.

DAIRY: Use dairy-free yogurt. Opt for an allergy-friendly granola bar, as some granola bars with chocolate contain dairy.

TODDLER TIP

Your toddler might love this lunch—yogurt, banana, granola bar, all the favorites! (For many toddlers at least!)

PICKY EATING TIP

Sometimes kids prefer to eat a "snack" instead of something we call a "meal." If this is your kid, simply rebranding dinner as a "dinner snack" can go a long way! This lunch contains a lot of foods kids see at snack time, so you might have more success with reluctant eaters because it feels like a "lunch snack."

CONTAINER: Responsible Products Compostable Sandwich Bags

Chicken Salad Croissant

Your kid loves chicken salad? Put it on a croissant! The croissant's buttery flavor and soft texture pair amazingly well with creamy chicken salad, and even though this is a very simple sandwich, it might feel fancy for a midweek lunch.

Chicken salad croissant

Grapes,
quartered lengthwise

Steamed broccoli and baby carrots

Goldfish crackers

White chocolate chips

PREP TIP
If the container is very deep, take a napkin or paper towel and fold it on top of the sandwich before closing the lid to help keep the sandwich in place.

"I CAN'T EVEN" TIP
Serve thinly sliced raw carrots and broccoli if you don't have steamed leftover veggies.

ALLERGY TIPS
WHEAT: Use gluten-free bread, tortilla, or pita instead of the croissant. Sub gluten-free cheesy crackers for the Goldfish crackers. Check out our Allergy Guide QR code (page 42) for brand recommendations.

DAIRY: Use dairy-free white chocolate chips instead of traditional white chocolate chips. Use dairy-free crackers instead of the Goldfish crackers.

EGG: Make chicken salad at home using vegan mayo instead of store-bought chicken salad, which might contain egg.

TODDLER TIPS
If this type of sandwich is tough for your toddler to eat, deconstruct it and send the croissant separately from the chicken salad (with a fork).

Check your chicken salad for whole grapes, whole nuts, or large celery pieces, since they can be choking hazards.

PICKY EATING TIP
This lunch looks visually appealing because it has so many colors. Chefs pay attention to colors on the plate because we eat with our eyes, and when there are a few different colors, we're more enthusiastic about our meal. We don't have to offer the whole rainbow with every lunch—quite the contrary, actually—but serving a few different colors in your kiddo's meal is a simple way to make it more visually appetizing.

VEGETARIAN SWAP
Use chickpea "chicken" salad or a plant-based deli meat substitute instead of the chicken salad.

CONTAINER: PlanetBox Rover

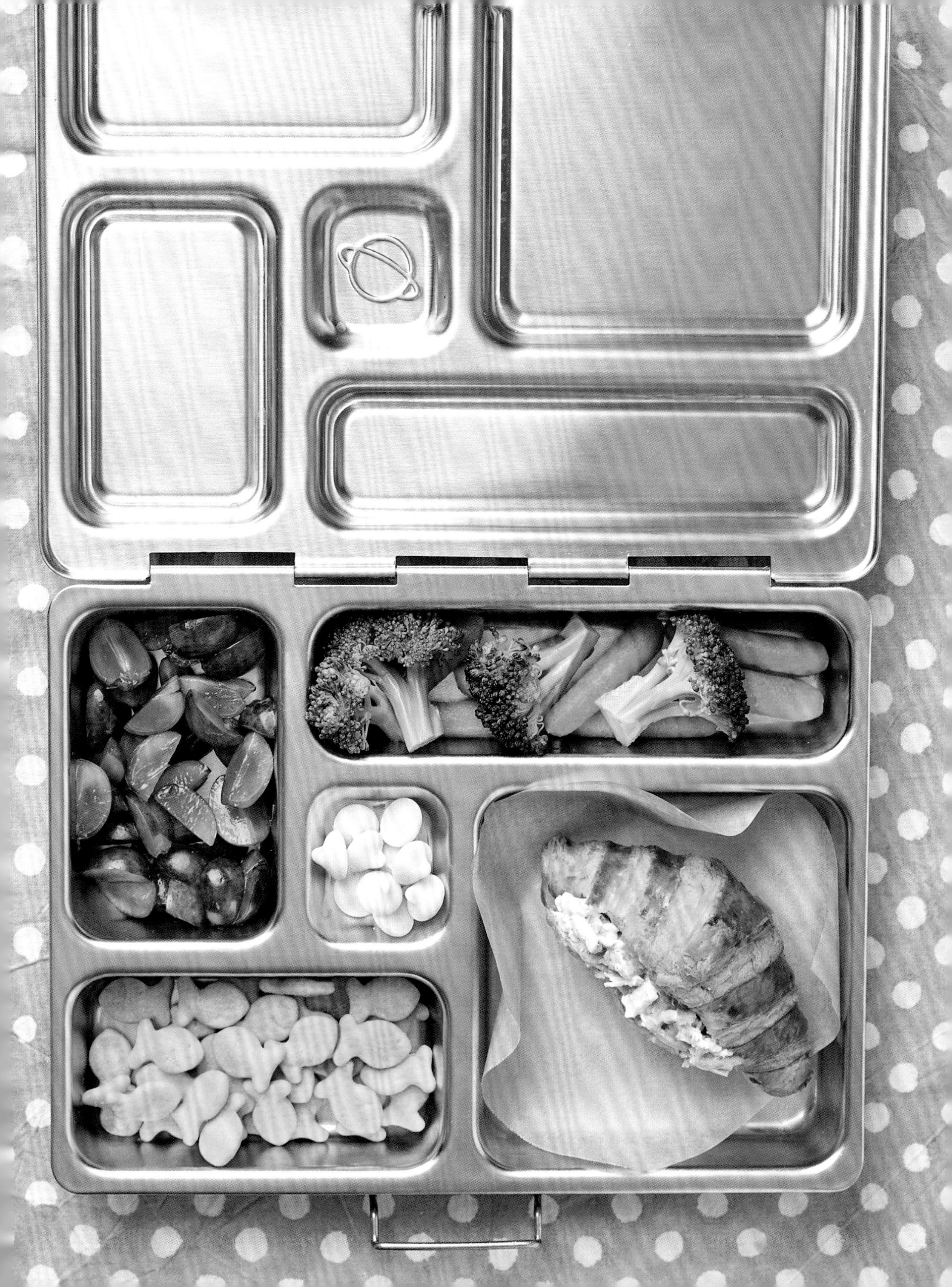

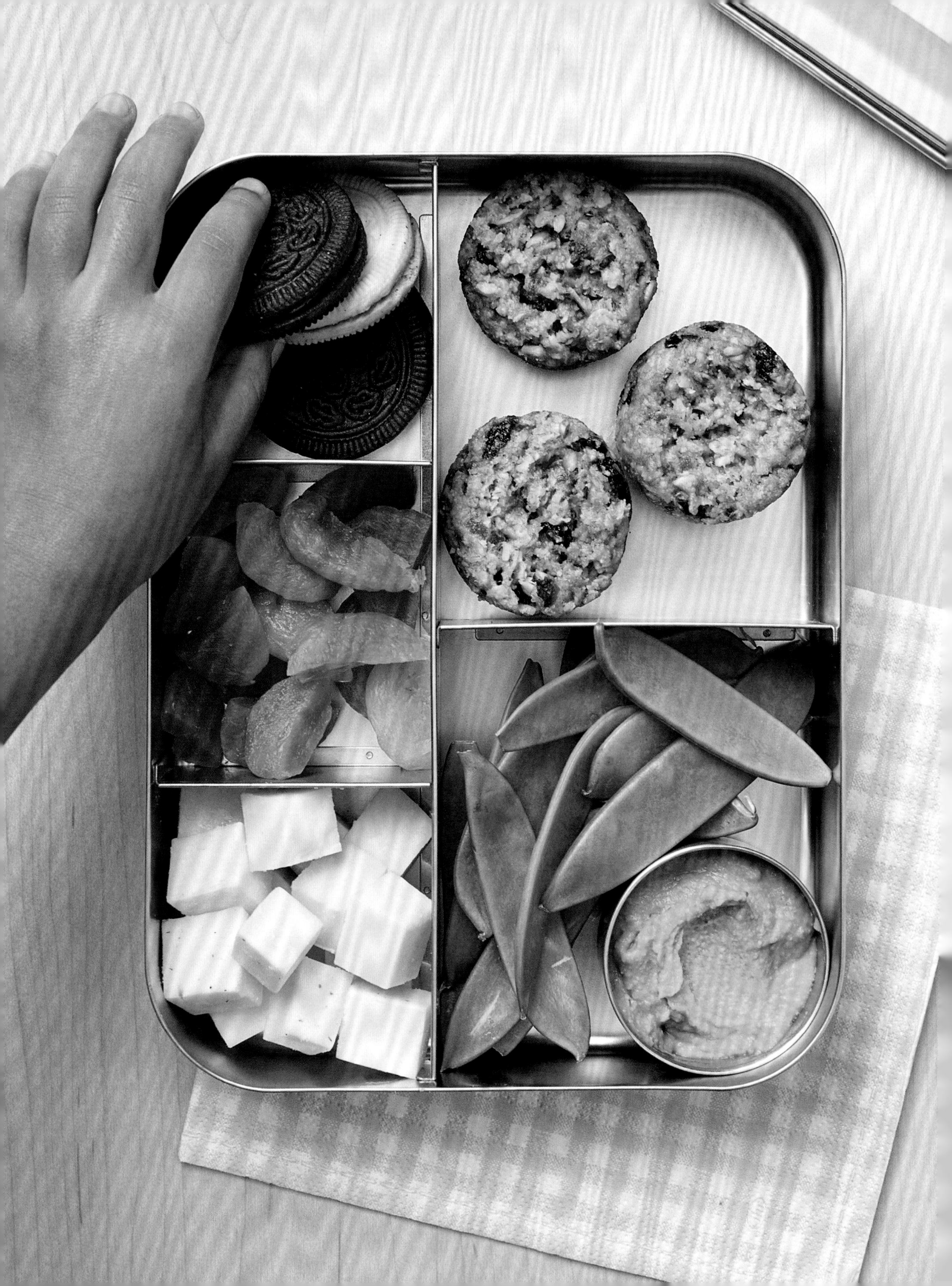

Granola Bites Snack Box

This lunch is another example of a "snack-style" lunch that's still nutritionally balanced and inviting to kids of all ages. (Many adults love lunches like this too!) Plus, it's super easy to pack with minimal prep required.

Aussie Bites
(granola bites)

Dried apricots

Snap peas

White cheddar cheese cubes

Sandwich cookies

Roasted red pepper hummus

ALLERGY TIPS

WHEAT: Use gluten-free sandwich cookies instead of traditional cookies. (Aussie Bites are wheat-free, but always check labels.)

DAIRY: Send a hard-boiled egg, tofu, kidney beans, or edamame instead of cheese for an alternative protein source. Aussie Bites are made with butter so they are not dairy-free. Use allergy-friendly granola bites or a granola bar instead.

TODDLER TIP

To help your toddler chew these dried apricots even better, consider cutting them into smaller pieces using kitchen shears.

PICKY EATING TIP

This lunch has some foods that might be unfamiliar to your child. Remember, this book is meant to inspire you, not stress you out. You don't have to serve everything shown here, or even most things shown here. Use it in a way that is helpful for *your* family. If only one or two components would work, combine them with other foods that your child is more into right now.

CONTAINER: LunchBots Large Cinco

Build-Your-Own Yogurt Parfaits

Yogurt on its own? Pretty good. Yogurt with toppings? *Awesome.* Many kids love yogurt, and doctoring it up with some delicious ingredients adds crunch, flavor, and nutrition. This is one of those lunches you probably never thought to send, but your kid might request it over and over again.

Greek yogurt
(sweetened or unsweetened)

Diced strawberries and pomegranate seeds

Carrot chips

Granola

Shredded coconut

ALLERGY TIPS

DAIRY: Use dairy-free yogurt instead of dairy-based yogurt.

TREE NUTS: Use nut-free granola.

TODDLER TIPS

Since pomegranate is a whole seed, it might pose a choking risk to toddlers. Omit for kids under four and simply send strawberries.

Break any big granola pieces into smaller pieces and pull out any whole nuts, as they might also be choking hazards.

PICKY EATING TIP

Your child might eat all these components separately, and that's totally OK. Sometimes mixed textures can be hard for kids. Practice making parfaits in clear glasses at home so they see how much fun it is to layer ingredients, but don't be surprised if they want to eat it deconstructed to start.

CONTAINER: **Bentgo Easyboxes 5-Compartment Meal Container (formerly EasyLunchboxes brand)**

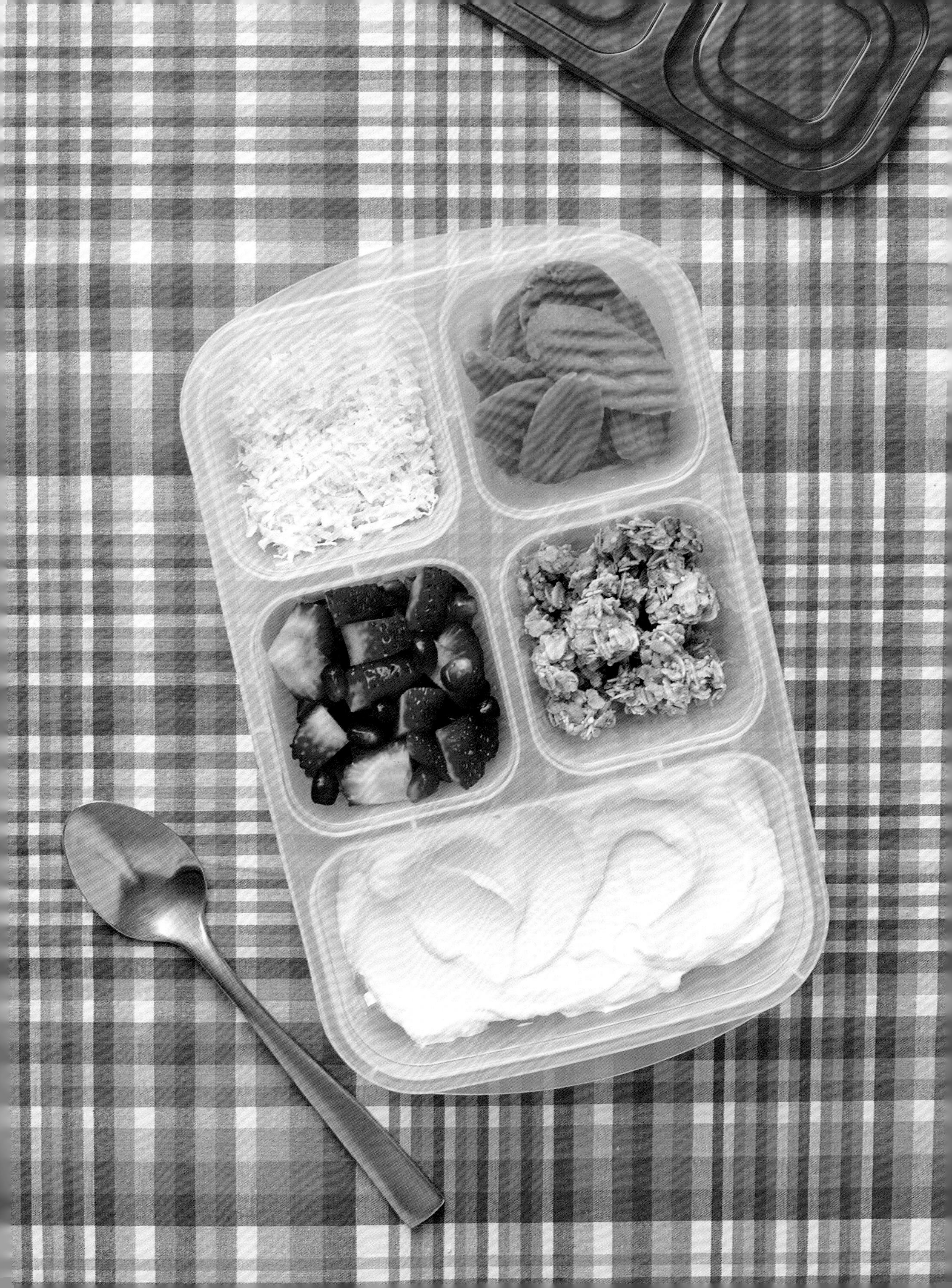

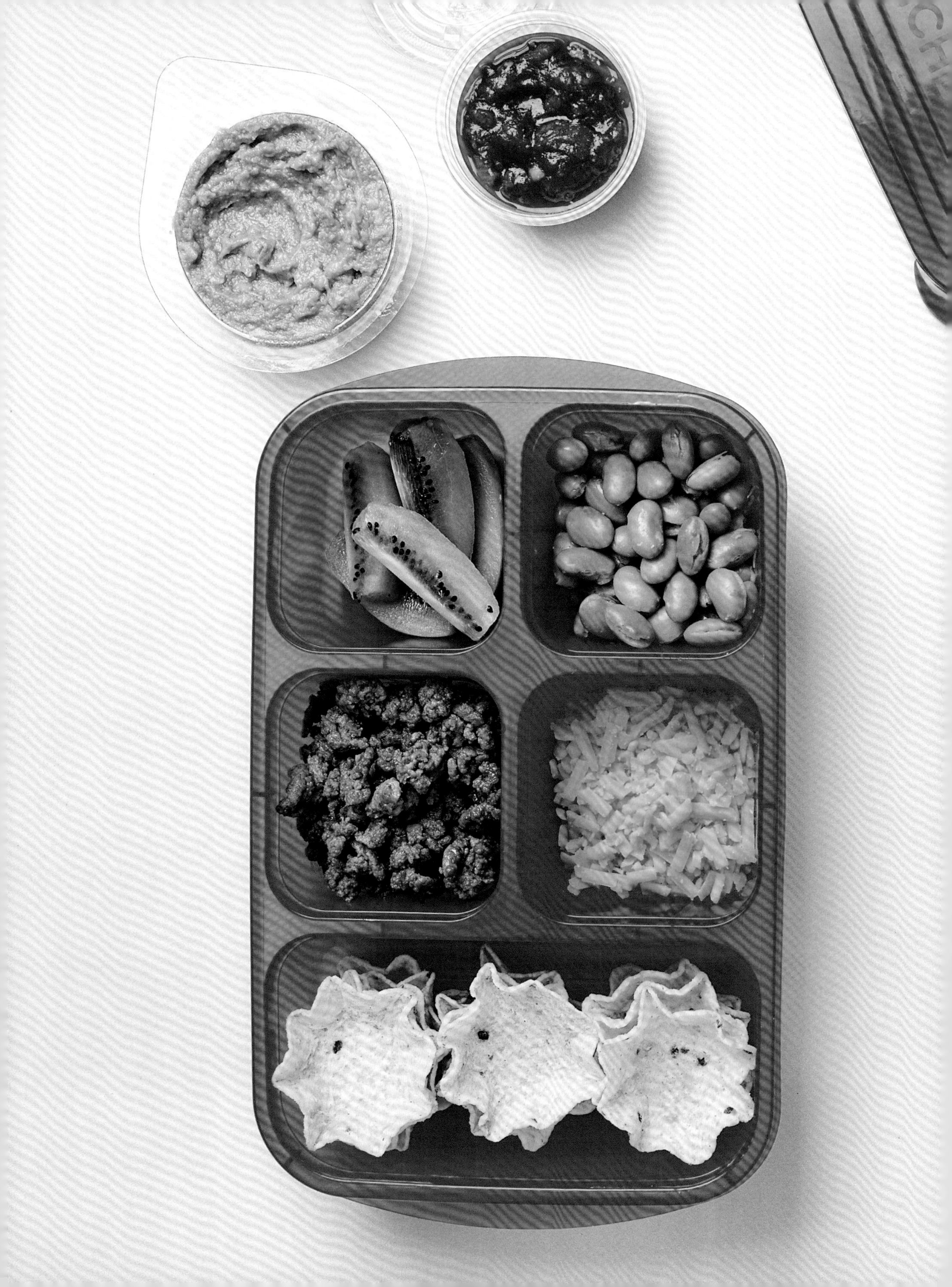

Nacho Bites

This lunch is one of our favorites in the whole book. Build-your-own nacho bites in little scoop chips? Sign us up! All four of our kids—Hannah, Mia, Prescott, and Elise—pointed this out as something they want to try.

Tortilla scoops

Leftover cooked ground beef
(can be made with taco seasoning)

Pinto beans

Shredded cheese

Kiwi

Dips: guacamole, salsa

PREP TIP This is truly a "choose your adventure" type of lunch. Swap out guac for sour cream, use black beans instead of pinto beans, omit the ground beef, or try grilled chicken instead. It's *all* good.

ALLERGY TIP **DAIRY:** Use dairy-free shredded cheese or dairy-free queso instead of dairy-based cheese.

TODDLER TIP Tortilla chips are considered a choking hazard by some governing bodies for kids under four, while other agencies consider them choking hazards for kids under three. Regardless, if you have a young eater, consider sending soft tortillas instead of tortilla chips.

PICKY EATING TIP Dips can make all the difference with this lunch. If your kid is really into sour cream, as many are, send that instead of the salsa or guac. Or, if you happen to have a spice lover, make sure the salsa has a little kick to it!

VEGETARIAN SWAP Omit ground beef or use a plant-based ground beef alternative.

CONTAINER: Bentgo Easyboxes 5-Compartment Meal Container (formerly EasyLunchboxes brand)

Sunflower Seed Butter and Honey Sandwich

Do you forget about honey as a deliciously sweet sandwich spread? If you have a honey lover, this might be a meal they really enjoy. It's also shelf-stable and has both antioxidant and anti-inflammatory benefits.

Sunflower seed butter and honey sandwich on whole-wheat bread,
cut in half

Mandarin orange cup

Snow peas

Frozen yogurt tube

Oatmeal cookie

PREP TIP

Most of this lunch is shelf-stable—only the snow peas need an ice source. If you need to pack a fully shelf-stable lunch, substitute freeze-dried broccoli for the snow peas.

ALLERGY TIPS

WHEAT: Use gluten-free bread and serve a gluten-free cookie.

DAIRY: Use dairy-free yogurt instead of traditional yogurt. Serve a dairy-free cookie.

TODDLER TIP

Although honey isn't suitable for babies because of the small risk of infant botulism, kids twelve months and older can safely enjoy honey.

PICKY EATING TIP

Your child might enjoy jarred mandarin oranges even if they don't like fresh ones. These have a different flavor and texture, and it's worth trying to see if your kiddo enjoys them. Just remember—it can take ten to fifteen-plus exposures to any given food for your child to like it, so don't get discouraged if it's a "no" for now.

CONTAINER: **EcoSoul Compostable Resealable Bags**

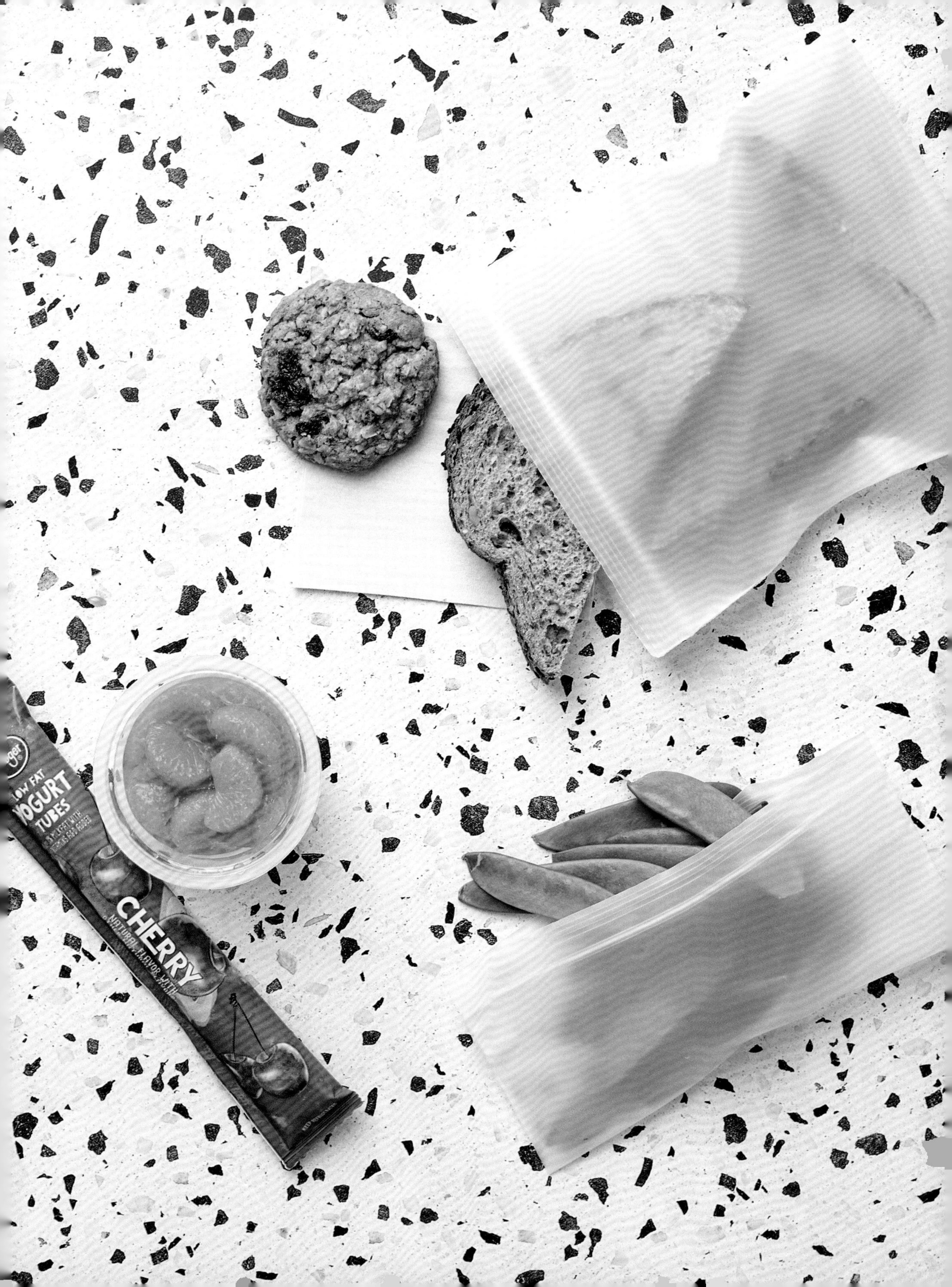
TUBES
CHERRY

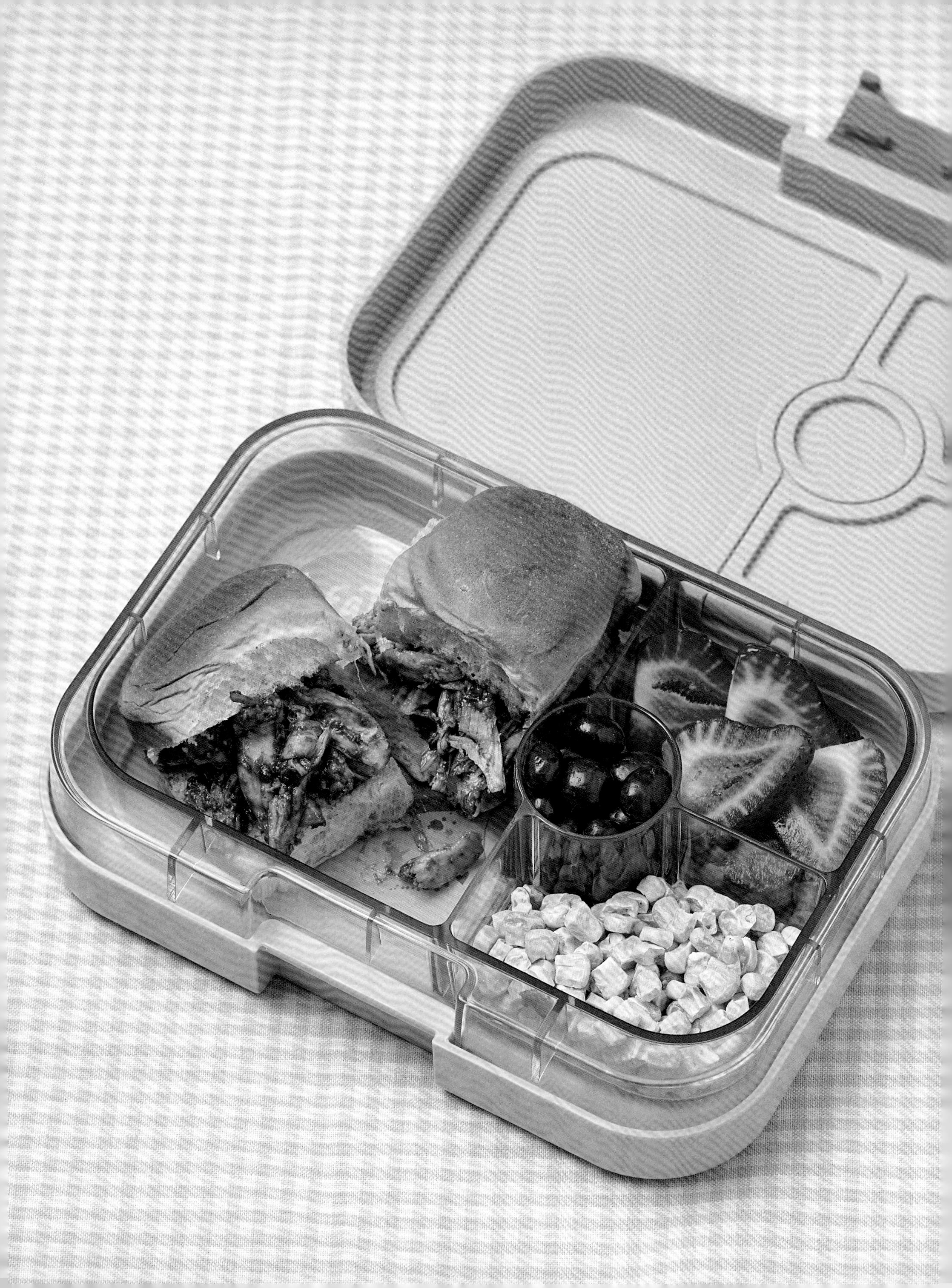

Hawaiian Roll BBQ Chicken Sliders

Have some leftover chicken but not sure what to do with it? Toss it in BBQ sauce and put it in a Hawaiian roll! This also works with premade rotisserie chicken from the grocery store. You'll feel great that you used up leftovers and sent something delicious and satisfying to school.

Hawaiian roll slider with leftover BBQ chicken

Strawberry slices

Freeze-dried corn

Chocolate-covered raisins

"I CAN'T EVEN" TIP

Use leftover grocery store rotisserie chicken—no cooking required!

ALLERGY TIPS

WHEAT: Use gluten-free buns instead of Hawaiian rolls. Make sure your BBQ sauce is wheat-free.

DAIRY: Send plain raisins, dairy-free chocolate chips, or another allergy-friendly dessert instead of chocolate-covered raisins. See our Allergy Guide QR code (page 42) for brand recommendations.

TODDLER TIP

Flatten these sandwiches a bit with your hand to make them easier for your toddler to bite into.

PICKY EATING TIP

A lot of really adventurous eaters (Megan included) despise raisins, and this is a good reminder that even if we dislike a food, it's still great to expose our kids to it. They might have completely different taste preferences than we do. Chocolate helps cut some of the raisin taste—your kid might really enjoy these, even if you don't.

VEGETARIAN SWAP

Use tofu tossed in BBQ sauce or BBQ chick'n instead of chicken.

CONTAINER: Yumbox Panino

Mini Pancakes and Sausage

Pancakes for lunch? Sign us up! You can find mini pancakes in the frozen section of many stores, or you can make them at home for breakfast and pop them in your kid's lunch box. They might get a kick out of seeing something new and unique.

Mini pancakes

Breakfast sausage patties

Blueberries

Pomegranate seeds

Cucumber spears

Nutella

PREP TIP

Toast the pancakes and cook the sausage per package directions before packing them in your kid's lunch box.

ALLERGY TIPS

WHEAT: Use a gluten-free pancake or toaster waffle instead of a wheat-based pancake.

DAIRY: Omit Nutella (it contains milk) or serve a dairy-free chocolate sunflower seed butter spread instead.

TREE NUTS: Nutella contains hazelnuts, making it inappropriate for tree nut–free schools. Use a chocolate-flavored sunflower seed butter as a suitable alternative.

TODDLER TIP

Because pomegranate seeds are technically a large seed, they're considered a choking hazard for kids under four. Try strawberries or raspberries instead or omit them entirely since this lunch already contains fruit.

PICKY EATING TIP

A sweet spread like Nutella (or an allergy-friendly alternative) may make all the difference with a reluctant eater. Remember, eating begets eating. Even if some of these foods are less familiar, if your child sees their beloved Nutella and pancakes, they might just eat everything else in their lunch box.

CONTAINER: **PlanetBox Rover**

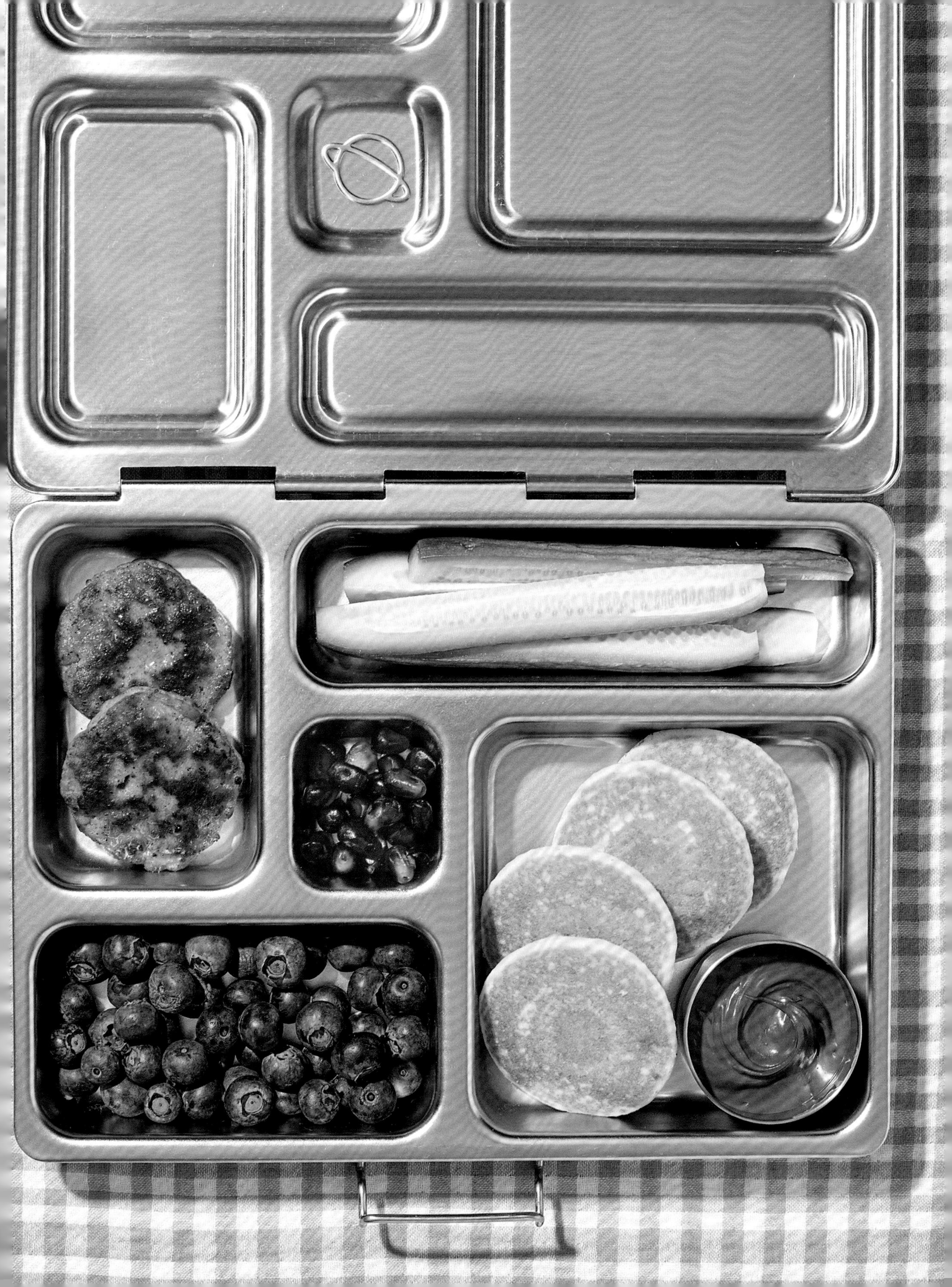

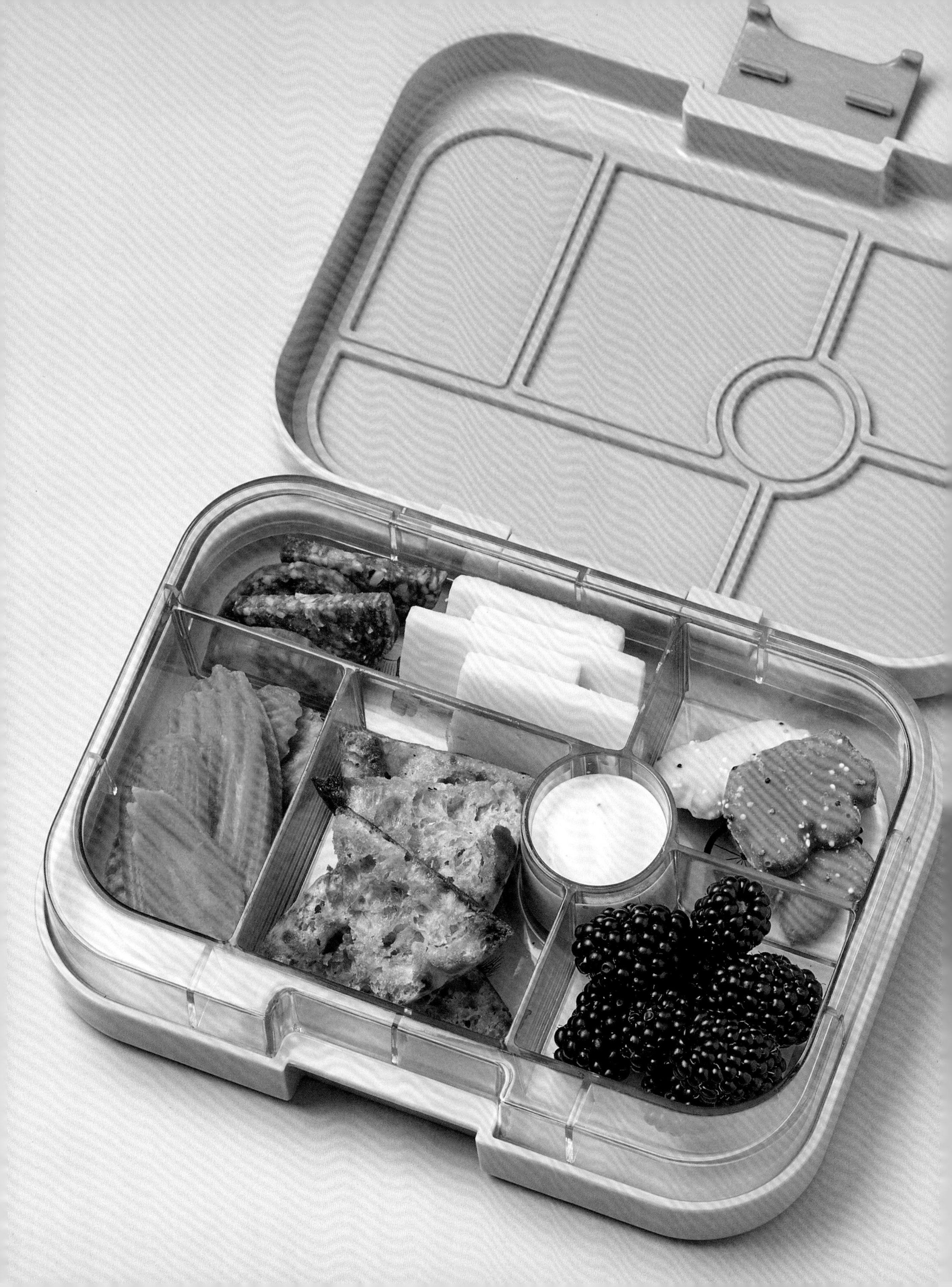

Deli Lunch Kit

This lunch appeals to many types of eaters: Some kids (and adults) will stack the salami and cheese on the pita chips. Others will eat them all separately. Regardless, this is a fun lunch that is slightly unique but still contains foods many kids prefer.

Sliced salami

Sliced white cheddar cheese

Pita chips
(use whole grain if available)

Blackberries

Carrot chips

Circus animal cookies

Ranch dressing

"I CAN'T EVEN" TIP

Buy carrot chips precut like this. They're available in the precut veggie section of many grocery stores.

ALLERGY TIPS

WHEAT: Use gluten-free pita or tortilla chips instead of wheat-based pita chips. Sub gluten-free animal crackers for the frosted animal cookies.

DAIRY: Omit cheese or sub it with another side (pickles, roasted chickpeas). Most commercially available frosted animal crackers are dairy-free, but always check labels. Use dairy-free ranch dressing. Additionally, salami may contain dairy; sub with pepperoni.

EGG: Use egg-free ranch dressing.

SOY: Use soy-free ranch dressing.

TODDLER TIP

Judy recommends quartering blackberries lengthwise to make them extra safe for toddlers to eat, although they're not traditionally a choking hazard food. See more about choking hazards on page 35.

PICKY EATING TIP

Build-your-own lunches like this are awesome for reluctant eaters who don't necessarily want all their food mixed or touching. Your child might eat all these components separately, but with more time and exposure they might start to eat the cheese and salami together, for example. This helps them become more comfortable with mixed-texture foods.

VEGETARIAN SWAP

Omit the salami or use a plant-based deli meat alternative.

CONTAINER: Yumbox Original

Build-Your-Own Naan Pizza

Naan is a favorite pizza base in many recipes because it's soft, flavorful, and sometimes easier to work with than pizza dough. In fact, one of our favorite recipes in our cookbook, *Feeding Littles & Beyond,* is Refried Bean Flatbreads made with frozen naan. (We want to give props to our co-author Ali Maffucci for that brilliant recipe!) These build-your-own pizzas are inspired by Ali's recipe and use fresh, ready-to-eat naan that can be purchased at many grocery stores.

Naan,
cut into wedges

Pepperoni

Shredded mozzarella cheese

Marinara or pizza sauce

Kiwi wedges

Sliced black olives

Brookie
(a brownie cookie you can usually get store-bought)

PREP TIP

Make sure to pack the sauce in a container or compartment where it won't leak. We nestled two smaller containers inside this larger one (packed with lids), but use whatever containers you have.

ALLERGY TIPS

WHEAT: Use gluten-free naan or pita instead of wheat-based naan. Serve a gluten-free brownie or another type of wheat-free dessert instead of the brookie.

DAIRY: Serve dairy-free cheese instead of the mozzarella cheese. Store-bought brookies might contain dairy, so sub in a dairy-free dessert.

EGG: Store-bought brookies might contain egg, so sub in your favorite safe dessert.

TODDLER TIP

Your toddler might eat all these components on their own, and that's OK! They'll learn how to assemble foods as they get older and practice with more foods.

PICKY EATING TIP

Olives are another highly polarizing food. Some people love them; others despise them. Even if your child hasn't tried them before, it's OK to send them in small quantities, like this. Your child might actually try them in a different environment.

VEGETARIAN SWAP

Omit pepperoni or use a plant-based pepperoni alternative.

CONTAINER: **LunchBots Large Cinco and LunchBots 1.5-oz Dip**

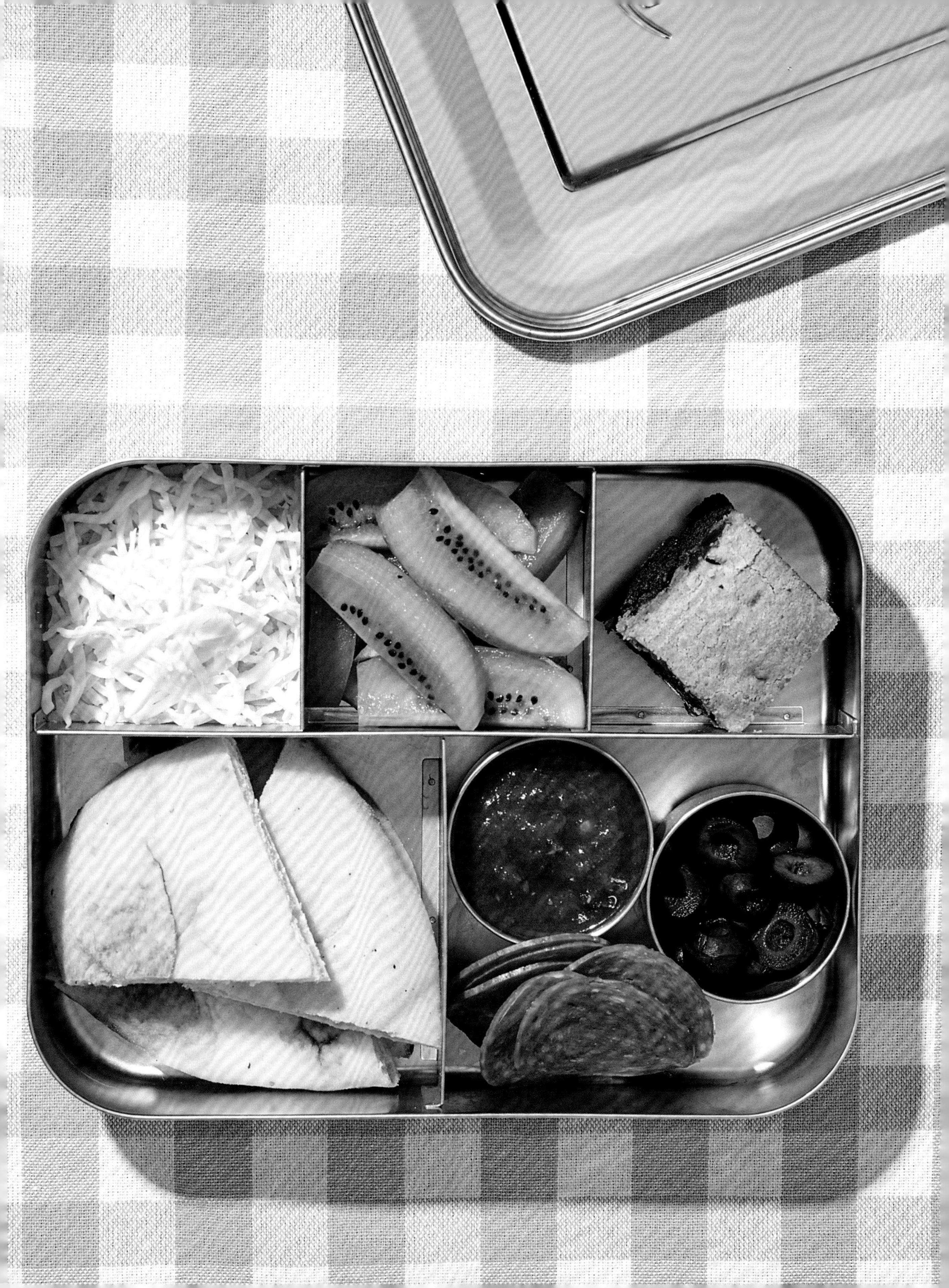

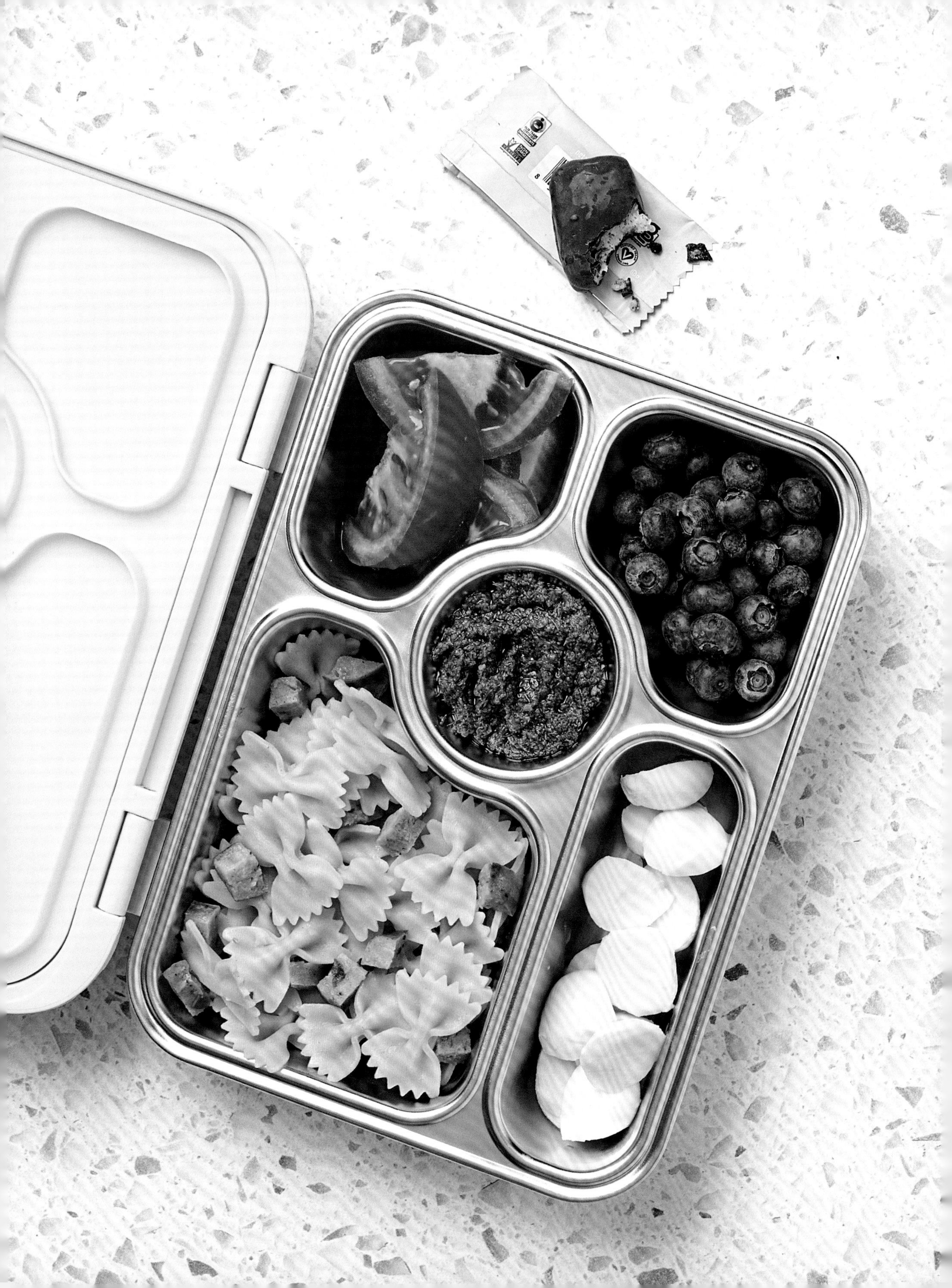

Chicken Sausage Bow Tie Pasta with Pesto

Bow tie pasta looks like little butterflies, and because of their unique shape, many kids enjoy eating them. Our employee Leah puts leftover bow tie pasta from dinner straight in her daughter's lunch box for the next day—no extra cooking required!

Leftover bow tie pasta with pesto

Diced chicken sausage

Blueberries

Tomato wedges

Halved fresh mozzarella balls

Chocolate coconut bar
(Unreal brand)

CONTAINER: Yumbox Presto

PREP TIP

Chicken sausage is typically fully cooked, so you can dice it and put it directly in your child's lunch straight from the package.

ALLERGY TIPS

WHEAT: Serve gluten-free bow tie pasta (or another pasta shape if bow tie is not available). Some gluten-free pasta doesn't hold up well as cold leftovers, so consider making this lunch at home.

DAIRY: Omit mozzarella balls or swap with another fruit or vegetable. Use a dairy-free, store-bought, or homemade pesto, or serve marinara sauce instead.

TREE NUTS: Pesto often contains pine nuts and is not appropriate for a tree nut–free school. Opt for a nut-free, store-bought (or homemade) pesto, or serve marinara sauce instead.

TODDLER TIP

Quarter the mozzarella balls to make them extra safe for young eaters.

PICKY EATING TIP

It's common for particular eaters to prefer starch (like noodles) and fruit. If this lunch comes back only half eaten, that's OK—remember that exposure and consistency help kids become familiar with new foods. If they don't ever see them in their lunch, it can be harder for them to learn to eat them.

VEGETARIAN SWAP

Replace sausage with a plant-based sausage alternative, tofu, or beans.

Spaghetti and Meatballs

Make spaghetti and meatballs for dinner, serve the leftovers in your child's lunch container, and add fruit on the side. Boom, done.

Meatballs
(meat-, poultry-, or plant-based)

Leftover spaghetti with sauce

Cantaloupe slices

"I CAN'T EVEN" TIP

Fully cooked refrigerated meatballs like Trader Joe's chicken meatballs are *amazing* for lunches like this (and the dinners that precede them)! They also happen to be gluten- and dairy-free.

ALLERGY TIPS

WHEAT: Serve gluten-free spaghetti and gluten-free meatballs instead of wheat-based pasta and traditional meatballs.

DAIRY: Check your meatball package/recipe for dairy.

TODDLER TIP

Spaghetti is a notoriously messy food for kids of all ages. Your toddler might be wearing some of this sauce when they come home. If you worry about this getting too messy with your young child, wait until they're older to send it.

PICKY EATING TIP

This is the perfect lunch to send with a fun or unique utensil—consider sending a fork in your child's favorite color or one made with a material they haven't seen before (like bamboo). Even an old-school spork might be interesting enough to intrigue your reluctant eater.

VEGE-TARIAN SWAP

Replace meatballs with a plant-based meatball substitute or shredded cheese.

CONTAINER: **PackIt Mod Lunch Bento**

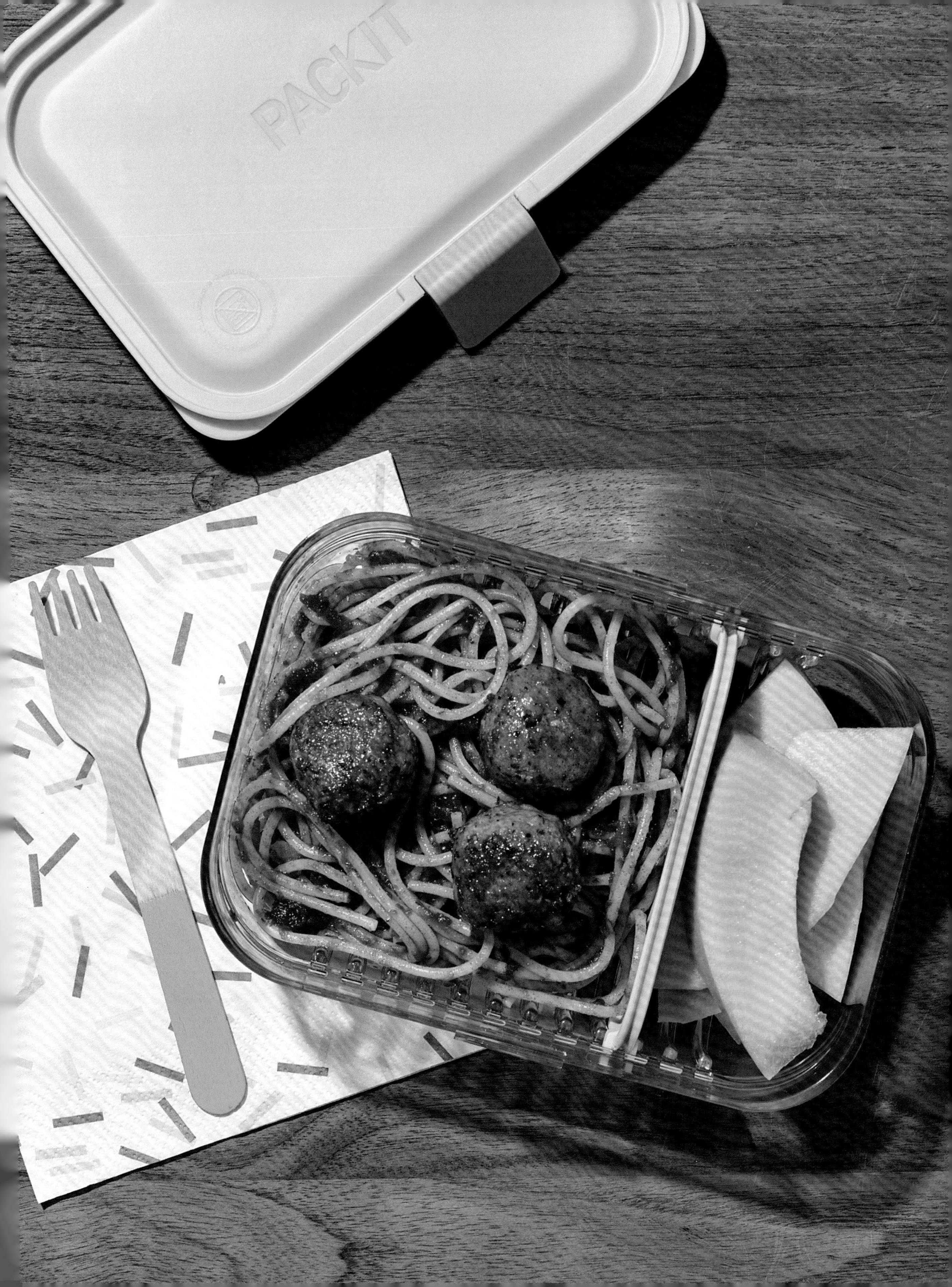
PACKIT

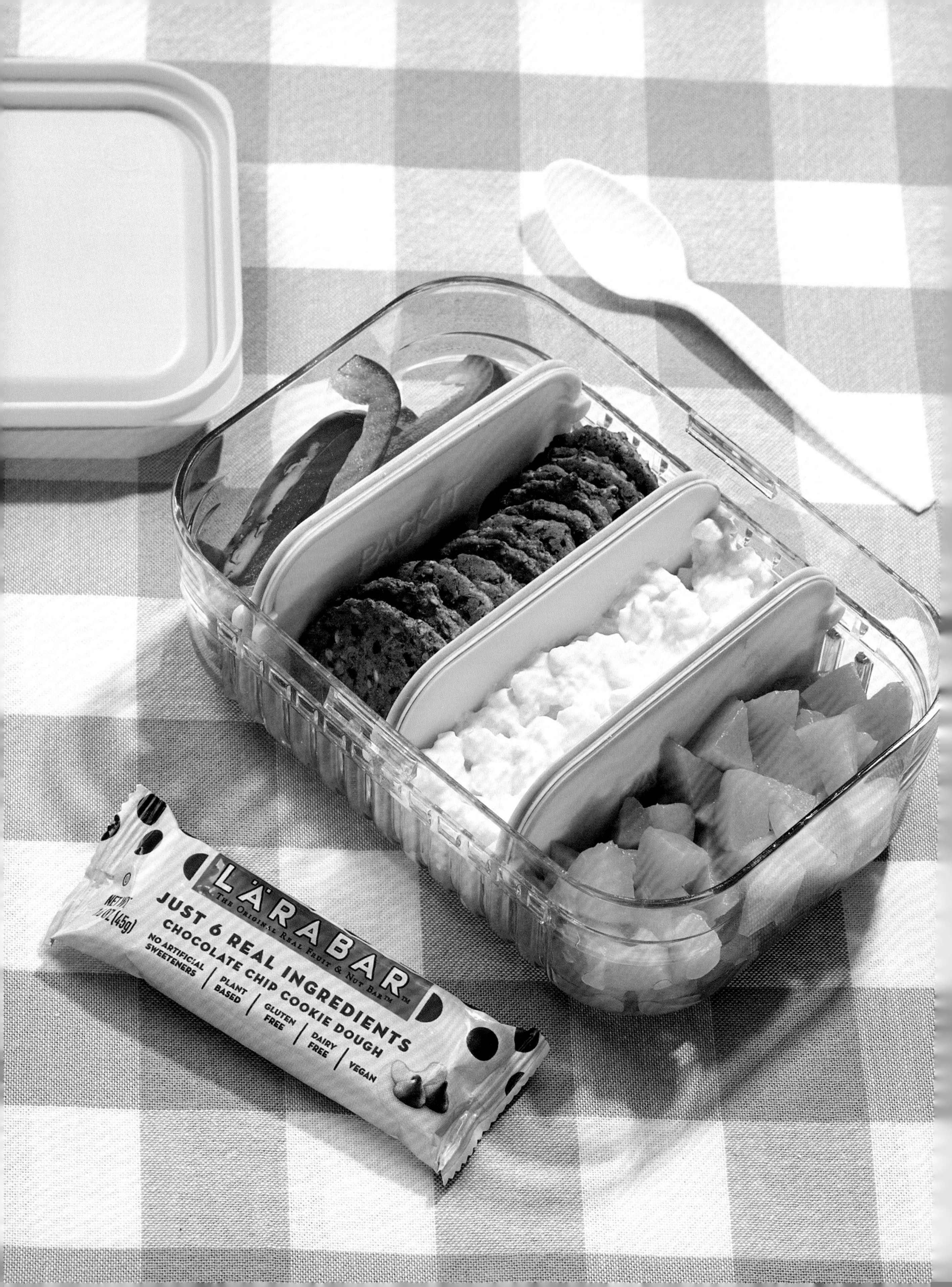
LÄRABAR
THE ORIGINAL REAL FRUIT & NUT BAR™
JUST 6 REAL INGREDIENTS
CHOCOLATE CHIP COOKIE DOUGH
NO ARTIFICIAL SWEETENERS
PLANT BASED
GLUTEN FREE
DAIRY FREE
VEGAN

Cottage Cheese, Peaches, and Crackers

Not everyone loves cottage cheese (or putting peaches in it), but for those of you who do, this one's for you. The best part? If you have a PackIt Mod Lunch Bento box like the one shown here, simply lift the separator between the cottage cheese and the peaches to combine them. Mind. Blown.

Cottage cheese
(our favorite brand is Good Culture, but any brand will do)

Hearty whole-grain crackers

Canned/jarred peaches

Red bell pepper slices

Lärabar or energy bar
(on the side)

ALLERGY TIPS

WHEAT: Serve gluten-free crackers instead of wheat-based crackers. (The crackers shown here are Mary's Gone Crackers brand, and they're gluten-free.)

DAIRY: There isn't a great commercially available dairy-free cottage cheese, although you can find some soy-based cottage cheese recipes online. Instead, send cubed turkey or chicken.

PEANUTS/TREE NUTS: Most Lärabars contain tree nuts or peanuts. If your child has a tree nut or peanut allergy or your school is peanut/tree nut–free, send an allergy-friendly energy bar or a granola bar.

TODDLER TIP

Send soft whole-grain crackers that are easy for your child to chew. If they're super crunchy and hard, they might be a choking hazard.

Some Lärabars contain large chunks of nuts, so consider sending a soft granola or energy bar instead.

PICKY EATING TIP

Not all cottage cheese is created equal. Megan discovered the Good Culture brand a few years ago and has recommended it to many clients who were not cottage cheese fans. Guess what? A bunch of them really like it and will only get this brand. It also happens to be a good source of probiotics. Try it with your reluctant eater—they might be down! Otherwise, sub out yogurt for cottage cheese.

CONTAINER: PackIt Mod Lunch Bento

Falafel, Pita, and Tzatziki

This lunch can really shake you out of your rut and is especially great if you serve falafel for dinner the night before and send the leftovers to school the next day.

Falafel
(from frozen)

Pita wedges
(or mini pockets)

Tzatziki

Freeze-dried strawberries

Cucumber sticks

Annie's brand Birthday Cake Bunny Grahams

PREP TIP

Fully cook falafel per package instructions before putting it in your child's lunch.

ALLERGY TIPS

WHEAT: Falafel likely contains wheat, so opt for a gluten-free frozen option. Send a gluten-free cookie or dessert instead of Annie's Birthday Cake Bunny Grahams.

DAIRY: Annie's Birthday Cake Bunny Grahams may contain milk. Use a safe-for-you alternative. Sub hummus for tzatziki.

SOY: Annie's Birthday Cake Bunny Grahams may contain soy.

TODDLER TIP

This lunch is already modified for choking hazards, but consider cutting the falafel into smaller pieces that might be easier for your toddler to pick up.

PICKY EATING TIP

We don't specify a lot of brands in this book because everyone has access to different things, but these Birthday Cake Bunny Grahams are pretty delicious. Your child might love seeing them in their lunch, especially if there are other new or less familiar foods there. Remember, sending at least one preferred or beloved food can make all the difference in your child's willingness to eat their lunch. Any other small cookie will work if you don't have access to this brand.

CONTAINER: Bentgo Kids Stainless Steel

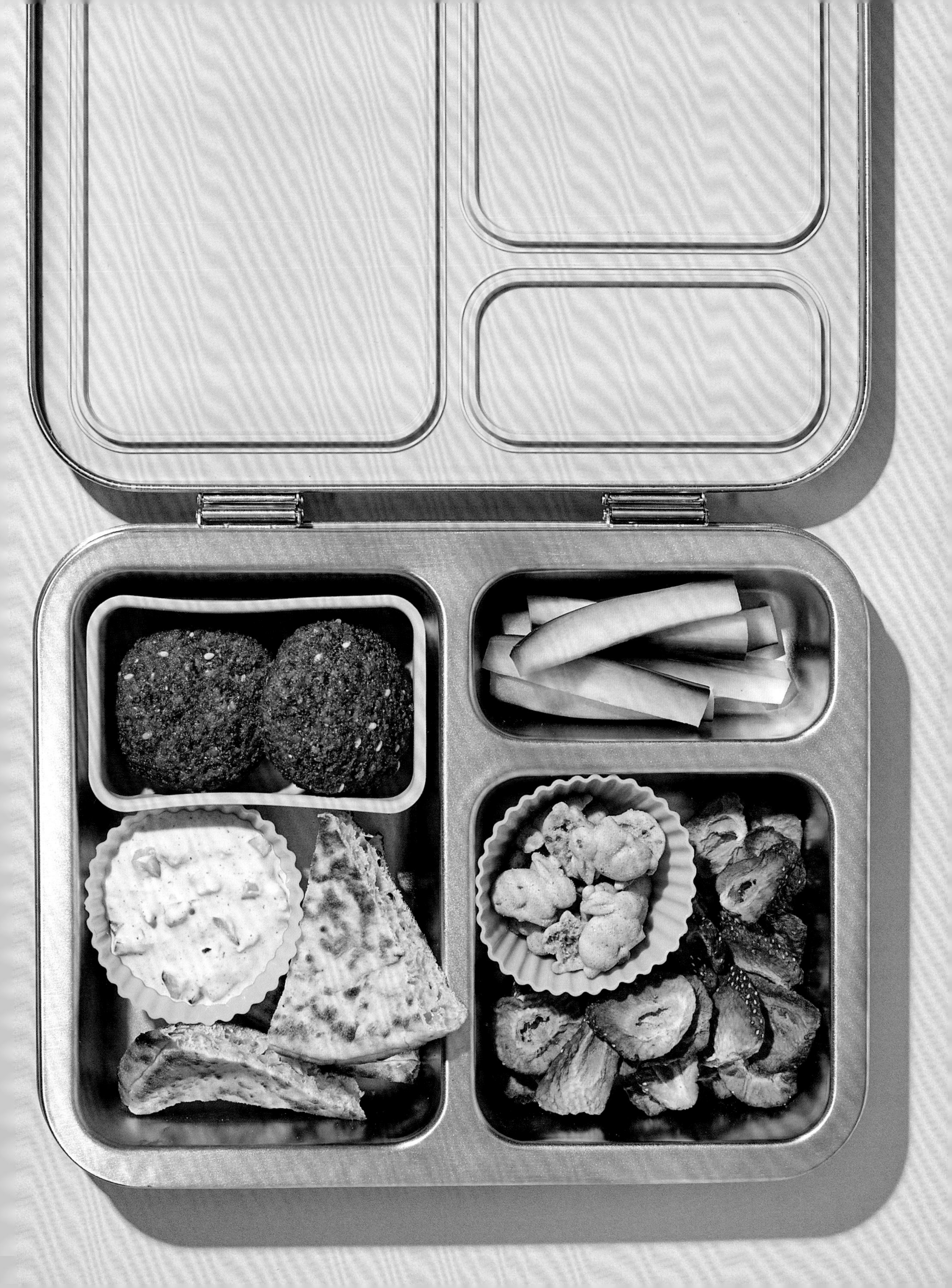

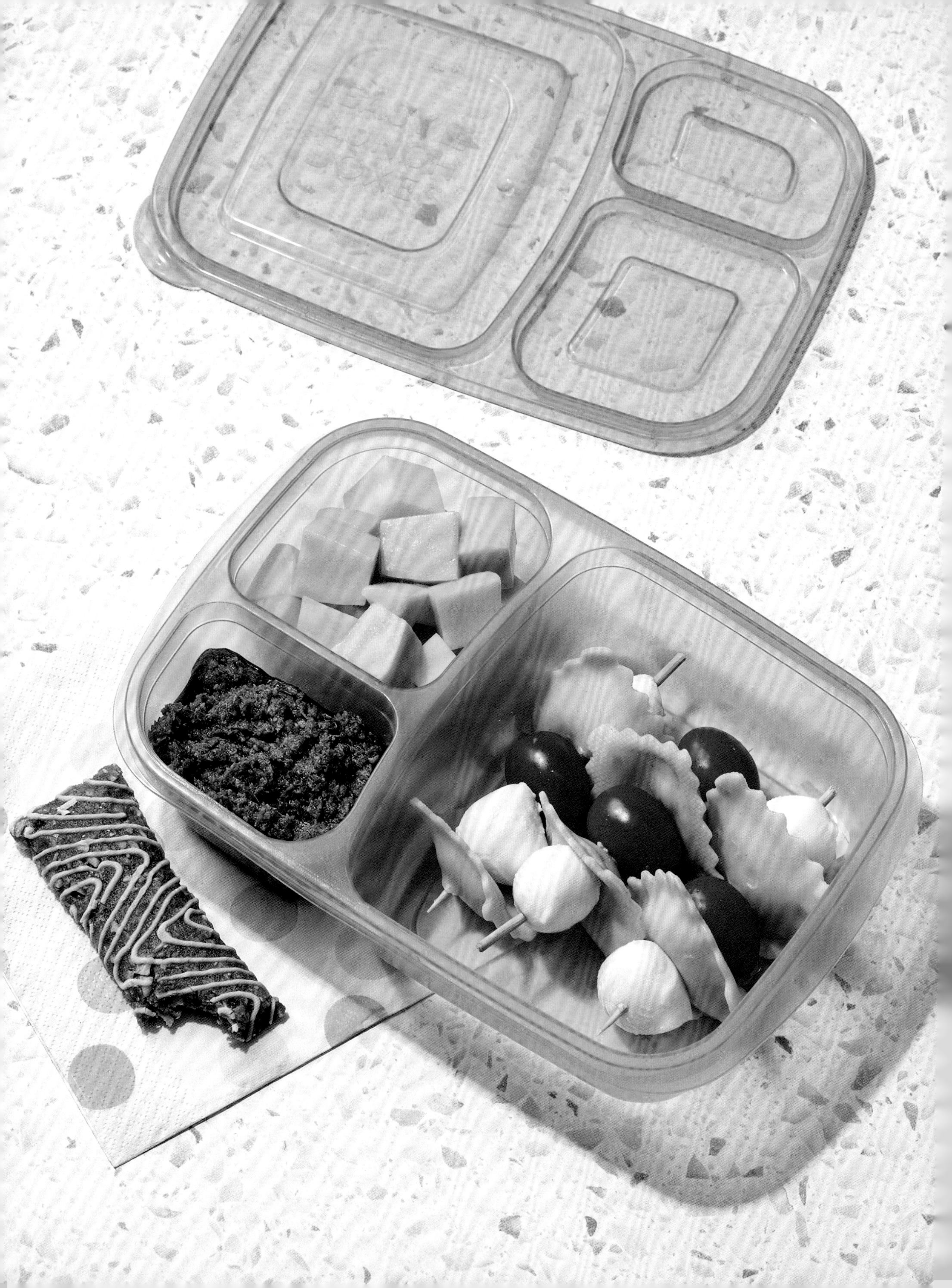

Ravioli Skewers

We promised nothing cutesy with this book, and we're really pushing the limit with skewers. But hear us out: Kids love stuff on sticks, as do adults. This takes a little extra time to prep, but it can exponentially increase the chance that your kid will eat it. If you make (packaged) ravioli for dinner and have some left over, this lunch takes just a few minutes to pack.

Ravioli skewers—fresh mozzarella balls, cherry tomatoes, and cooked ravioli

Diced mango

Kids' energy bar

Pesto

PREP TIP

Cut bamboo skewers with sharp kitchen shears to fit into your kiddo's lunch box. Remove any sharp ends with your shears as well.

ALLERGY TIPS

WHEAT: Use gluten-free ravioli instead of traditional ravioli. However, it might not skewer appropriately, so send it on its own. Send a wheat-free energy bar or granola bar.

DAIRY: Use dairy-free ravioli instead of traditional ravioli. Use your favorite dairy-free cheese instead of the mozzarella balls. Send a dairy-free energy bar or granola bar.

TREE NUTS: Most pesto contains pine nuts, a type of tree nut. Use nut-free pesto (premade or homemade), or send marinara sauce instead—check our Allergy Guide QR code (page 42) for a recipe. Make sure your energy bar is nut-free.

TODDLER TIPS

Skewers might be too sharp for a young toddler, so consider serving the ravioli, mozzarella, and tomatoes mixed together with or without dipping sauce.

Quarter the tomatoes and mozzarella balls lengthwise to reduce choking risk.

PICKY EATING TIP

Using skewers is one of Judy's favorite techniques with reluctant eaters because most kids—and adults—find it fun to eat food on a stick. Even if you don't make this for lunch, try serving food on a stick at home. Your kid might surprise you with what they're willing to try!

CONTAINER: Bentgo Easyboxes 3-Compartment Meal Container (formerly EasyLunchboxes brand)

Salami Cheddar Skewers

Here's another skewer option, but we swear we aren't going all Pinterest Parent on you! These skewers are salty and savory and are a big hit with pickle lovers. They're also fun to eat, as are the mini toasts featured.

Salami cheddar skewers—cheddar cubes, pickle slices, salami

Canned pear slices

Snow peas

Brioche toasts

PREP TIP

Cut bamboo skewers with sharp kitchen shears to fit into your kid's lunch box. Remove any sharp ends with your shears as well.

ALLERGY TIPS

WHEAT: Use gluten-free crackers instead of brioche toasts. Alternatively, consider a gluten- or grain-free baguette.

DAIRY: Swap cheese cubes for dairy-free cheese cubes. Alternatively, you can sub with cubed turkey. Some salami brands contain milk—sub with pepperoni.

TODDLER TIP

Skewers might be too sharp for a young toddler, so consider serving the salami (cut into small pieces), cheese, and pickle pieces mixed together.

PICKY EATING TIP

These skewers are super adaptable. You can put whatever you like on them—pepperoni, turkey, chicken pieces, tofu, etc. Let your kiddo help you make them the night before so they know what to expect in their lunch!

VEGETARIAN SWAP

Try plant-based "salami" or another deli meat alternative, or use cubed tofu.

CONTAINER: PackIt Mod Lunch Bento

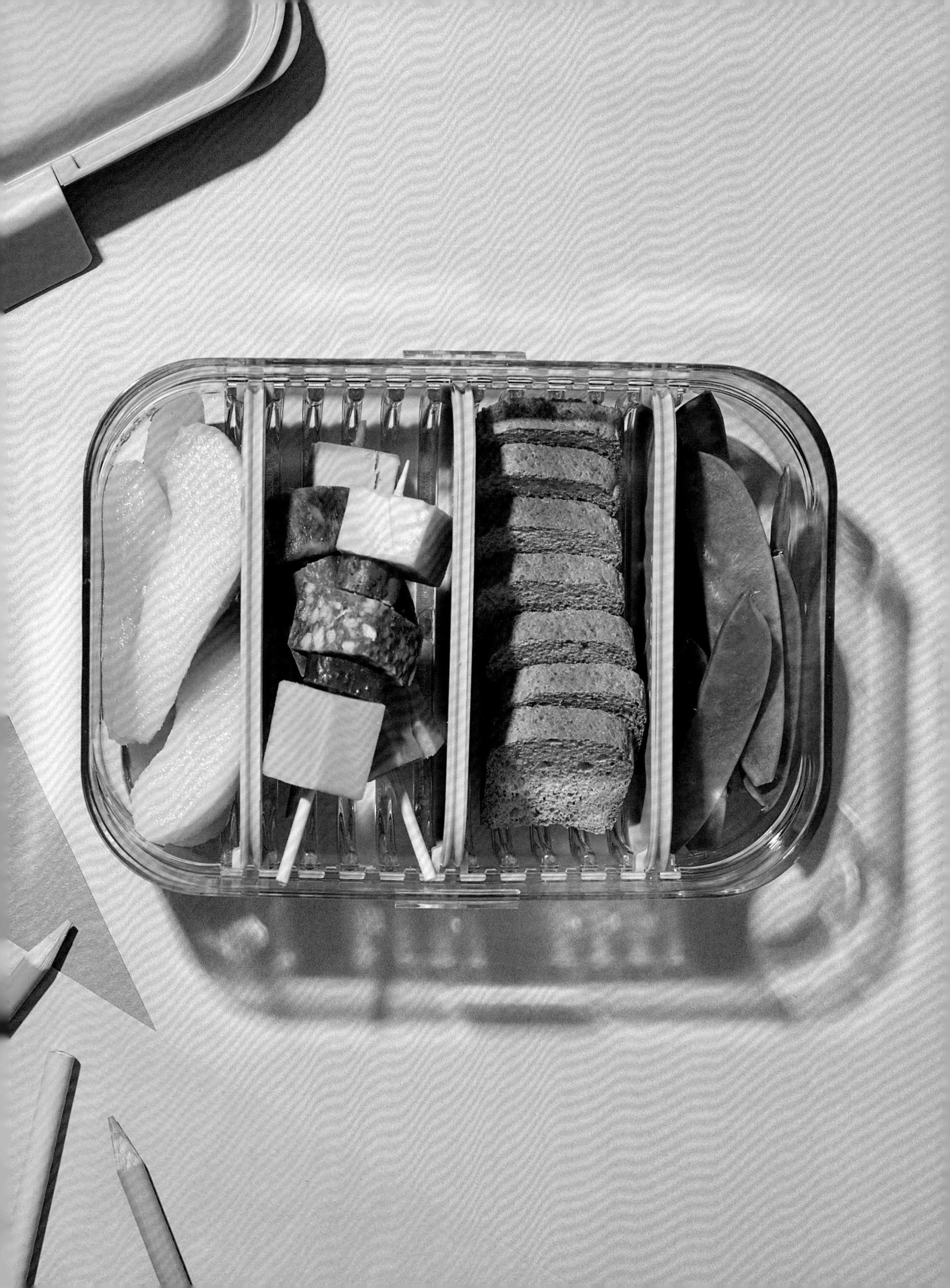

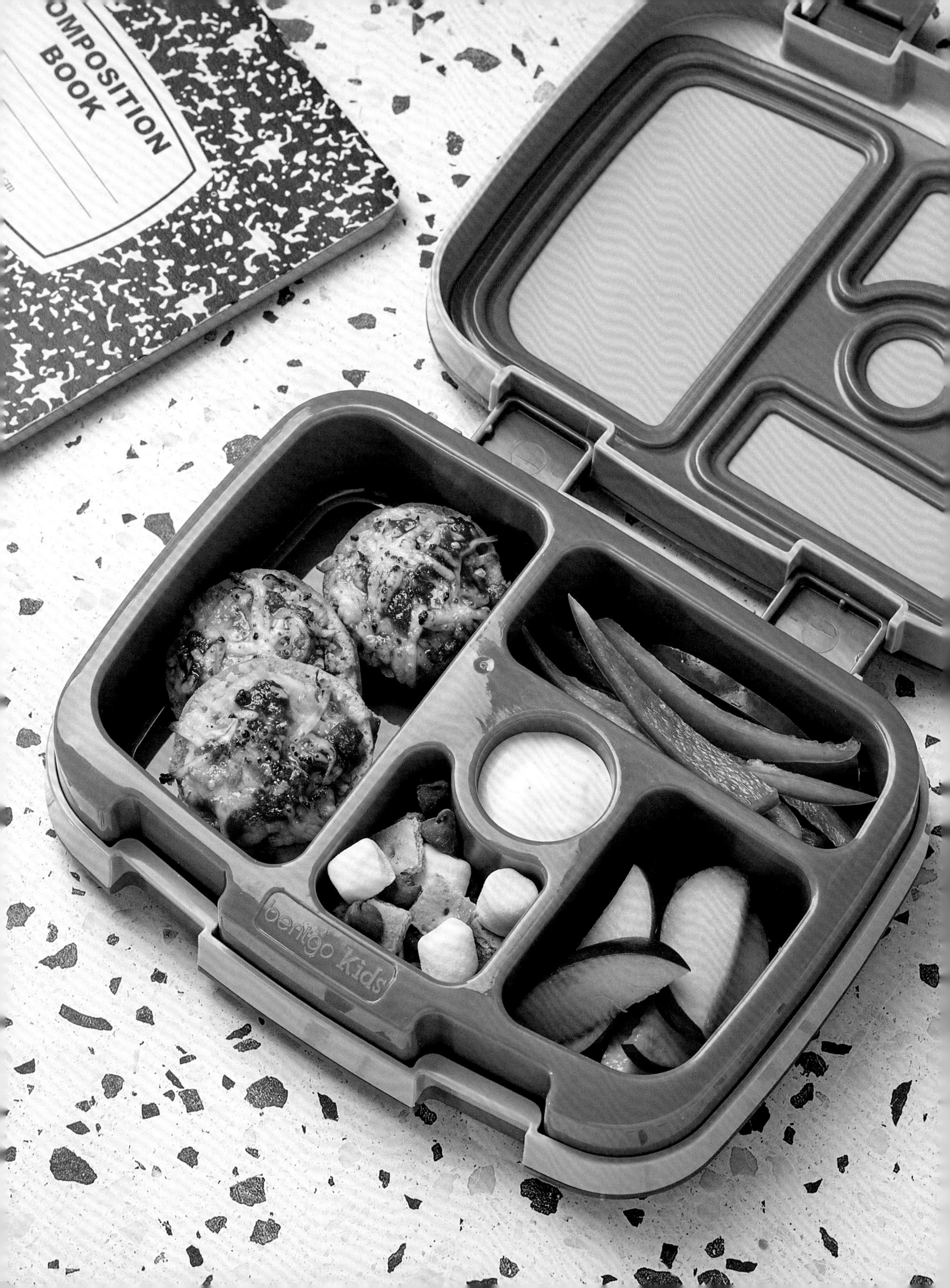
OMPOSITION
BOOK
bentgo Kids

Pizza Bagels

Pizza bagels were a hit in the '90s and are still popular with kids today. Megan's family really loves Annie's brand, although there are many options on the market. We've paired them with a s'mores mix that is a huge hit with all the kids we've tested them on. We hope this will be a fan favorite in your house!

Pizza bagels
(from frozen)

Nectarine slices

Green bell pepper strips

Mini s'mores mix—chocolate chips, broken-up graham crackers, and mini marshmallows

Ranch dressing

PREP TIP

Cook pizza bagels per package instructions before packing them in your child's lunch. If you have access to a microwave or are eating them at home, enjoy them hot.

ALLERGY TIPS

WHEAT: You might be able to find gluten-free pizza bagels, but if not, try gluten-free pizza bites. Use gluten-free graham crackers in the s'mores mix.

DAIRY: Try frozen cheese pizza snacks, which are like pizza bites. Use dairy-free chocolate chips in the s'mores mix.

EGG: Use egg-free ranch dressing.

SOY: Use soy-free ranch dressing.

TODDLER TIP

Marshmallows are technically a choking hazard for kids under four. Omit them and just send graham crackers and chocolate chips.

PICKY EATING TIP

If pizza bagels are a huge hit in your house, your reluctant eater might really love these! Plus, they're easy to throw together as an "I Can't Even" lunch at home.

CONTAINER: **Bentgo Kids**

Tofu and Rice

If you make tofu, rice, and broccoli for dinner, set some aside to pop in your kiddo's lunch box. In just a few minutes you'll have a fully packed lunch with minimal extra work!

Sliced tofu

Brown rice

Mango

Steamed broccoli

Teriyaki sauce

Fortune cookie

Dried seaweed snack
(optional)

PREP TIP

We show teriyaki sauce here as a dip option, although you can also put it directly on the tofu and rice as well.

ALLERGY TIPS

WHEAT: Use gluten-free teriyaki sauce instead of standard teriyaki sauce, as it might contain wheat. Sub a gluten-free dessert for the fortune cookie.

SOY: Use soy-free teriyaki sauce and chicken instead of tofu, and opt for a different dessert if your fortune cookie contains soy, as many do.

SESAME: Since teriyaki sauce is usually made with sesame oil, try ponzu sauce, hoisin sauce, soy sauce, or coconut aminos instead.

TODDLER TIPS

If you think the fortune cookie is too hard for your young toddler to chew, break it into smaller pieces.

The dried seaweed snack can be tricky for toddlers to chew; omit if your child struggles with it.

PICKY EATING TIP

Some kids love tofu while others have never seen it (or willingly eaten it) before. If your kid is in the latter group, try this with a more familiar protein option, like chicken or beef, first. If they love teriyaki sauce, they might really enjoy it!

CONTAINER: Bentgo Kids

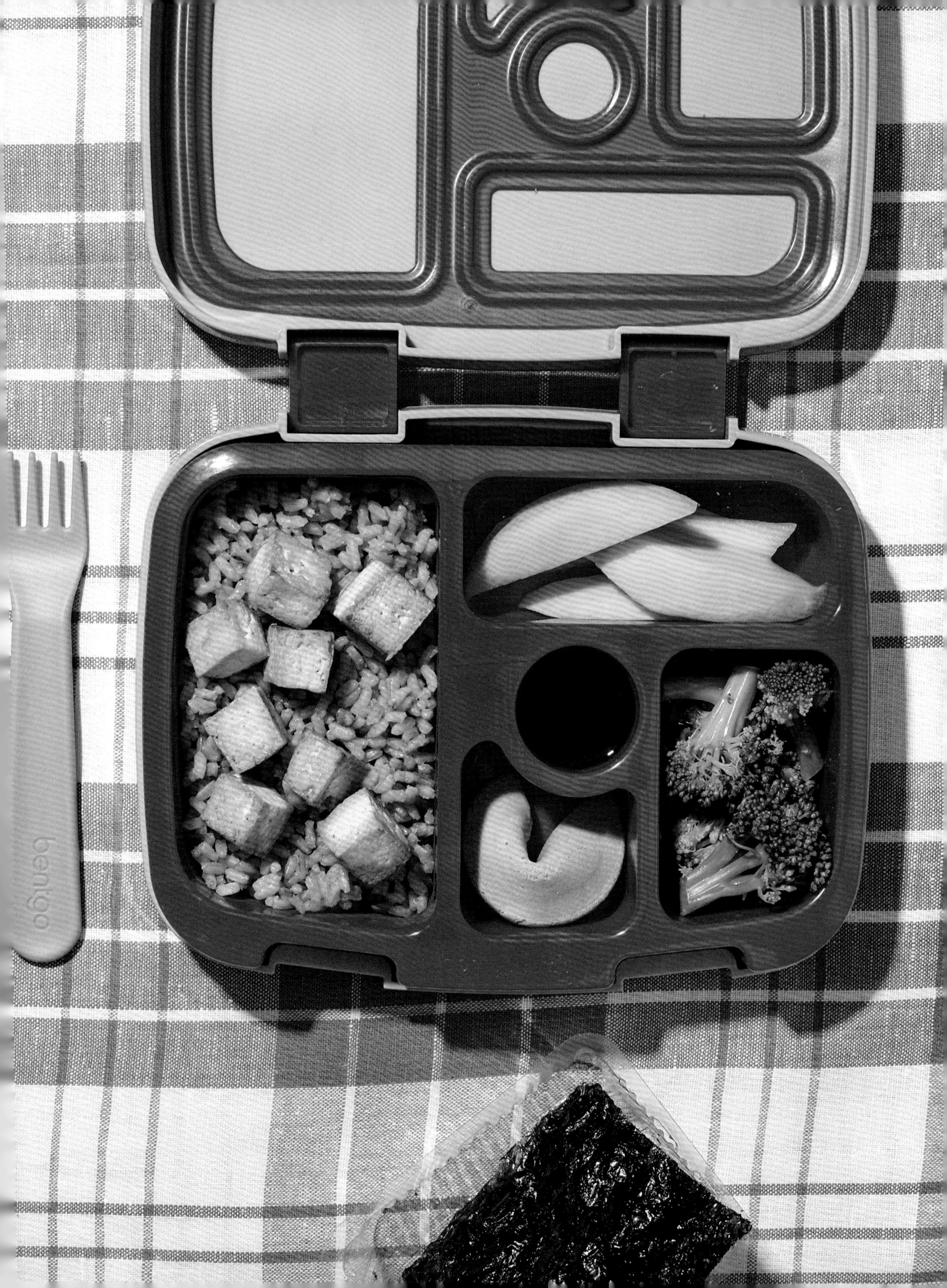
bentgo

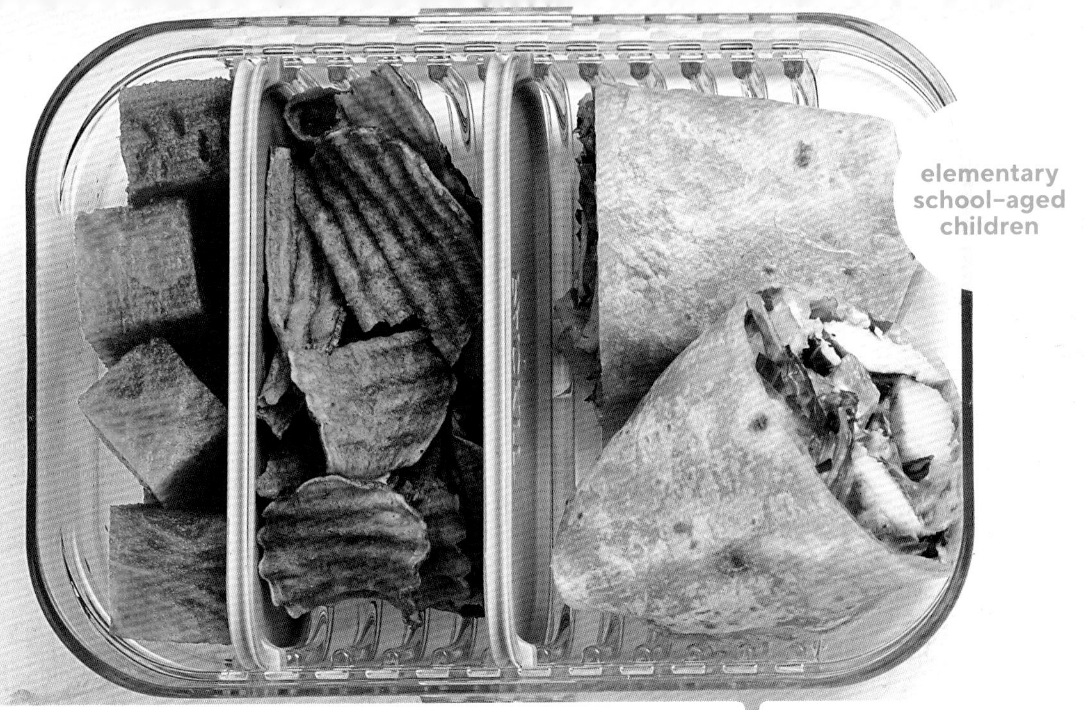

Chicken Caesar Wrap

We wanted to show an example of a lunch packed for three different age groups: toddlers/preschoolers, elementary school–aged kids, and teenagers/adults. As you can see, they all contain mostly the same ingredients, just modified for appetite, eating skill, and choking hazards. All the lunches in this book are just like this—you can change the quantity or presentation to make them work for any age.

Chicken Caesar wrap
(whole or deconstructed)

Watermelon pieces

Sweet potato chips
(or veggie straws for toddlers)

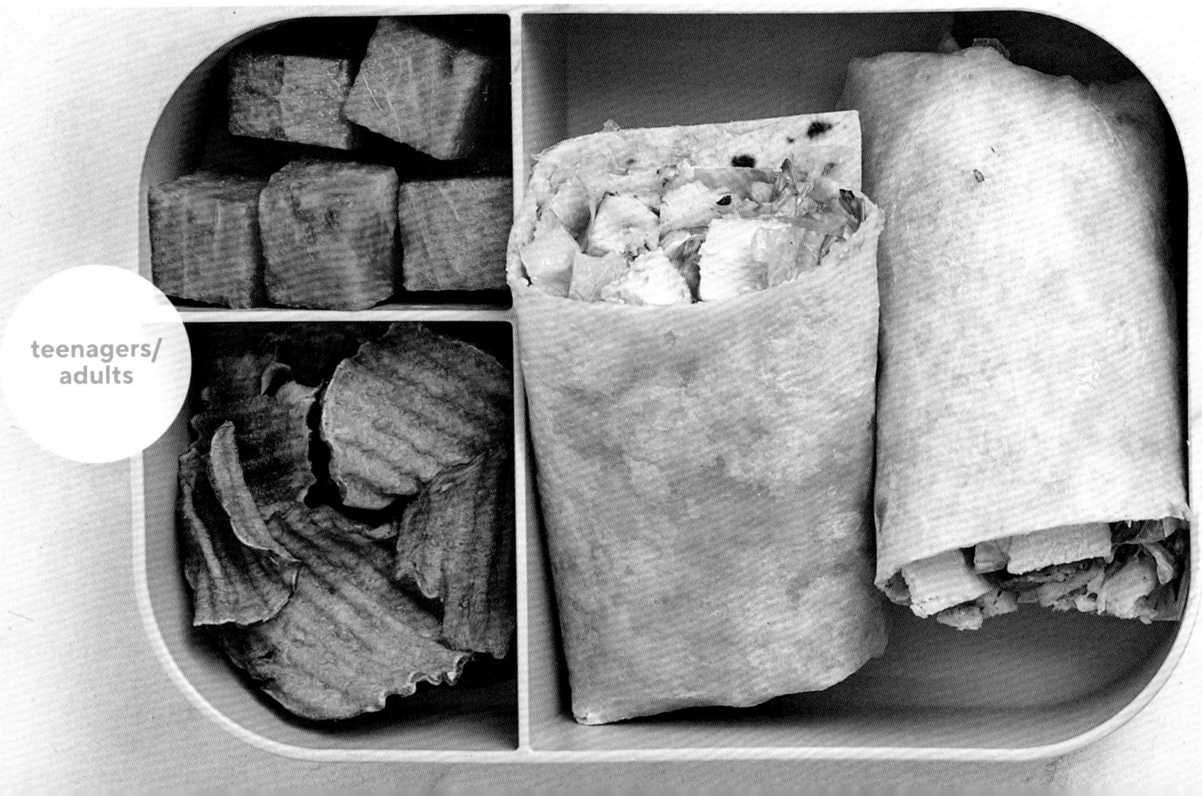

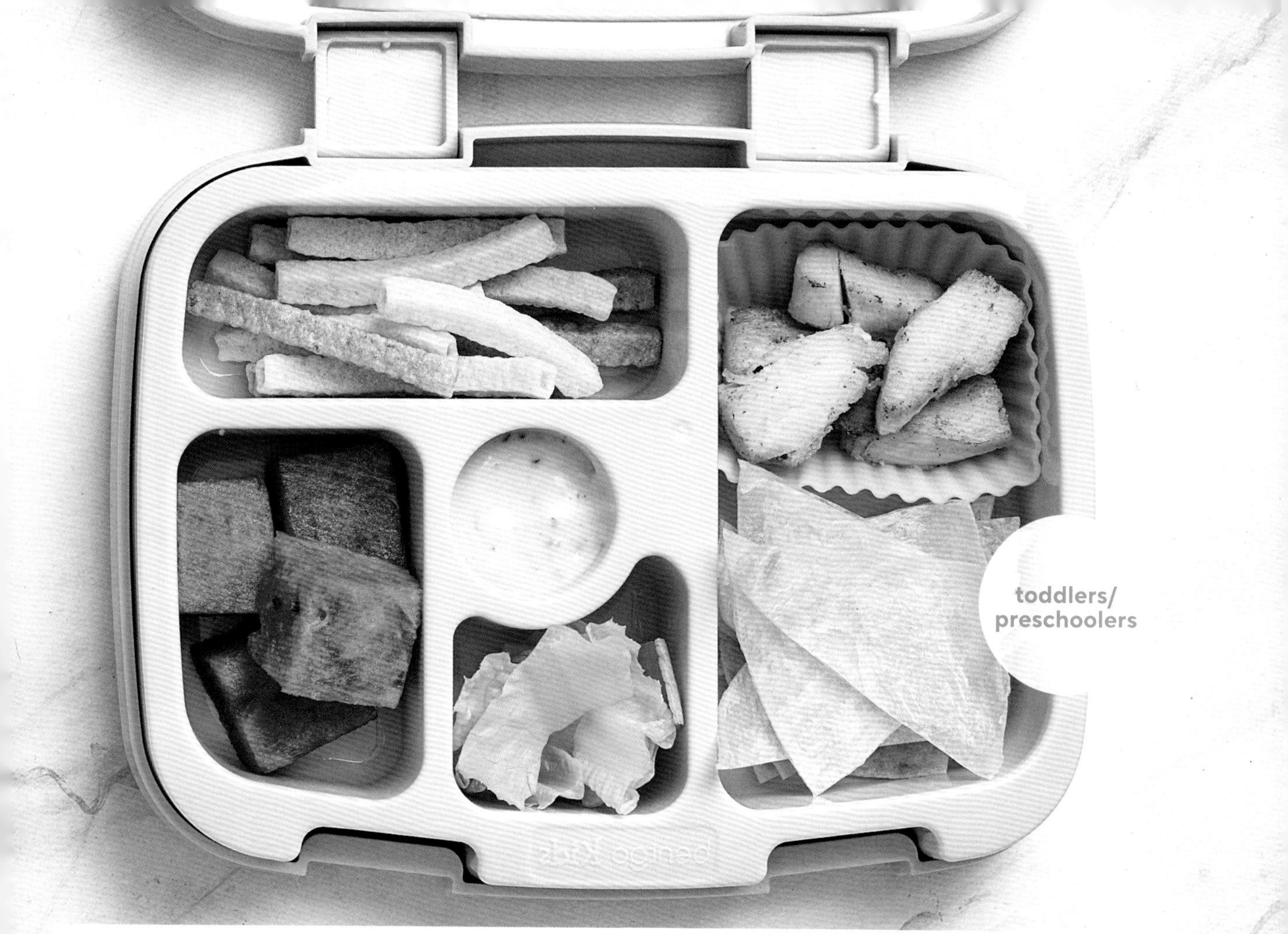

PREP TIP

Use bagged Caesar salad or make homemade Caesar salad with romaine lettuce, shaved Parmesan, and Caesar dressing. Add leftover sliced or diced chicken. Wrap it up in a large tortilla and cut it in half. This meal is best packed the morning you send it to school, not the night before, as the lettuce can wilt easily.

ALLERGY TIPS

WHEAT: Use a gluten-free tortilla.

DAIRY: Make this salad with romaine and ranch dressing (many store-bought ranch brands are dairy-free, but check labels). It will still taste creamy and tangy without the cheese or Caesar dressing. You can still use dairy-free cheese.

EGG: Use an egg-free Caesar dressing.

SOY: Use a soy-free Caesar dressing.

TODDLER TIP

This lunch is best deconstructed for your toddler. Serve crunchy romaine pieces with Caesar dressing as a dip, and cut the soft tortilla into wedges to eat alongside strips of chicken. Serve shaved Parmesan on the side, if desired (not shown here). We subbed veggie straws for sweet potato chips, as chips can be a choking hazard for kids under four.

PICKY EATING TIP

Caesar salad is a "gateway salad" for many kids. Learning to like salad can take a long time, but we've found that Caesar salad tends to be the first salad kids consistently eat.

VEGETARIAN SWAP

Use tofu, seitan, or plant-based "chicken" instead of the chicken. You can also omit the chicken and add extra Parmesan.

CONTAINERS (CLOCKWISE FROM TOP LEFT):
PackIt Mod Lunch Bento, Bentgo Kids, and Bentgo Modern

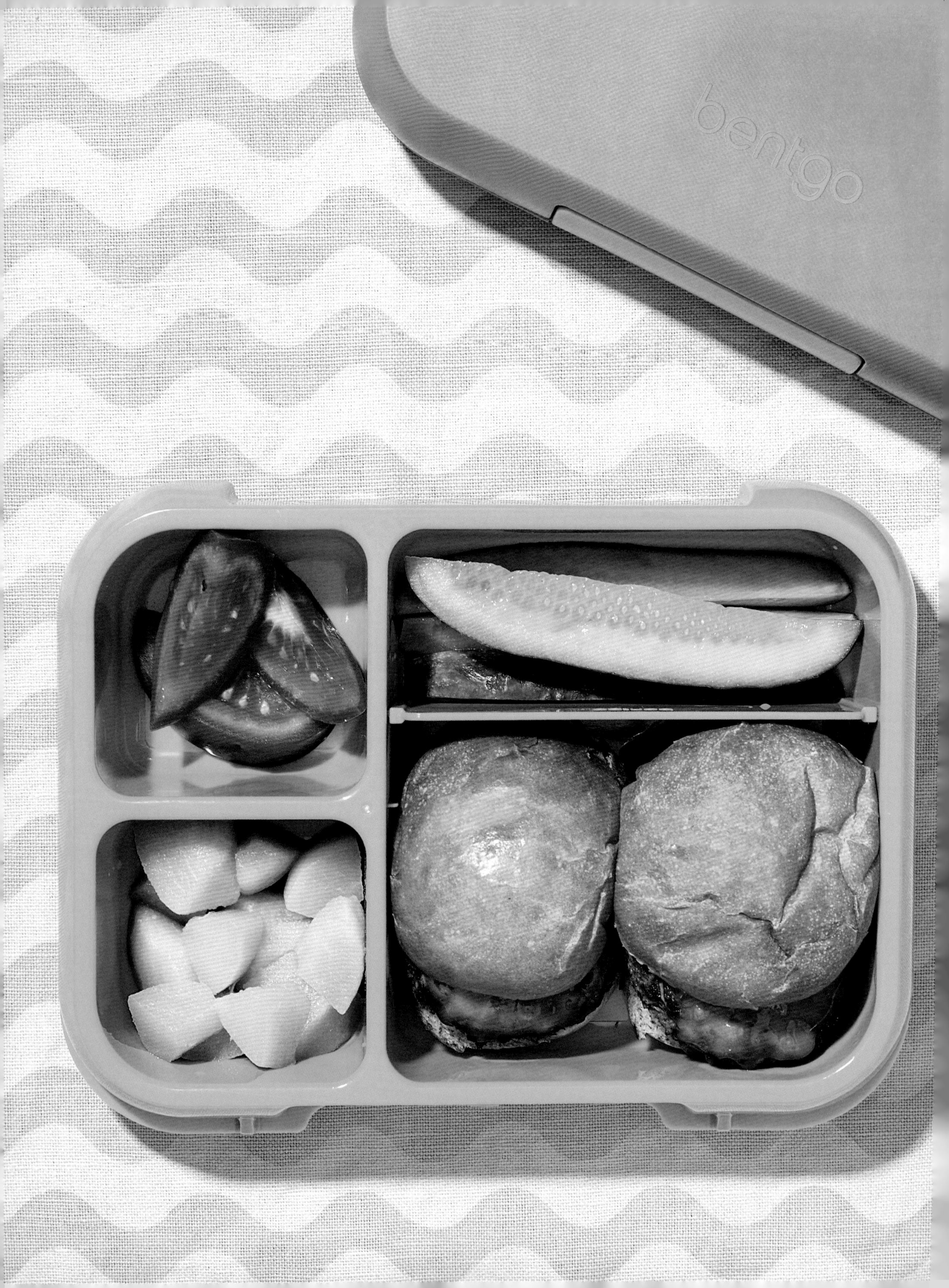
bentgo

Leftover Burger Mini Sliders

If you grill burgers for dinner and make a few extra, save them for your kid's lunch the next day. Megan's girls love this—cold burgers are surprisingly good and can be sent with a slew of toppings and sides.

Leftover cheeseburger patty on mini buns

Diced canned pear

Tomato wedges

Pickle spears

Condiments: ketchup, mayo, mustard
(optional)

PREP TIP

If you can remember to, make smaller patties when you're grilling your burgers—they'll fit better on the mini buns. If all you have are full-size patties, that works too. Just cut them to fit the buns and use the scraps to top a salad or enjoy as a snack.

ALLERGY TIPS

WHEAT: Use gluten-free buns.

DAIRY: Omit cheese or use your favorite dairy-free cheese on the burgers.

TODDLER TIP

If you think your toddler will struggle to pick this up and eat it assembled, take the burgers apart and serve deconstructed or cut them into quarters.

PICKY EATING TIP

This lunch might seem a little unexpected, but cold burgers can actually be really tasty. Let your child add their favorite condiments while you're packing them (or put condiments on the side) so they have some favorite flavors with their sliders.

VEGETARIAN SWAP

Serve a black bean or veggie burger instead of a beef burger.

CONTAINER: Bentgo Pop

Ravioli with Parmesan

This lunch is a reminder that simple can be delicious. It's also an awesome way to use up leftover cooked ravioli when you don't know what to do with it.

Ravioli topped with Parmesan cheese

Orange segments

Blueberries

Cherry tomatoes, quartered lengthwise

Chocolate chunks

PREP TIP Try butternut squash ravioli for a little sweet flavor.

ALLERGY TIPS

WHEAT: Use gluten-free ravioli.

DAIRY: Use dairy-free ravioli and top with dairy-free cheese.

TODDLER TIP This lunch is great for toddlers since all the components are easy to pick up.

PICKY EATING TIP If your child loves fruit but shies away from veggies, know that they're still getting lots of nutrition! Some families choose to pack more fruits because that's what their kid eats, and that's great too. This lunch has two different fruits, a great option if you have a fruit lover in the house.

CONTAINER: Bentgo Kids

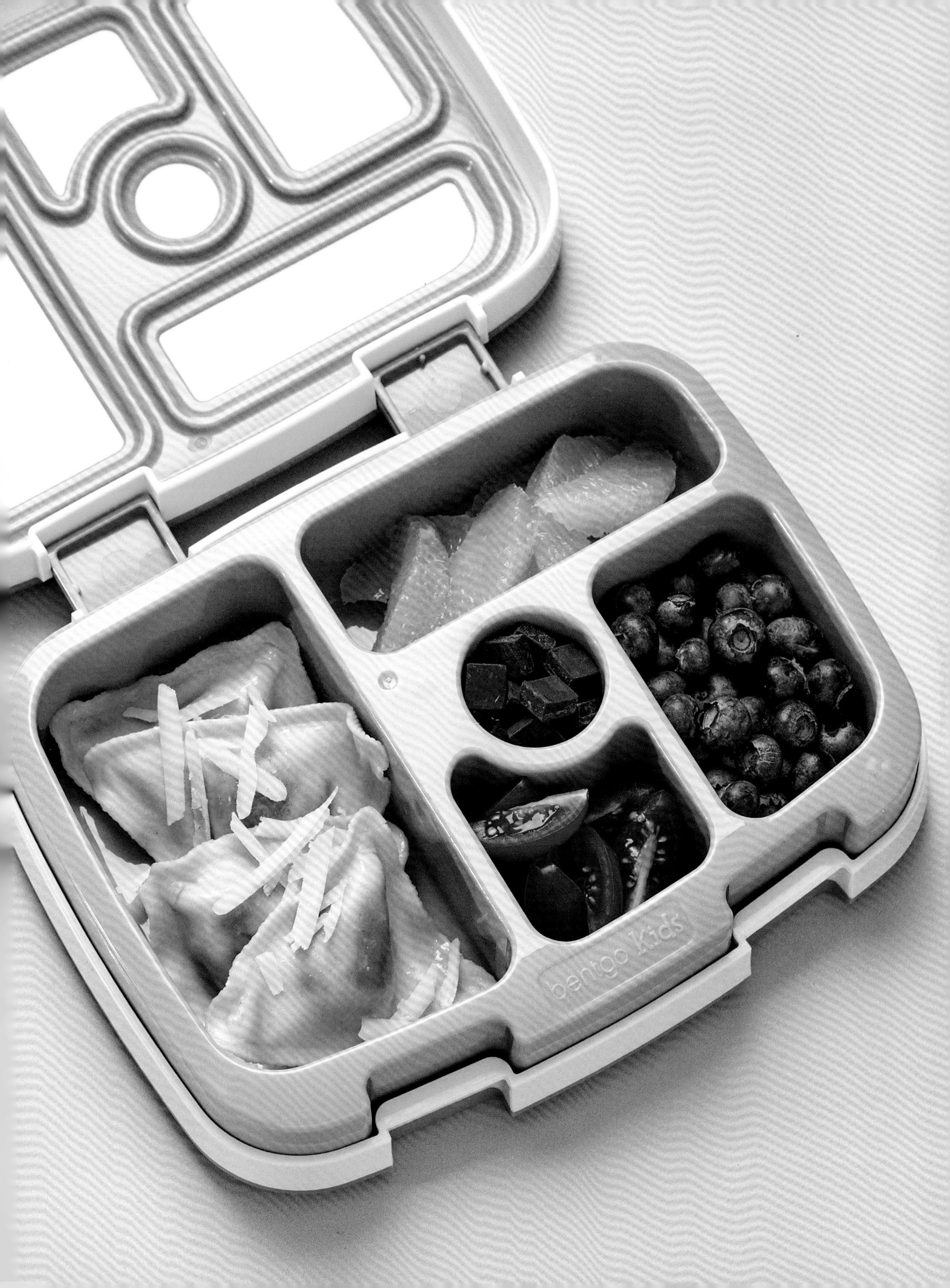
bentgo kids

Chicken Wontons

Another delicious-served-cold food? Wontons! This is a fan favorite in the home of one of our Feeding Littles team members. Oh, and see this little handwritten note? Before you roll your eyes . . . we popped it in here as a reminder that you can add a note if you have no idea what to put in part of their lunch box. Check out page 61 for some cute ideas, or skip on through if that's definitely not your thing!

Chicken wontons
(from frozen)

Edamame

Canned/ jarred mandarin oranges

Pocky sticks
(chocolate-dipped bread sticks)

Soy sauce

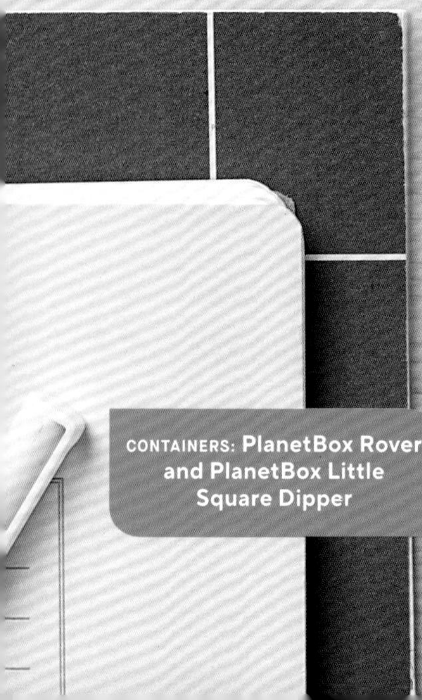

CONTAINERS: PlanetBox Rover and PlanetBox Little Square Dipper

PREP TIP

Heat the wontons per package instructions and then let them cool a bit before placing them in your child's lunch box.

ALLERGY TIPS

WHEAT: Use gluten-free wontons or pot stickers instead of traditional wontons. Use a wheat-free dessert instead of Pocky sticks.

SOY: Soy is tricky when it comes to premade wontons because they almost always contain soy sauce. Sub with chicken and rice topped with coconut aminos, and use hoisin or ponzu sauce instead of soy sauce. Pocky sticks also contain soy, so sub for a soy-free chocolate.

SESAME: Some frozen wontons contain sesame oil and seeds, while others do not. Read the package labels carefully.

TODDLER TIP

This is a fun, bite-size lunch for toddlers. The soy sauce might get a little messy at preschool or day care, so consider omitting it. If you're not ready to send dessert with your toddler, add another serving of fruit or omit dessert entirely.

PICKY EATING TIP

We've mentioned dips as an amazing way to help reluctant eaters try new foods, but what if your child *isn't* into dips? Try a favorite dipper with any dip you offer—for example, offer a dip with pretzels if your child is a pretzel lover. One more Judy technique to try? Play with slime, Play-Doh, and Silly Putty *away* from mealtime. This can help them become more comfortable with dip-like textures in their hands. Tolerating it on their hands leads to tolerating it in their mouth one day! Cool, right?

VEGETARIAN SWAP

Serve vegetable wontons instead of chicken wontons.

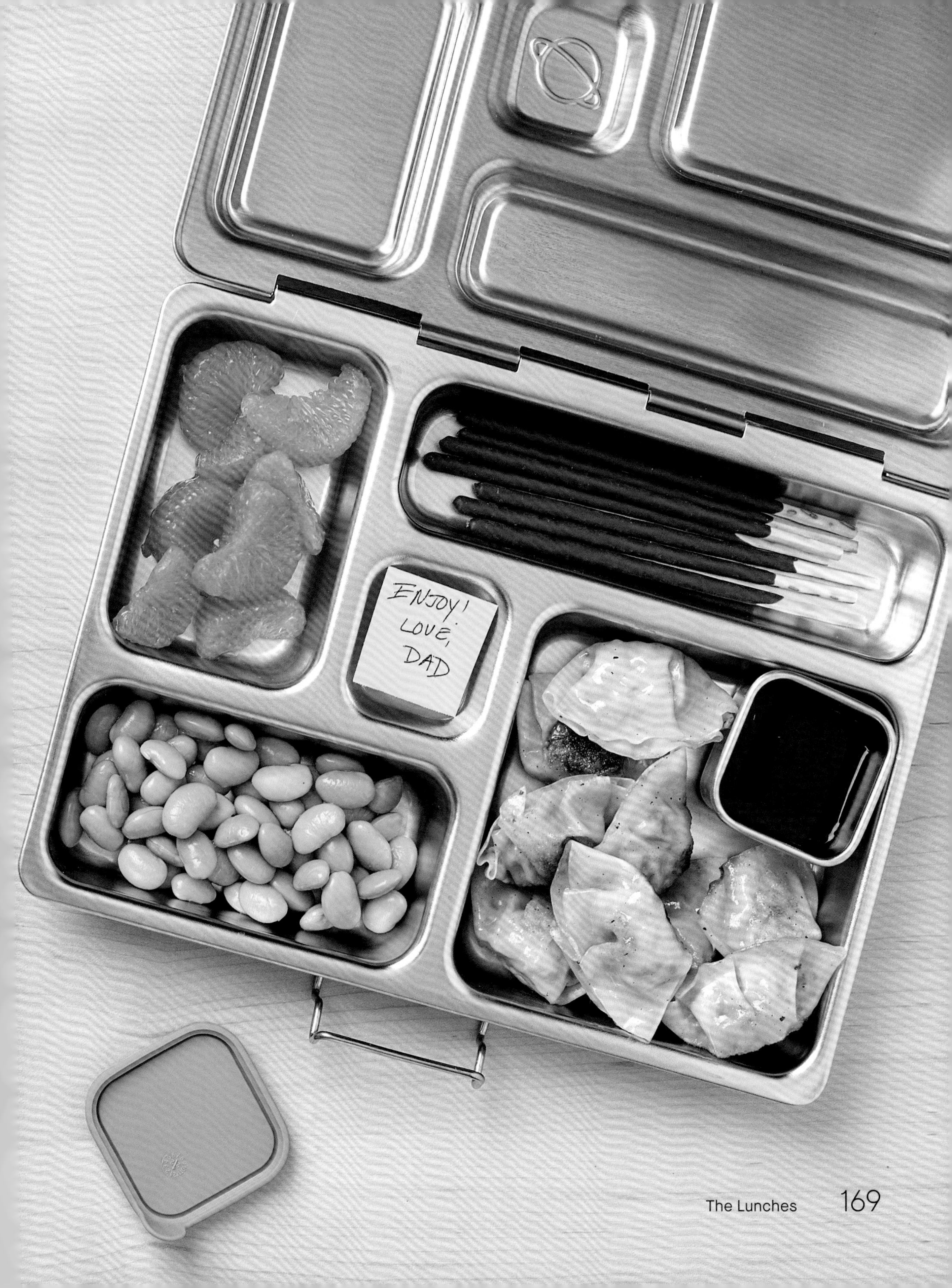
ENJOY!
LOVE,
DAD

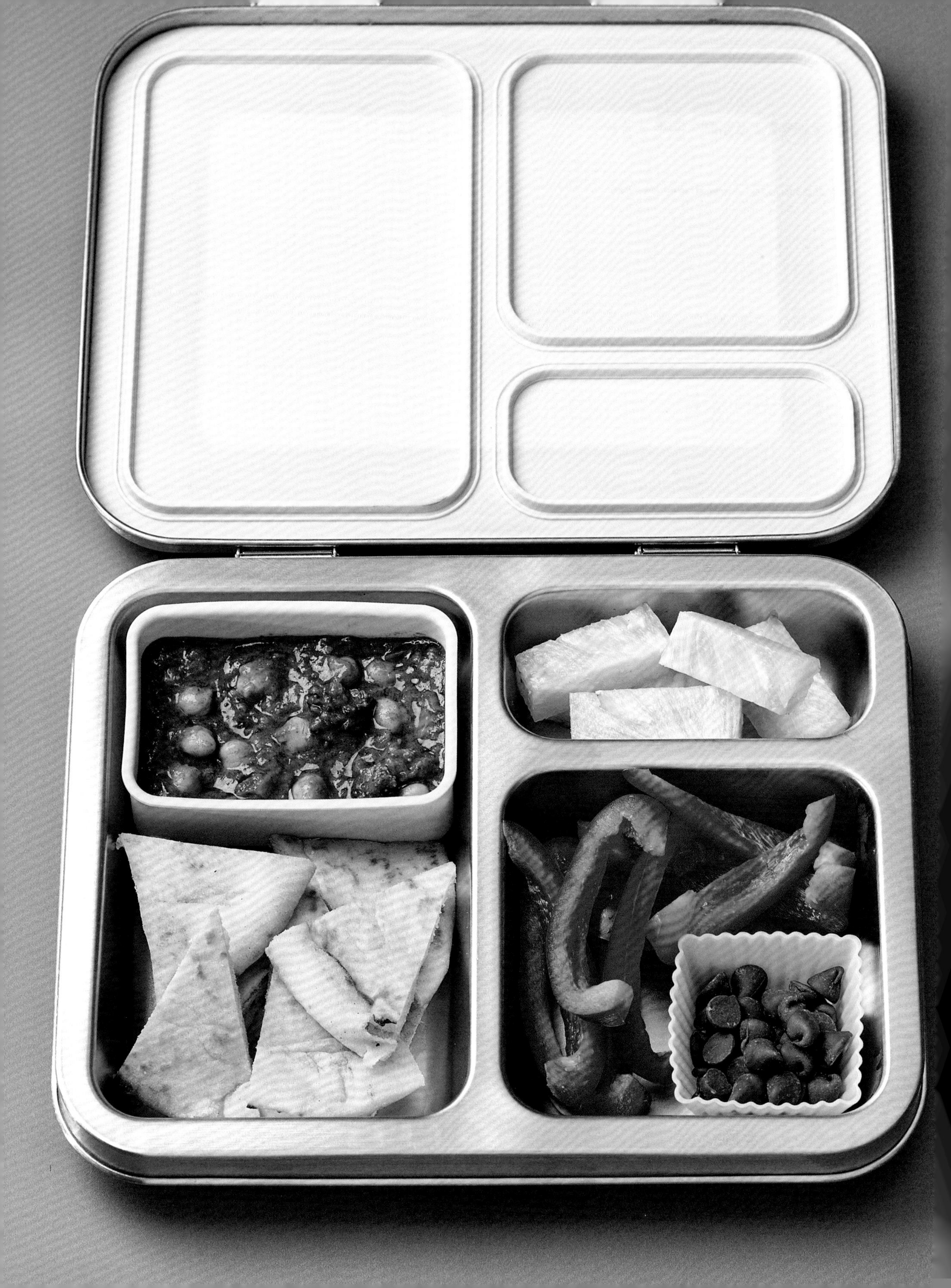

Leftover Vegetable Curry with Naan

Does your family love curry? Make a little extra for dinner and serve leftovers in your child's lunch the next day. This is great served hot or cold, but if you want to enjoy it hot, send it in an insulated container for hot food separately from the cold sides. Alternatively, put it in a container that can be microwaved at school.

Leftover vegetable curry

Naan

Pineapple chunks

Red bell pepper strips

Chocolate chips

ALLERGY TIPS

WHEAT: Use gluten-free naan.

DAIRY: Some premade curry or curry recipes contain dairy, so make sure to check labels and recipes carefully. Use dairy-free chocolate chips instead of milk-containing chocolate chips.

SOY: Some premade curry or curry recipes contain soy, so make sure to check labels and recipes carefully.

TODDLER TIP

We commonly think toddlers don't like spicy food—and don't get us wrong, many of them don't—but some kids really enjoy it. If you have a spice lover, sending some curry with a kick might be a welcome change to their lunch rotation.

PICKY EATING TIP

Your family might eat curry often, or perhaps it's a new food for your child. Because curry is so flavorful, it might be best served at home before sending it to school.

CONTAINER: Bentgo Kids Stainless Steel

Mini Pancake Sammies

Miniature food is always more fun to eat, and these mini pancakes are no exception. You can find them in most grocery store frozen-food sections or make them from scratch at home and send leftovers in your kid's lunch. Add jelly (or your child's favorite topping) for an extra boost of flavor.

Mini pancake sammies
(mini pancakes with jelly in the middle; grape jelly shown here)

Raspberries

Jicama

Tillamook cheese
(in the package, placed in the same compartment as the pancake sammies)

ALLERGY TIPS

WHEAT: Use gluten-free frozen pancakes. If you can't find mini pancakes, try a full-size pancake sandwich.

DAIRY: Send dairy-free or plant-based frozen pancakes, or make them from scratch. This meal is low in protein without the cheese, so send a dairy-free protein food like soy-based yogurt or a sausage patty.

TODDLER TIP

Isn't it amazing how messy kids get when they eat? They'll probably get jelly stripes on the side of their mouth from eating these mini sandwiches, and that's actually a good thing. When kids get messy as they eat, they're teaching their body to tolerate that specific texture or temperature of food. Don't worry—your day-care and preschool teachers are very experienced at helping kids clean up after mealtime!

PICKY EATING TIP

The great thing about mini pancake sammies is that you can put a bunch of different toppings on them to accommodate your child's taste preferences. Jelly, honey, butter, sunflower seed butter, Nutella, cream cheese, granola butter . . . they're all great options! Take it one step further and have your child make the sandwiches themselves. When they're involved in the prep, they're more likely to eat the food.

CONTAINER: **Bentgo Easyboxes 3-Compartment Meal Container (formerly EasyLunchboxes brand)**

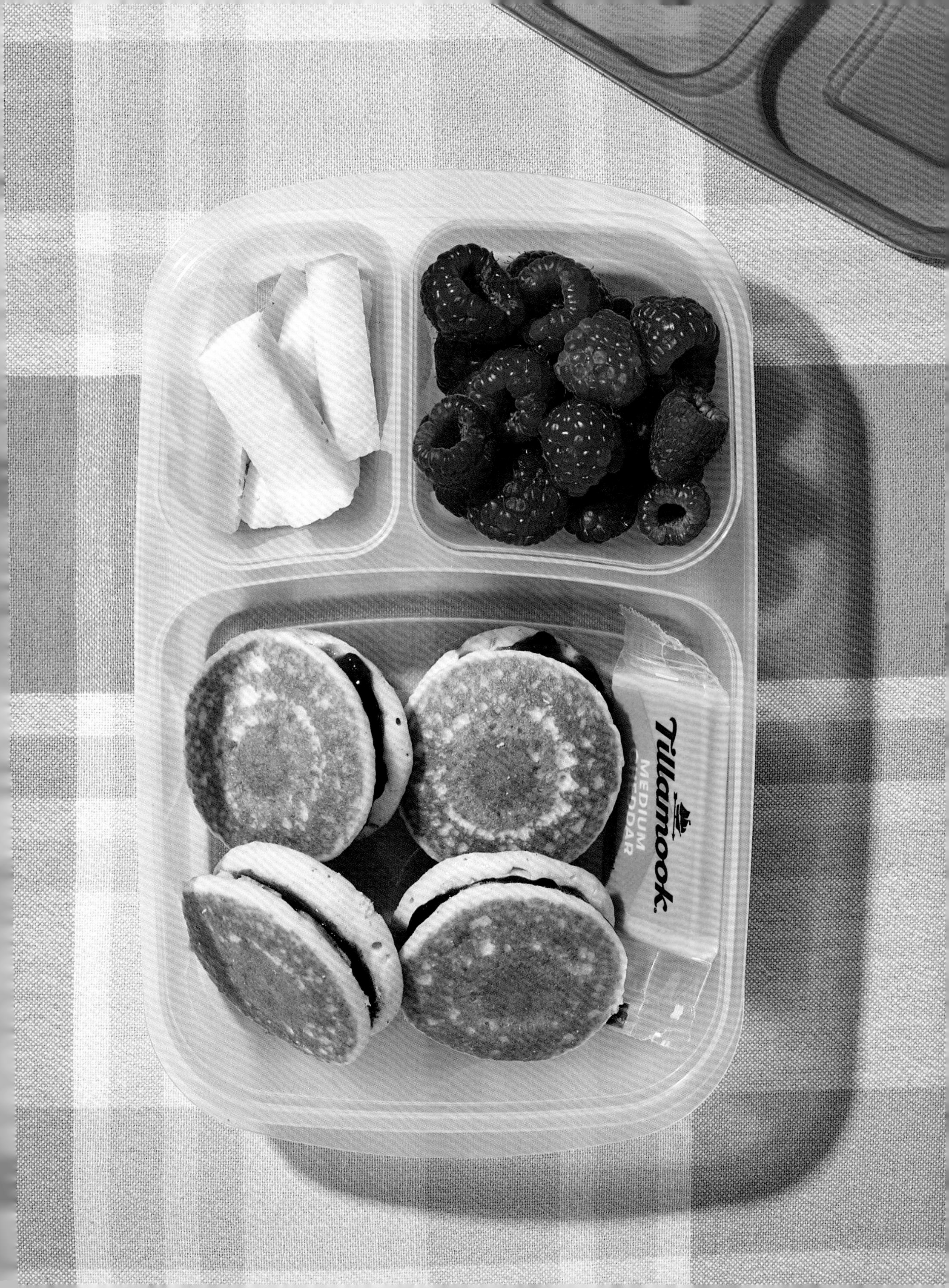
Tillamook
MEDIUM

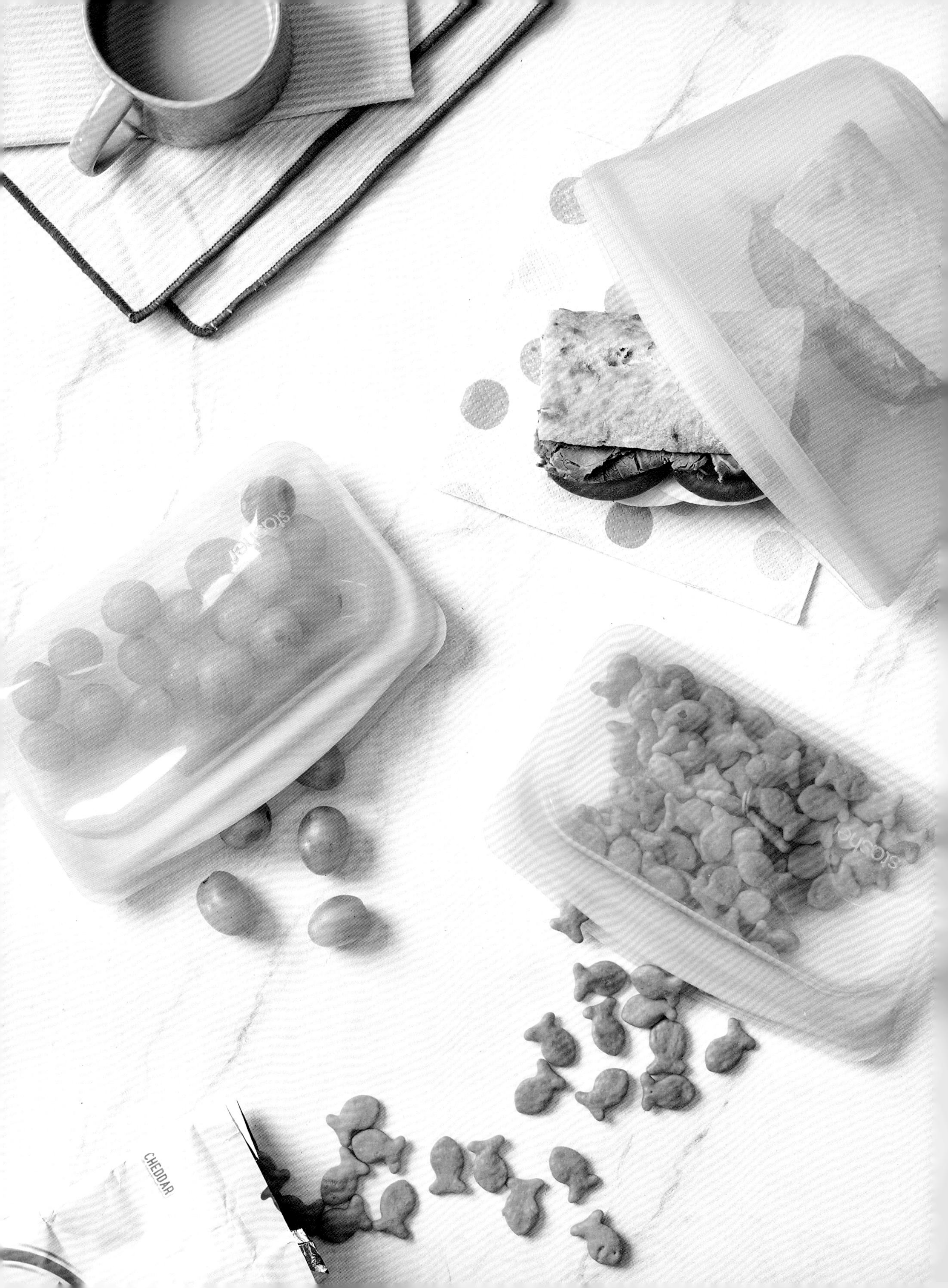

CHEDDAR

Sub Sandwich

Sub sandwiches aren't always a favorite among the younger kid crowd, but as children get older many of them grow to love this hearty lunch option. Customize it with whichever fillings your child enjoys. We use roast beef, tomato, and cheese here, but there are so many options: vegetarian, different deli meats or cheeses, pickles, avocado, green bell peppers, sliced black olives, and so on!

Sub sandwich
on long sub roll with roast beef, tomato, and cheese

Whole green grapes

Goldfish crackers

PREP TIPS

Opt for whole-grain bread whenever possible.

Try to get deli meat without added nitrates/nitrites if available.

ALLERGY TIPS

WHEAT: Use a gluten-free sub roll instead of a wheat-based roll. Send gluten-free crackers or an additional fruit/veggie side instead of Goldfish crackers.

DAIRY: Omit cheese on the sandwich and send a dairy-free cracker (or another side) instead of Goldfish crackers.

TODDLER TIPS

Cut the sub into four pieces so it's easier for your toddler to hold.

Conversely, deconstruct the sub and serve the components separately.

Quarter grapes lengthwise to reduce choking risk.

PICKY EATING TIP

It took Megan's kids years to want to eat sub sandwiches. It finally clicked when they went to a sub shop where they could choose their own toppings. Having some control over the process made it less intimidating for them. Now they request sub sandwiches for lunch!

VEGETARIAN SWAP

Send a meat-free sub or swap plant-based deli meat for roast beef.

CONTAINER: Stasher Bags (Snack and Bowl Sizes)

Muffin Snack Box

Here's another easy lunch that is balanced and filling yet feels like snack time to your child. Use store-bought or homemade muffins. If your child has allergies, check online for homemade muffin recipes that accommodate their needs. There are so many amazing recipes, and you can freeze them for quick lunch options!

Honey wheat pretzel sticks

Zucchini muffin

Strawberry slices

Thinly sliced celery sticks

Small peanut butter cup
(or sunflower seed butter cup)

Greek yogurt with peanut butter or sunflower seed butter mixed in

PREP TIP

Peanut butter or sunflower seed butter mixed into Greek yogurt creates a tasty dip for pretzels and strawberries while adding a boost of protein. If you're serving plain Greek yogurt, you can add a little sweetness with a drizzle of honey (optional).

ALLERGY TIPS

PEANUTS: Use sunflower seed butter instead of peanut butter.

WHEAT: Send gluten-free pretzels and a gluten-free muffin.

DAIRY: Serve dairy-free yogurt. Check muffin ingredients for dairy.

EGG: Send a vegan muffin, since many traditional baked goods contain egg.

TODDLER TIP

Like raw carrots, raw celery is a commonly forgotten choking hazard for kids under four. Steam to soften it or send it very thinly cut to keep it safe for your toddler. For more choking hazard tips, check out page 35.

PICKY EATING TIP

Zucchini muffins are a less intimidating way to get your child comfortable with the zucchini flavor. However, they might not be into it yet. Send whichever muffin flavor works for your kid right now—try banana, blueberry, chocolate chip, poppy seed, lemon, oat, etc.

CONTAINER: Bentgo Kids

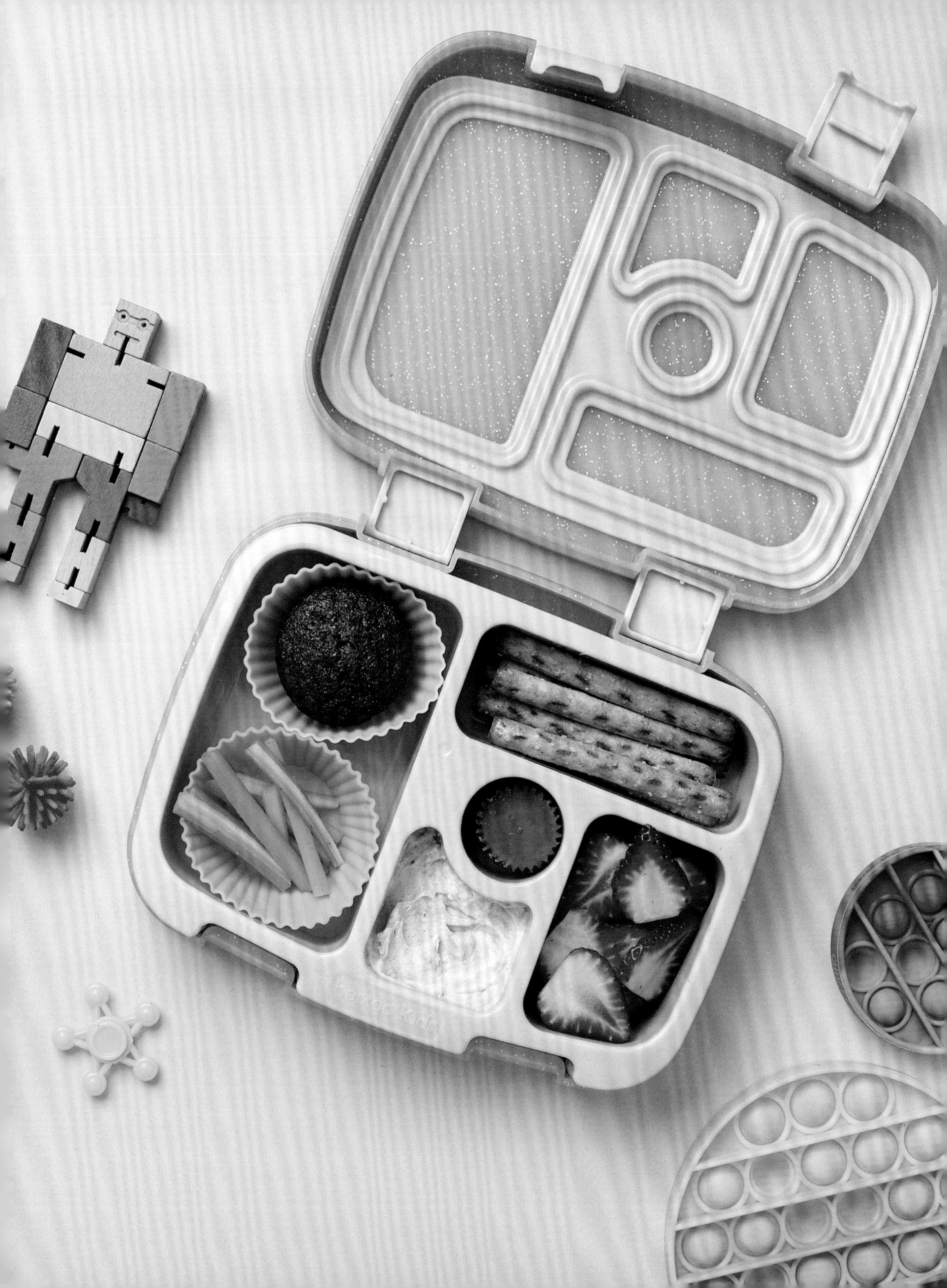

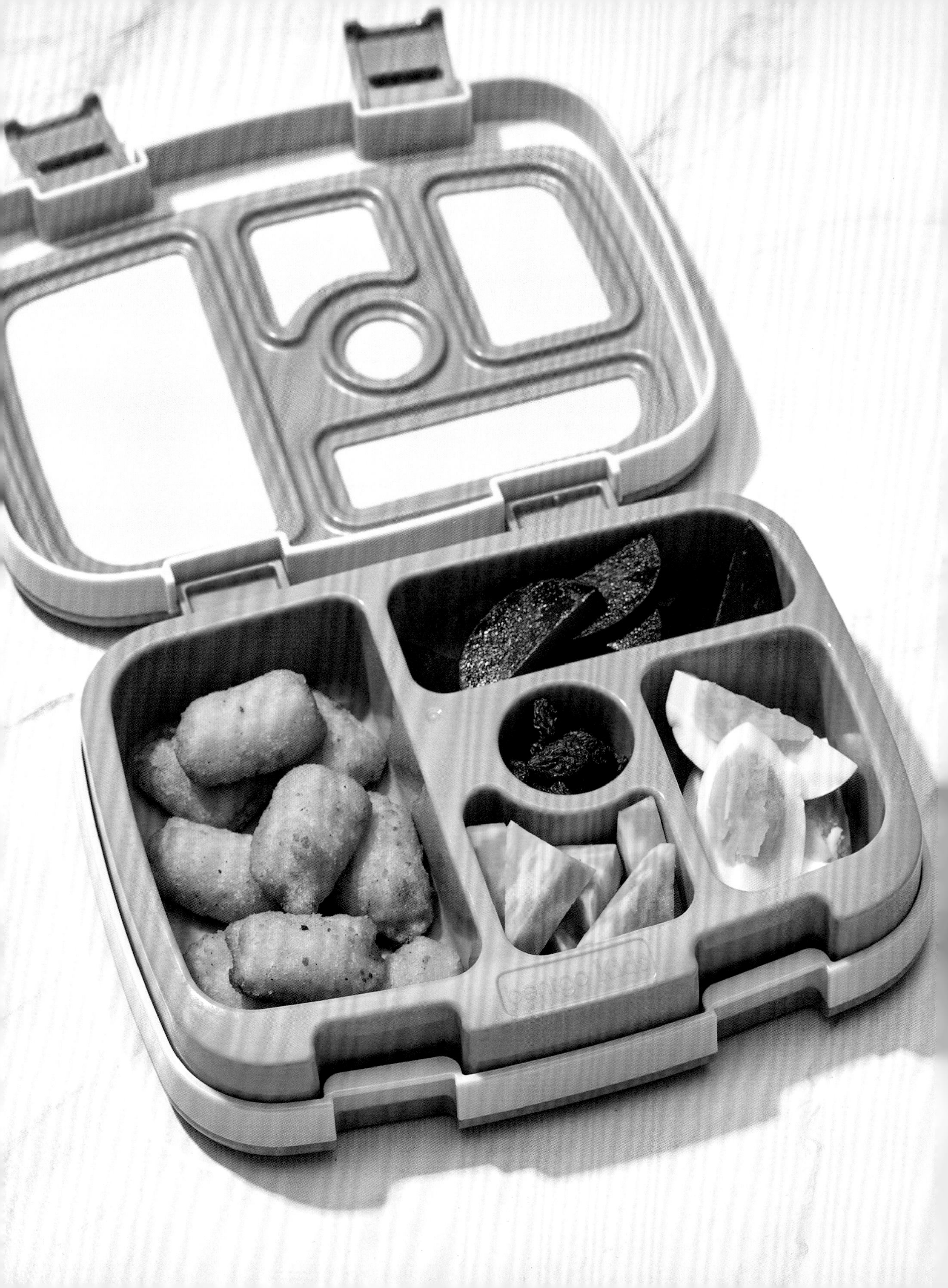
bentgo kids

Veggie Tots

Have veggie tots always been a thing? Judy and Megan didn't know about them when their kids were toddlers, but they're delicious! They can be found in the freezer section of most grocery stores, or you can make some from scratch. (We have an easy recipe in our cookbook *Feeding Littles & Beyond,* but store-bought works just fine here!)

Frozen veggie tots

Hard-boiled egg wedges

Plum slices

Sliced Colby Jack cheese triangles

Raisins

PREP TIP

Cook the veggie tots per package instructions, then let cool before adding them to your child's lunch box. We like popping them in the air fryer at 375°F for about seven minutes—cook time will vary depending on which tots you use.

"I CAN'T EVEN" TIP

Buy premade hard-boiled eggs.

ALLERGY TIPS

WHEAT: Opt for a gluten-free veggie tot (search for "vegetable nuggets").

DAIRY: Send a dairy-free veggie tot, although these might be hard to find.

EGG: Some veggie tots contain egg; check our Allergy Guide QR code (page 42) for specific brand recommendations. Send cheese, cubed chicken, edamame or other beans, or tofu instead of a hard-boiled egg.

SOY: Many veggie tots contain soy, so read labels carefully.

TODDLER TIP

This lunch is full of finger foods that are easy for toddlers to enjoy. Just make sure that the raisins are soft, as some can get difficult to chew if they dry out too much.

PICKY EATING TIP

Veggie tots are a lifesaver for families dealing with picky eating. They help introduce kids to strong vegetable flavors, like broccoli and cauliflower, in a less overwhelming (and more familiar beige-looking) way. Of course, it's still really important for your child to see vegetables in their whole form, but veggie tots can be just one of many ways to enjoy them.

CONTAINER: Bentgo Kids

Deconstructed Chicken and Cheese Sandwich

Sandwiches can be hard for younger kids to eat, and some kids, no matter how young (or old) they are, just don't love them. This unique idea allows you to serve sandwich components in a disassembled way. You might be surprised by how much your child loves eating this, especially if they like all their foods separated.

Cubed whole-grain bread

Cubed Colby Jack cheese

Chopped leftover chicken

Nectarine cubes

Red bell pepper slices

"I CAN'T EVEN" TIP

Instead of using leftover chicken you cooked at home, buy store-made rotisserie chicken.

ALLERGY TIPS

WHEAT: Send gluten-free bread instead of wheat-based bread.

DAIRY: Send a dairy-free cheese instead of Colby Jack cheese, or replace the Colby Jack cheese with another fat source like sliced hard-boiled egg, olives, dairy-free yogurt, or cubed avocado (with lemon juice).

TODDLER TIP

A deconstructed sandwich is a great first step in helping toddlers eat sandwiches. If they do well with this, try an assembled sandwich with flattened bread cut into quarters.

PICKY EATING TIP

Has your child tried nectarines yet? If not, this might be a fun new fruit for their lunch box. Don't be surprised if they don't take to it right away, even if they usually love fruit. Kids need ten to fifteen-plus exposures to new foods to learn to love them.

VEGETARIAN SWAP

Send cubed tofu instead of cubed chicken.

CONTAINER: Bentgo Easyboxes 5-Compartment Meal Container (formerly EasyLunchboxes brand)

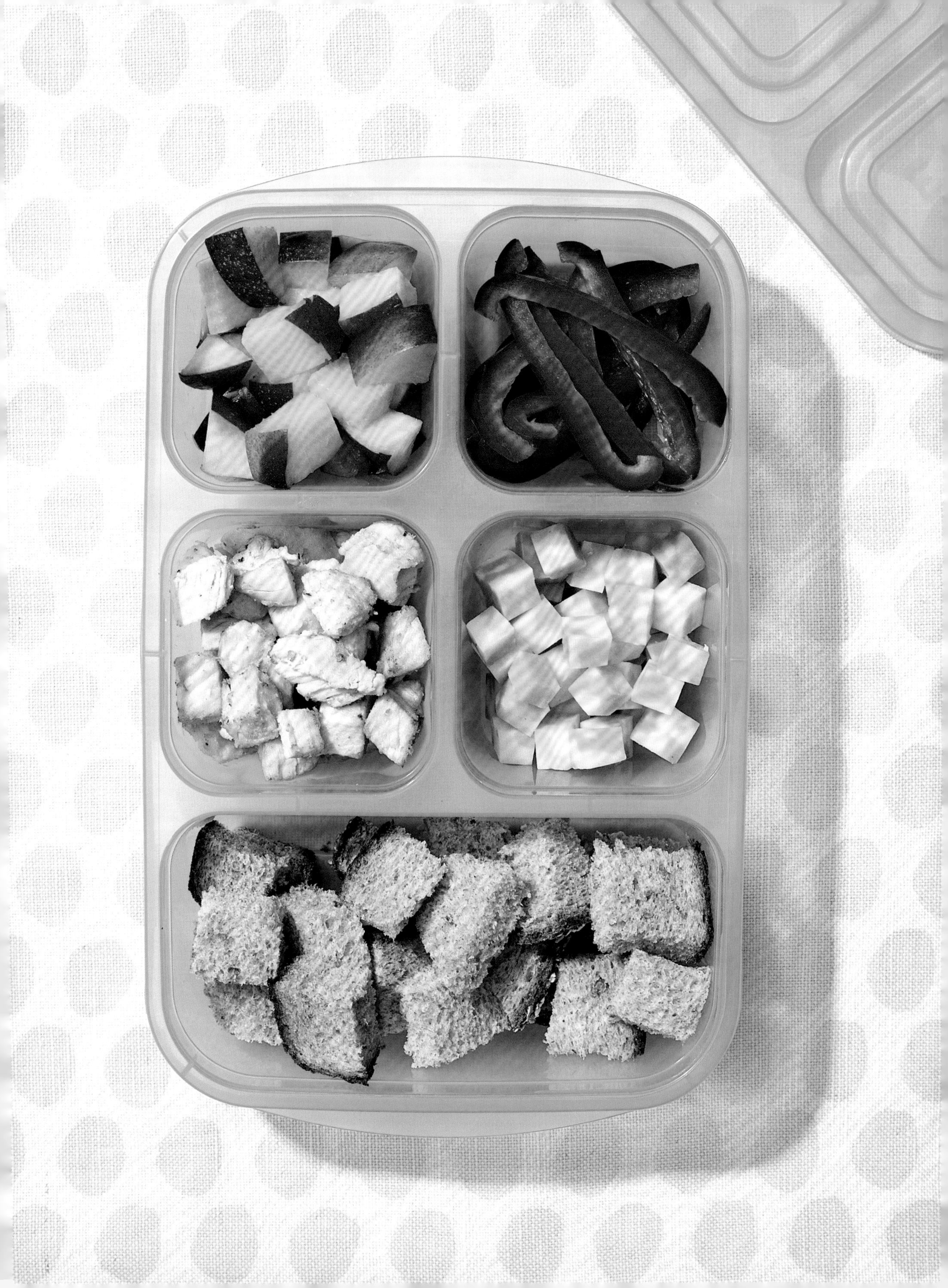

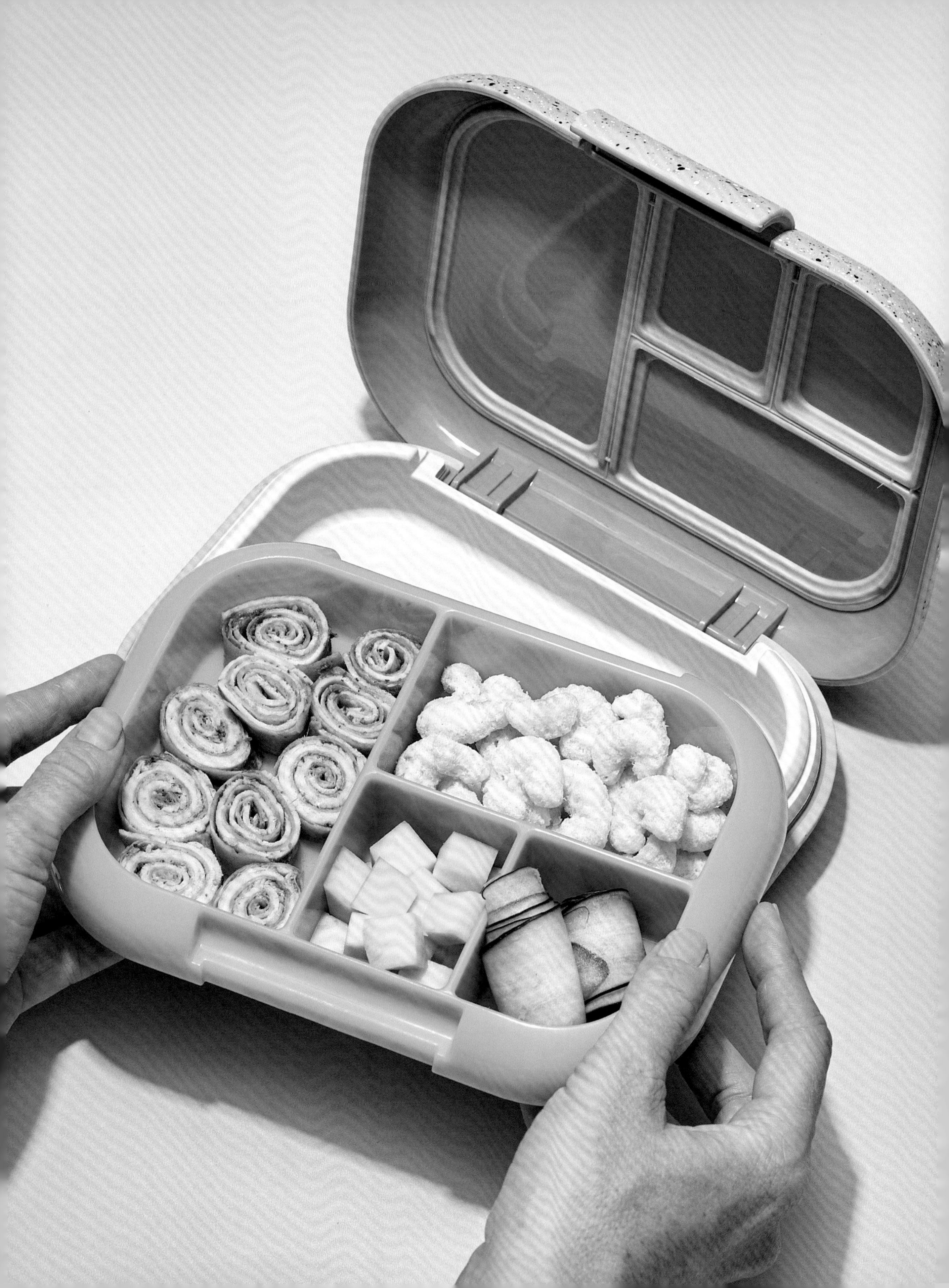

Pesto Turkey Wrap Rounds

If you have a few extra minutes, you can make these pesto turkey rounds. Simply spread pesto on a tortilla, layer it with turkey slices, roll it up, and cut! Your child might not have eaten a turkey pesto sandwich, but they might be totally down with these bite-size rounds. (Yes, kids are unpredictable.)

Pesto turkey wrap on whole-wheat tortilla

Diced mango

Cucumber ribbons
(use a mandoline or veggie peeler)

Puffed cheese snack

PREP TIP These cucumber ribbons look intimidating, but all you do is use a veggie peeler or mandoline to make a long strip of cucumber, then roll it up. It increases your kid's likelihood of eating it, and for you, it's just a bit more difficult than peeling and cutting cucumbers as usual.

ALLERGY TIPS

WHEAT: Use a gluten-free tortilla instead of a whole-wheat tortilla.

DAIRY: Pesto usually contains dairy. Instead, make these with hummus, mustard, or dairy-free cream cheese. Serve dairy-free puffs (like Hippeas or Spudsy brand) instead of a puffed cheese snack. (Note: Hippeas may be made on equipment shared with dairy.)

TREE NUTS: Pesto contains pine nuts, which are classified as a tree nut and are not allowed at tree nut–free schools. Use cream cheese, hummus, or mustard instead.

TODDLER TIP These little rounds are fun for toddlers to eat, but if you think your child will shove them into their mouth without chewing well, consider sending them deconstructed.

If you're worried about your child's chewing skills, cut the cucumbers into sticks instead of ribbons, which can be slippery.

PICKY EATING TIP We don't want you to miss this cucumber ribbon idea. It's such a novel way for kids to enjoy vegetables, and if your kid isn't really into cucumbers yet, give it a try! You can also make ribbons out of carrots and bell peppers.

VEGETARIAN SWAP Use cheese instead of turkey or try plant-based "turkey."

CONTAINER: Bentgo Kids Chill

Leftover Vegetarian Chili

This lunch is a great example of how to send a hot food like chili or soup to school without worrying about keeping the other foods cold. Since the freeze-dried raspberries, chips, and pretzels are shelf-stable, no ice packs are required! Follow your container's instructions for keeping food hot, and know that food with liquid, for example soups and stews, will stay hot much longer than dry foods. Note: You can use any type of chili you have left over.

Leftover vegetarian chili
(served hot)

Freeze-dried raspberries

Fritos chips or other corn chips

White chocolate pretzels

ALLERGY TIPS

Fritos chips are a surprisingly allergy-friendly snack for people who can tolerate corn, as they contain only corn, vegetable oil (corn or canola), and salt.

WHEAT: Send gluten-free white chocolate pretzels instead of traditional white chocolate pretzels.

DAIRY: Try a dairy-free dessert instead of white chocolate pretzels, which usually contain dairy.

TODDLER TIPS

Make sure your child can use a spoon well before sending this lunch to school.

Since chips can be a choking hazard for kids under four, try soft crackers instead.

PICKY EATING TIPS

Chili is extra delicious with corn chips poured in. If your kiddo loves crunchy foods, show them how to do this before school.

You can also send other favorite toppings, like shredded cheese or sour cream.

CONTAINERS: Yumbox Snack and Yumbox Zuppa Insulated Stainless Steel Thermal Food Jar

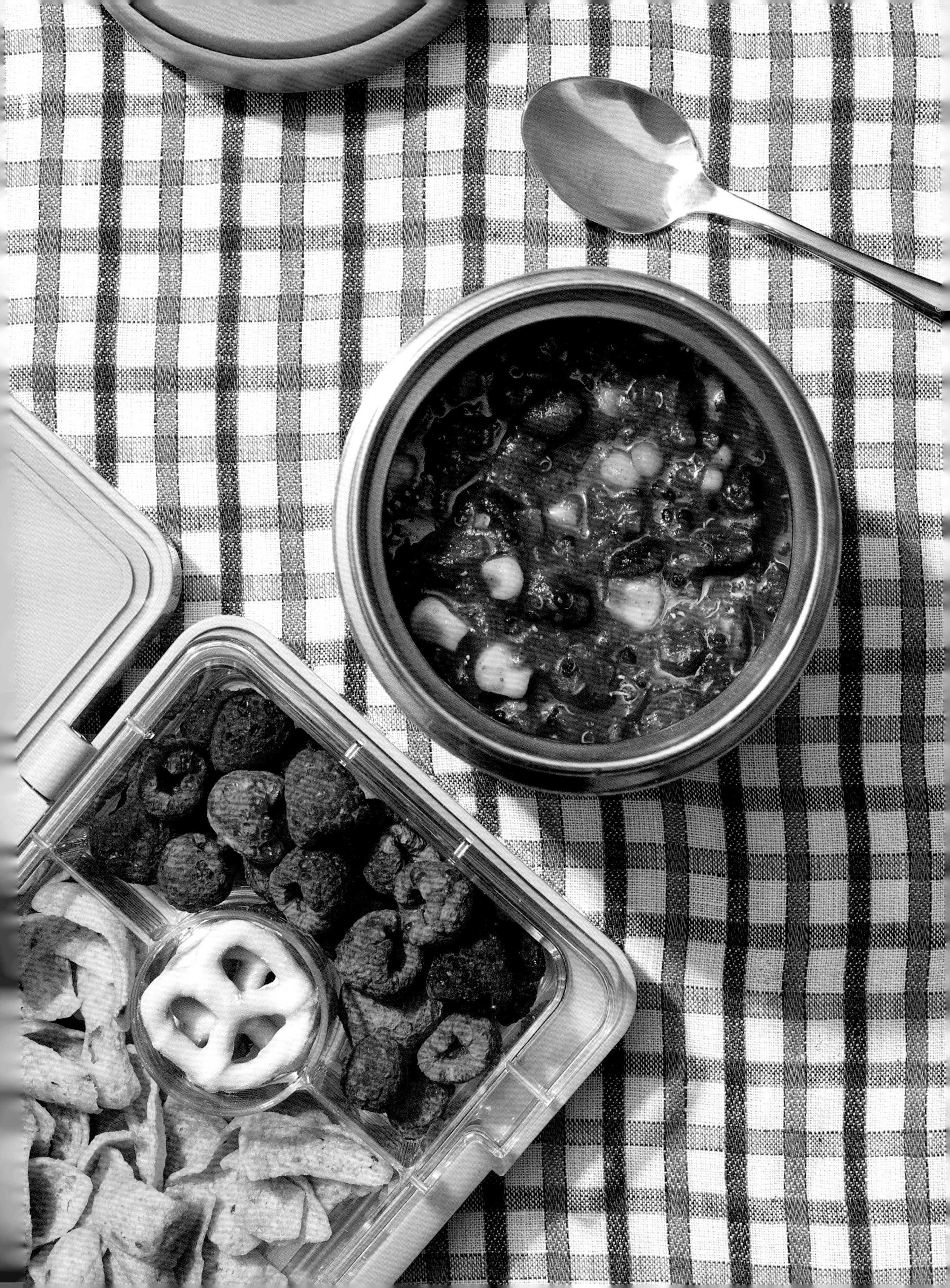

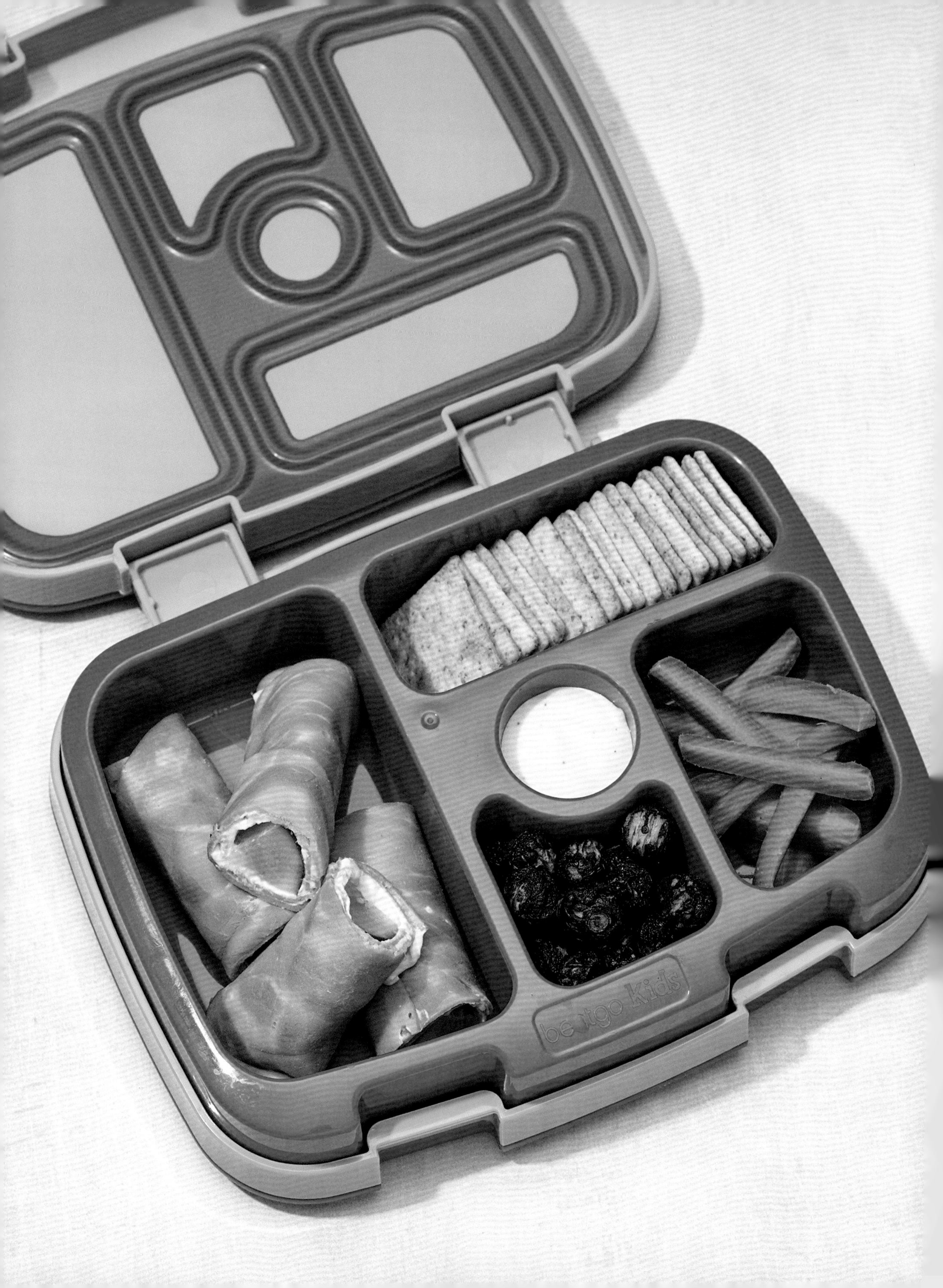
Kids

Ham, Cream Cheese, and Pickle Roll-Up

Judy and Megan both grew up in the Midwest, and ham and cream cheese rolled around a pickle was a *thing* at baby showers. They were typically served cut into bite-size pieces, but this is an easier version of the same salty, delicious snack. If you have a kid who loves pickles, this might just become their dream lunch. (Psst—this was *devoured* by all the adults during the photo shoot for this book!)

Ham and cream cheese roll-ups with pickle inside

Freeze-dried blueberries

Baby carrots,
cut lengthwise

Whole-grain crackers

Ranch dressing

PREP TIP

Spread cream cheese on a piece of deli ham laid on a flat surface. Roll up a dill pickle in the ham and cream cheese, creating a tight wrap around the pickle. Cut it in half. Shown here: two roll-ups, cut into two pieces each. Note: Opt for nitrate/nitrite-free ham whenever possible; turkey also works here.

ALLERGY TIPS

WHEAT: Choose gluten-free crackers instead of wheat-based crackers.

DAIRY: Use dairy-free cream cheese instead of traditional cream cheese, or replace the cream cheese with honey mustard or hummus. Use dairy-free ranch dressing.

EGG: Use egg-free ranch dressing.

SOY: Use soy-free ranch dressing.

TODDLER TIP

Freeze-dried fruits are hugely popular with toddlers. Just make sure that they're not really hard. If you can squish them between your fingers, your toddler can eat them too!

Cut the baby carrots into thin strips to minimize choking risk.

PICKY EATING TIP

Speaking of freeze-dried fruit, don't forget to try different types of fruit when you're dealing with picky eating! Freeze-dried fruits add a beloved crunch factor, but canned, dried, and frozen fruits can also appeal to your reluctant eater. You never know until you try!

VEGETARIAN SWAP

Use plant-based deli meat instead of ham.

CONTAINER: **Bentgo Kids**

Coffee Shop Protein Box

Do your kids love those expensive little protein boxes from your local coffee shop? Yup, ours do too, and this is a homemade option that will save you a few bucks. Take note that this lunch doesn't have a veggie in it because neither do these protein boxes. Even though we have veggies in our Lunch Formula, sometimes we don't serve them!

Cranberry snacking rounds
(or any whole-grain flatbread/round)

Hard-boiled egg slices

White cheddar cheese,
sliced into thicker pieces

Whole red grapes and green apple slices

Chocolate-covered raisins

Sunflower seed butter
(in plastic disposable cup)

PREP TIP

Whole apples are hard to serve cut up because they're likely to brown. Spritz them with lemon juice or cut them and then keep the slices packed tightly together to help prevent browning from oxygen exposure.

"I CAN'T EVEN" TIP

Use individually packed peanut or almond butter to save an extra step. Justin's brand has a few options. (Note: This is only an option if peanuts or tree nuts are allowed in your child's day care or school.)

ALLERGY TIPS

WHEAT: Send a gluten-free flatbread instead of a whole-grain flatbread.

DAIRY: Omit cheese—there are already a lot of protein sources in this lunch. Replace chocolate-covered raisins with dairy-free chocolate chips.

EGG: Use chopped turkey, chopped chicken, or cannellini beans instead of hard-boiled egg slices.

TODDLER TIPS

Apple slices are a choking hazard for toddlers under four unless they're thinly sliced. Consider sending applesauce instead.

Quarter grapes lengthwise to make them less of a choking hazard.

PICKY EATING TIP

Your kid might love spreading sunflower seed butter on their flatbread with a plastic, non-sharp knife or spreader. Prepping food can seem mundane to us adults, but kids love practicing the tasks they see us doing.

CONTAINER: **Bentgo Kids Stainless Steel**

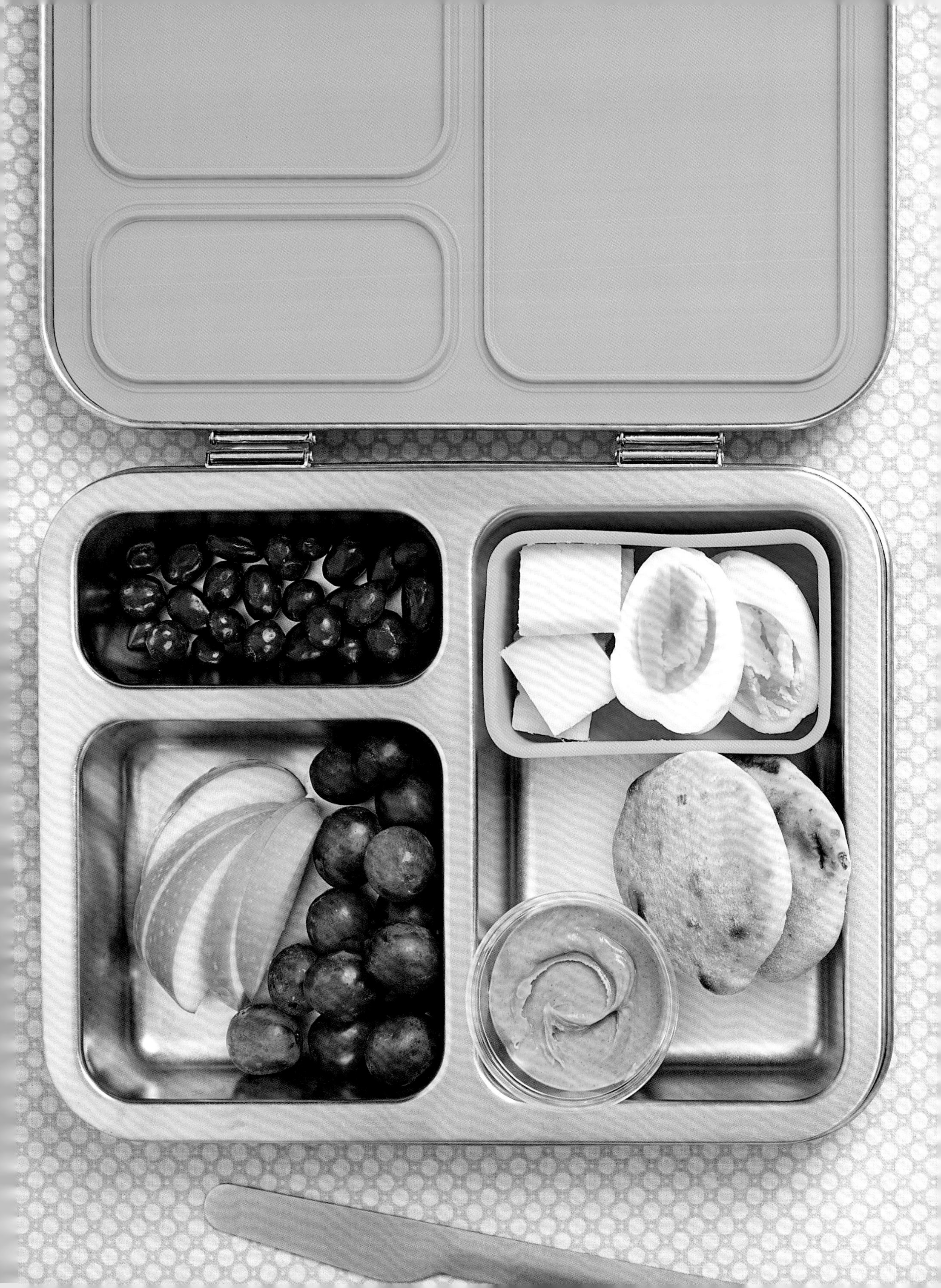

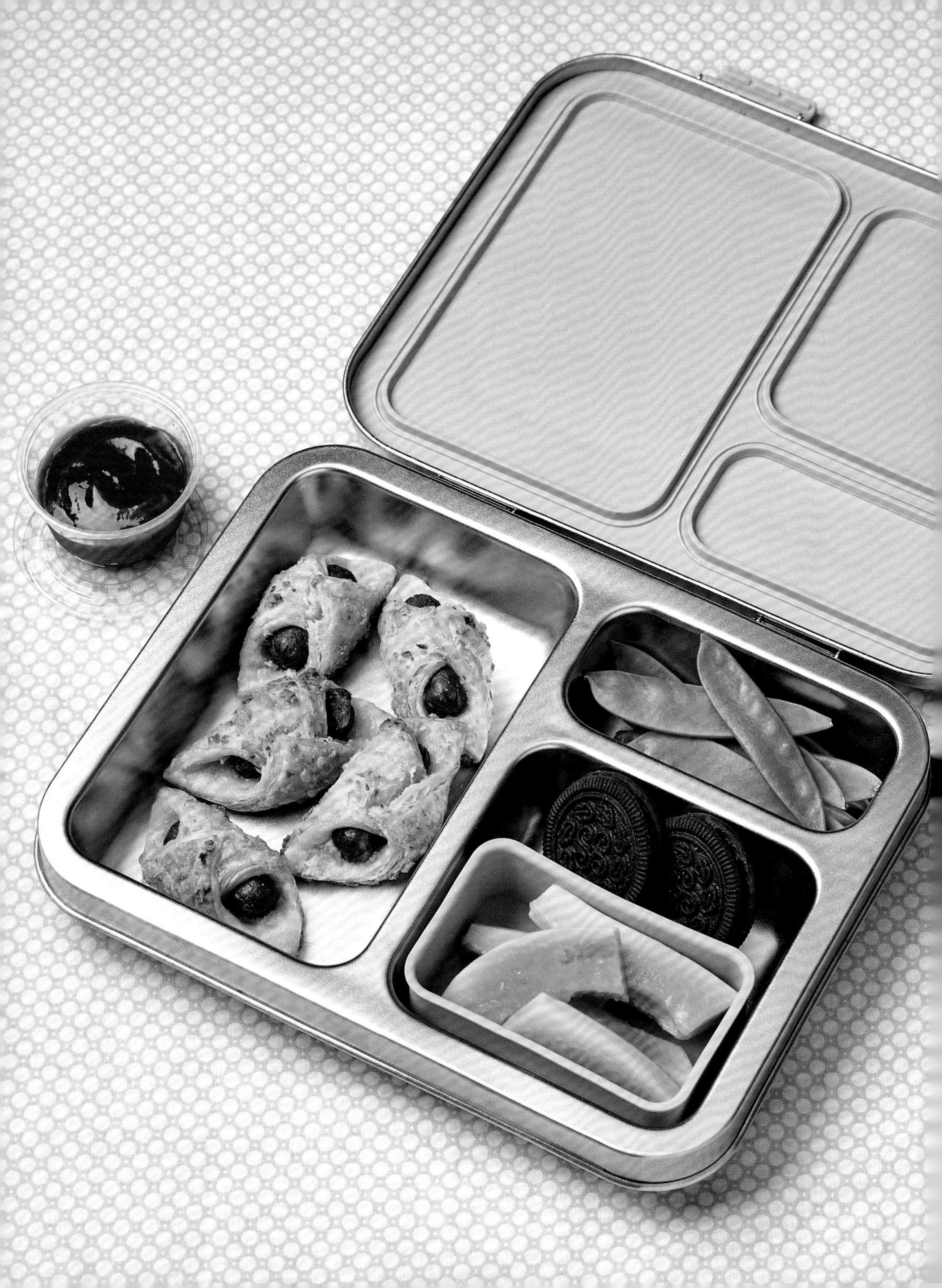

Pigs in a Blanket

Pigs in a blanket are another frozen appetizer that translates well to a lunch box meal. They are a fan favorite of reluctant eaters, so if you're feeling stuck or frustrated, give these a try.

Wrapped hot dog or "pigs in a blanket"
(from frozen)

Sliced papaya

Snap peas

Sandwich cookie

Ketchup
(in a plastic container)

PREP TIP Cook these pigs in a blanket per package instructions, then let cool before adding to your child's lunch box.

ALLERGY TIPS

WHEAT: Try gluten-free pigs in a blanket. Offer gluten-free sandwich cookies instead of traditional ones.

DAIRY: Try Hebrew National Franks in a Blanket.

EGG/SOY: Many pigs in a blanket products contain soy and egg. Serve all-beef hot dogs (diced) with tolerated whole-grain crackers instead.

TODDLER TIP Whole hot dogs are a choking hazard for kids under four. Cut these into small pieces for your young eater.

PICKY EATING TIP We haven't had a lot of chances to serve ketchup in this book, but ketchup is a staple for many particular eaters. It can actually be helpful—pair a less familiar food with their beloved ketchup and they're more likely to try it!

VEGETARIAN SWAP We're not aware of any commercially available vegetarian options, but you can send vegetarian "sausage" or a vegetarian "hot dog" with whole-grain crackers.

CONTAINER: Bentgo Kids Stainless Steel

Chicken Nugget Sliders

If you have a nugget fan at home, they may love trying these easy sliders. Simply save a few nugs from a meal the day before and pop them on Hawaiian rolls with BBQ sauce. Serve with canned green beans, a very underrated, inexpensive veggie; pineapple chunks; and some chocolate.

Chicken nugget sliders on Hawaiian rolls with BBQ sauce

Canned pineapple chunks

Canned green beans

Fun-size candy bar

PREP TIP

Cook your nuggets in the air fryer! Try 375°F for about seven to eight minutes, flipping halfway through. They're deliciously crispy like this. Choose nuggets made with whole grains whenever possible.

ALLERGY TIPS

WHEAT: Use gluten-free BBQ sauce, gluten-free nuggets, and a gluten-free roll.

DAIRY: Swap dairy-free chocolate for standard chocolate.

SOY: Many nuggets and BBQ sauces contain soybean oil, so check labels closely. If you can't find a safe alternative, use a sausage patty or a burger patty.

TODDLER TIP

Squish these sandwiches down a bit to flatten them and make them easier for your toddler to eat.

PICKY EATING TIP

If BBQ sauce is a no-go for your child, try ketchup, honey mustard, mayo, or another preferred sauce. These can also be made without any sauce.

VEGETARIAN SWAP

Use plant-based nuggets instead of chicken nuggets.

CONTAINER: **Bentgo Easyboxes 3-Compartment Meal Container (formerly EasyLunchboxes brand)**

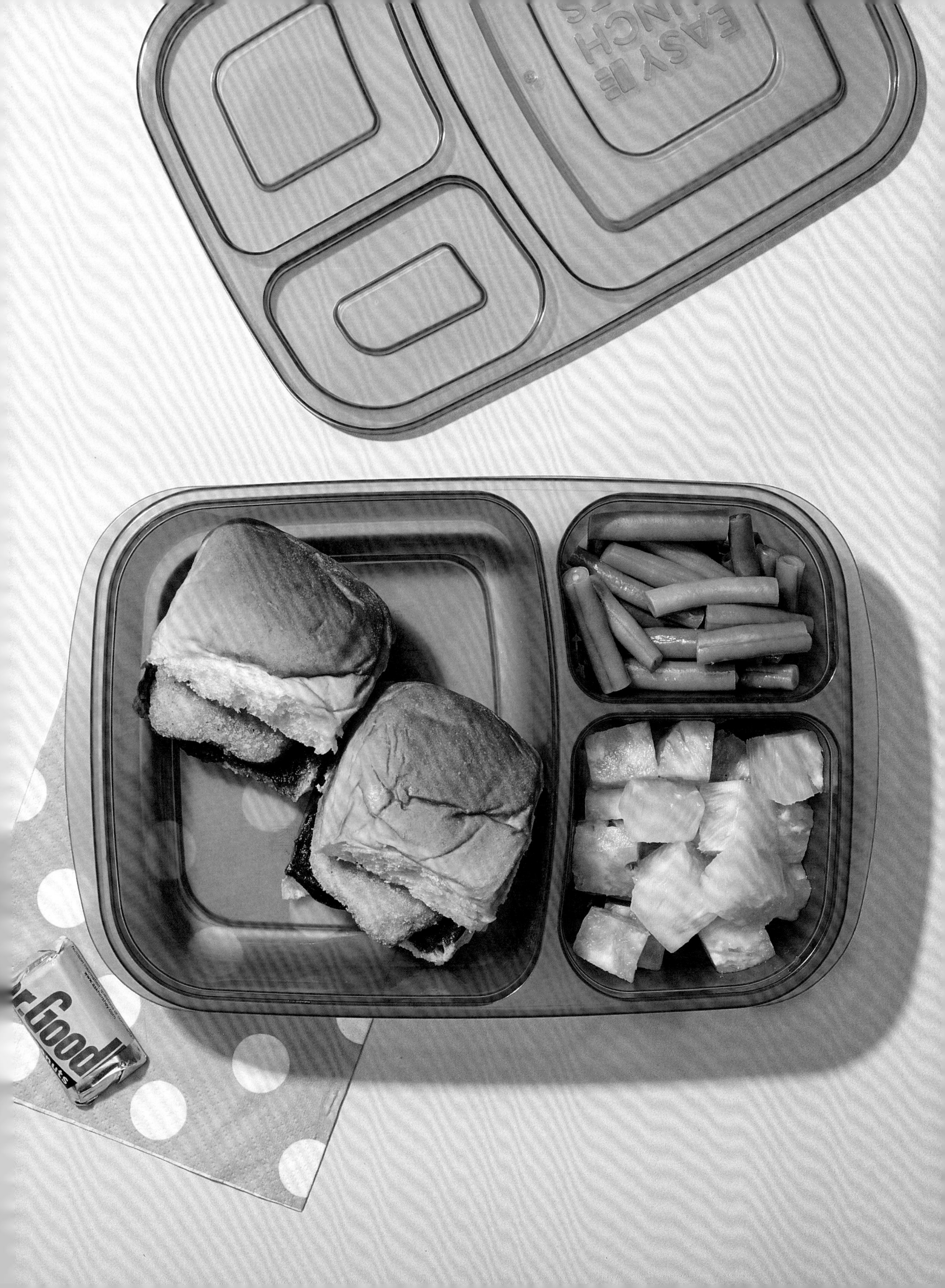

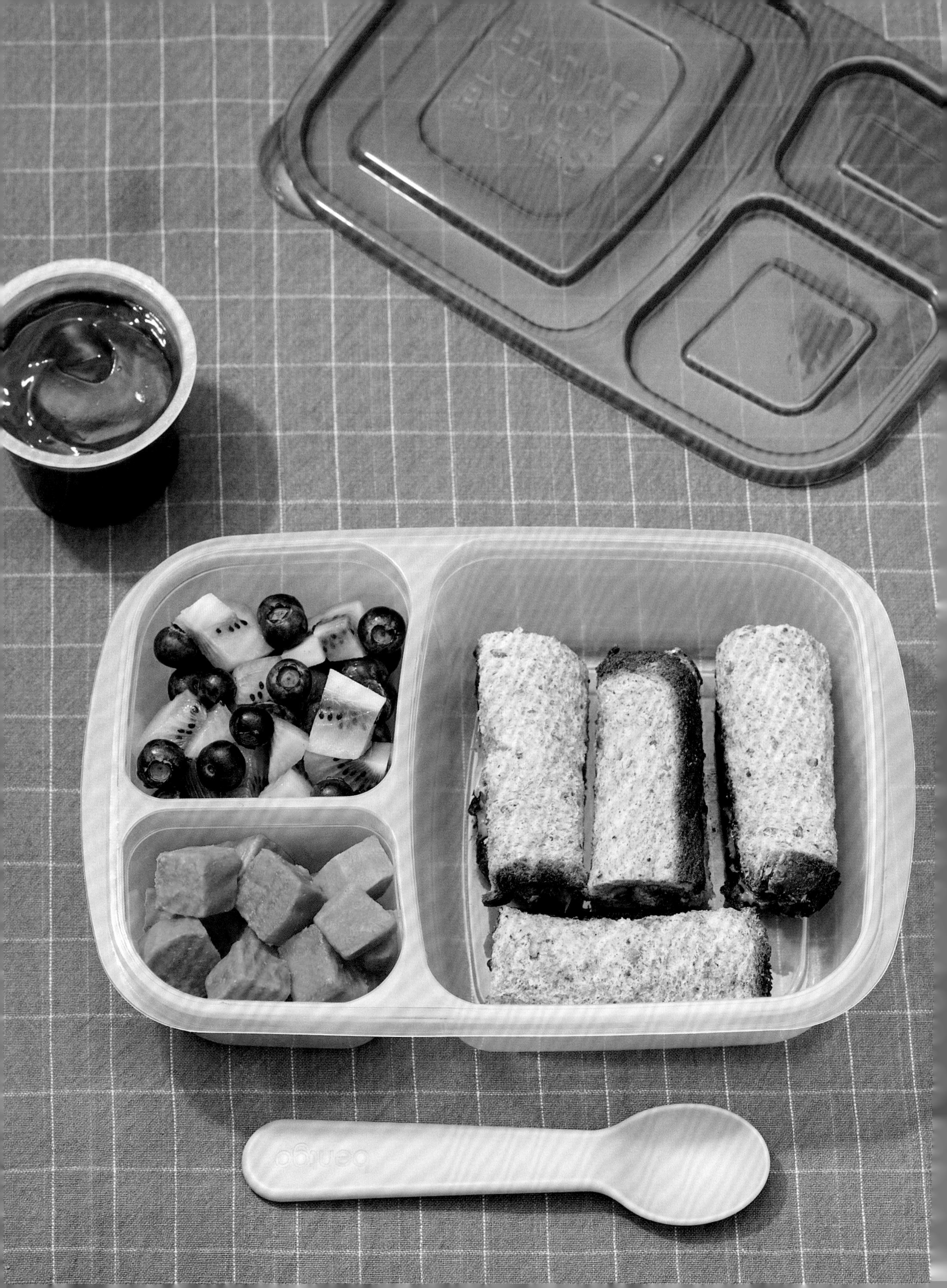

Rolled PB&J

Rolled PB&J is essentially one piece of flattened bread with peanut butter and jelly, all rolled up so it's easy to pick up and eat. Here we show two full pieces of bread, rolled up and cut in half, to make four total pieces. While they're an awesome option for a younger eater, kids of all ages who love PB&J will enjoy this fun twist on their favorite classic.

Rolled PB&J

Roasted sweet potato cubes

Blueberries and kiwi

Chocolate pudding

PREP TIP

Using a rolling pin, roll two pieces of soft whole-wheat bread until flattened. Apply a thin layer of peanut butter and jelly to each piece and roll them up separately. Cut in half to make four pieces.

ALLERGY TIPS

PEANUTS: Instead of peanut butter, use sunflower seed butter, granola butter, soy butter, or cream cheese.

WHEAT: Use gluten-free bread. Note: Some GF breads don't roll or hold their shape. If that's your bread, use a gluten-free tortilla instead. You might have to warm it up slightly before rolling it.

DAIRY: Send dairy-free chocolate pudding or dairy-free chocolate yogurt.

TODDLER TIP

This lunch is a toddler favorite, especially if they enjoy the sweet flavors of sweet potato and fruit. If you're not ready to send them with a dessert, offer cheese or yogurt instead.

PICKY EATING TIP

If cold, cubed sweet potatoes might not go over well, try sweet potato chips (for those four and over). Sweet potato chips and tots help kids get used to the flavor of sweet potatoes, even if they don't like eating them in their whole form yet.

CONTAINER: Bentgo Easyboxes 3-Compartment Meal Container (formerly EasyLunchboxes brand)

Turkey, Cheese, and Veggie Wrap

Wraps are great for packed lunch because they refrigerate well and offer a dense, satisfying mouthfeel on a busy day of play, learning, or work.

Wrap with turkey, cheese, lettuce, tomato, and mayo

Fresh cherries,
pitted, quartered lengthwise

Fresh steamed green beans

Hippeas snacks

PREP TIP

Place a large whole-wheat, white, gluten-free, or grain-free tortilla on a flat surface. Apply mayo, then add turkey, shredded lettuce, shredded cheese, and tomato slices. Roll into a wrap and cut in half.

"I CAN'T EVEN" TIP

A cherry pitter will be your best friend if you have fruit lovers in your house. Many cherry pitters pit multiple cherries at once!

ALLERGY TIPS

WHEAT: Use a gluten-free or grain-free tortilla. To help them roll better, warm them in the microwave for twenty to thirty seconds first.

DAIRY: Sub avocado for cheese or skip the cheese entirely. Try Hippeas or Spudsy instead. (Note: Hippeas may be made on equipment shared with dairy.)

EGG: Use vegan mayo.

TODDLER TIP

A thinner wrap will be easier for your toddler to bite into. If you go easy on the fillings, it will be smaller to wrap up.

PICKY EATING TIP

Add a pinch of salt or another seasoning to the steamed green beans for a little extra flavor. If your child likes "everything but the bagel" seasoning or a special spice, it might help them try these green beans.

CONTAINER: **PackIt Mod Lunch Bento**

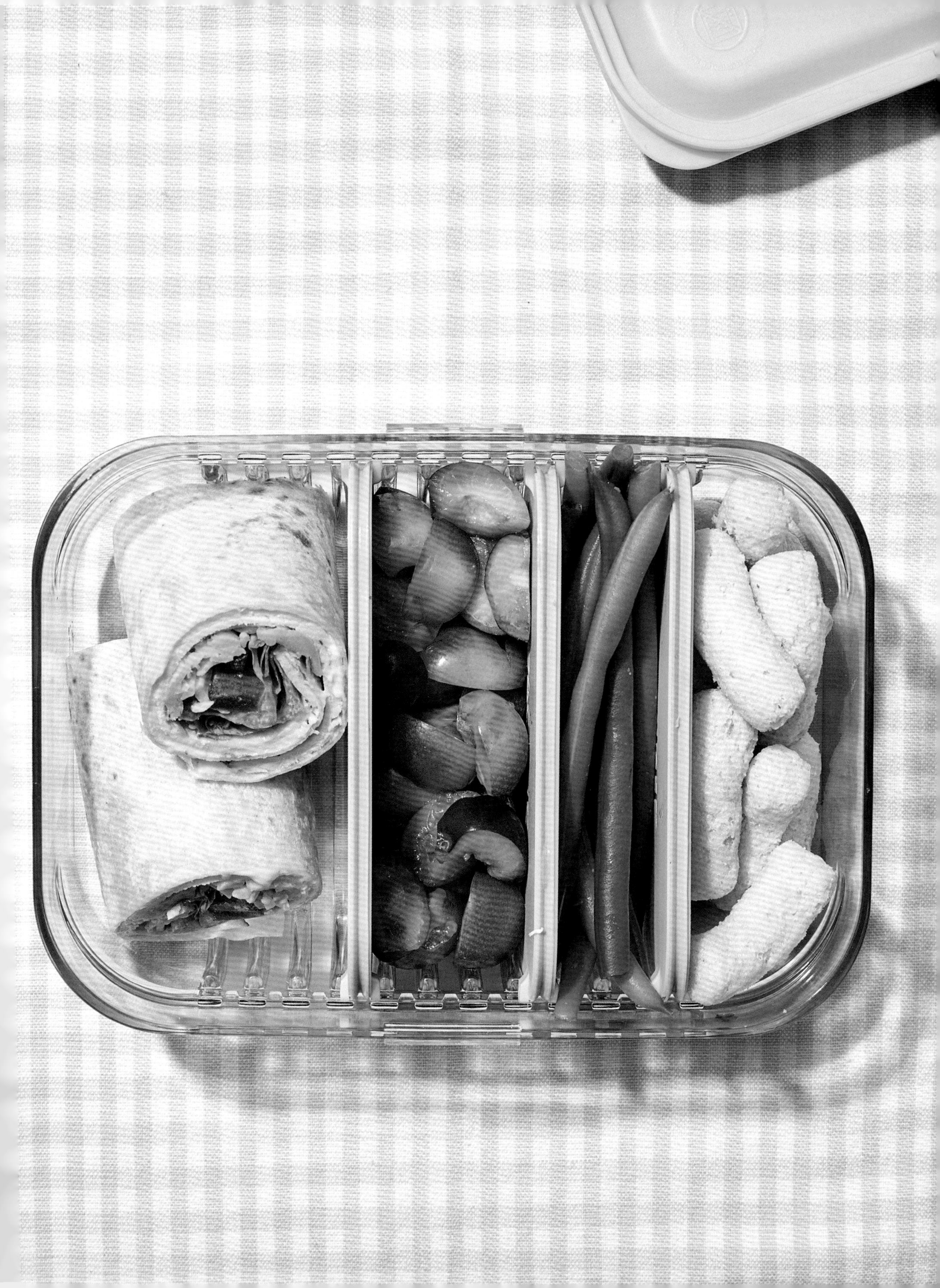

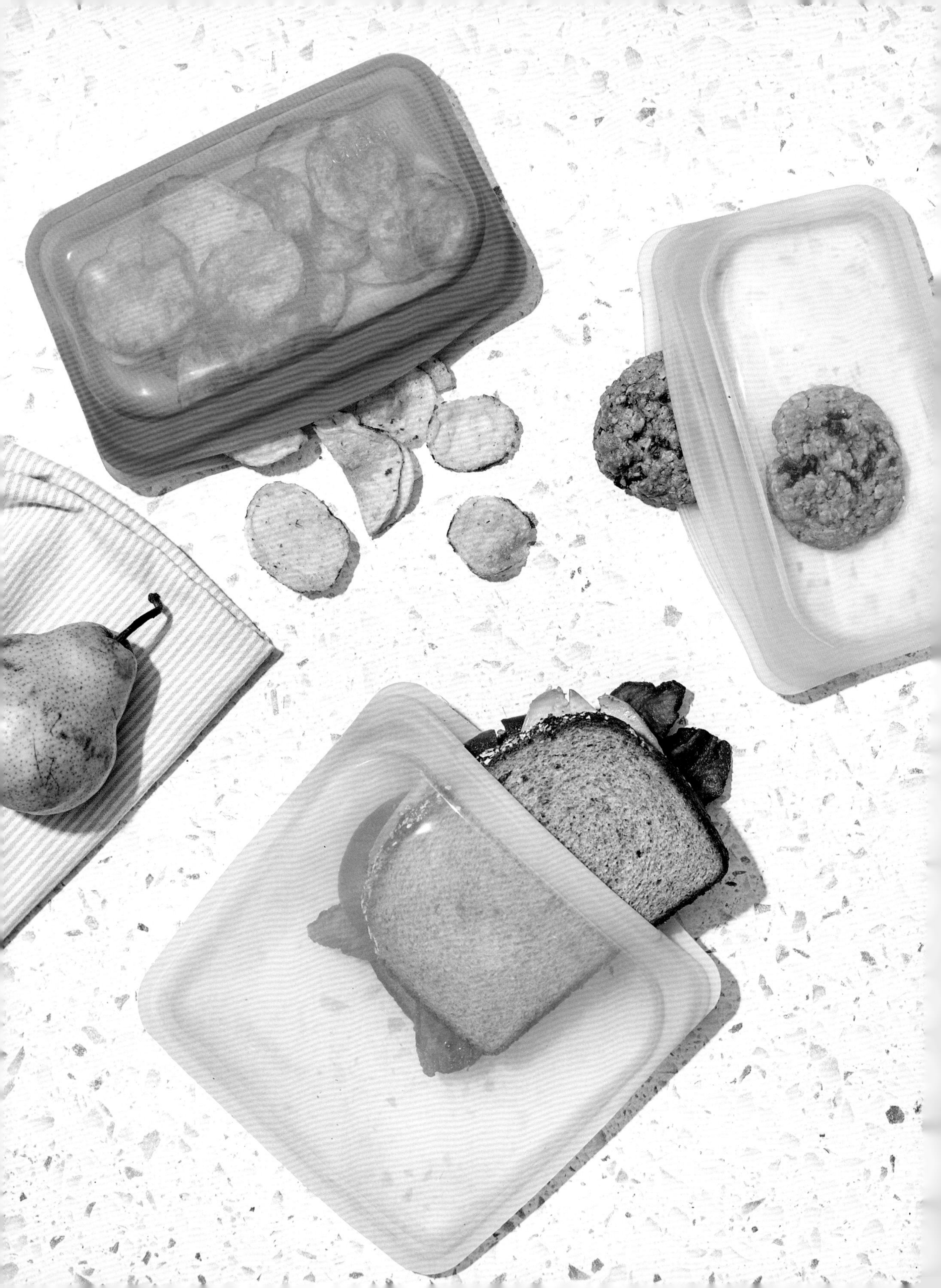

BAT Sandwich

You've heard of BLTs, but BATs are a delicious upgrade! Bacon, avocado, and tomato are amazing on a sandwich, and the avocado is less likely to brown if sandwiched between bread and other ingredients (with minimal exposure to the air). Use leftover bacon to make this a truly "I Can't Even" meal.

Whole-grain bread with leftover cooked bacon, sliced avocado, and sliced tomato

Fresh pear
(wrap in a kitchen towel to protect it)

Potato chips

Oatmeal cookie

PREP TIP Wrap this sandwich in an airtight container, like the one shown here, as soon as you make it to help reduce avocado browning. You can also send individually wrapped guacamole on the side for your kid to put on the sandwich at lunchtime.

ALLERGY TIPS

WHEAT: Use gluten-free bread and a gluten-free cookie.

DAIRY: Send a dairy-free dessert, since some oatmeal cookies contain butter.

TODDLER TIP Cut this sandwich into quarters to help your toddler eat it more effectively, or consider deconstructing it. Send veggie straws instead of chips (a choking hazard for kids under four).

PICKY EATING TIP These little Stasher bags are great for meals at school or snacks on the go. Your reluctant eater might be more willing to eat a new food out of a unique and novel container like this, so try sending them to school one day and see if it helps!

VEGETARIAN SWAP Use cheese or a plant-based "bacon" instead of bacon.

CONTAINER: **Stasher Bags (Snack and Sandwich Sizes)**

String Cheese Pizza Roll-Up

You might notice that we have a bunch of different pizza-like options in this book, and that's because it's a quintessential kid (and adult) favorite. This idea takes it up a notch with a string cheese roll-up. It's a really fun and easy way to send the flavors of pizza as a wrap.

String cheese rolled with marinara or pizza sauce and pepperoni in a Mediterranean flatbread

Blueberries

Thinly sliced rainbow baby carrots

Mini marshmallows

Ranch dressing

PREP TIP

Lay flatbread on a flat surface and cover it with marinara or pizza sauce. Lay down a few pieces of pepperoni, then add a string cheese stick. Roll it up, then cut it in half. If needed, use a non-sharp toothpick to keep the wrap in place.

ALLERGY TIPS

WHEAT: Use a gluten-free flatbread or tortilla instead of Mediterranean flatbread.

DAIRY: Use dairy-free string cheese of your choice instead of mozzarella string cheese. Use dairy-free ranch dressing.

EGG: Use egg-free ranch.

SOY: Use soy-free ranch.

TODDLER TIPS

Cut this into smaller, bite-size pieces if your toddler struggles to "bite and pull" from a sandwich or wrap.

Since marshmallows are a choking hazard for kids under four, omit them or replace them with another dessert or fruit.

PICKY EATING TIP

These wraps are fully customizable. If your reluctant eater doesn't like pepperoni (yet), omit it or serve it on the side.

VEGE-TARIAN SWAPS

Omit pepperoni or used plant-based pepperoni.

Use vegan marshmallows to avoid gelatin in most commercially available marshmallows.

CONTAINER: **Bentgo Kids**

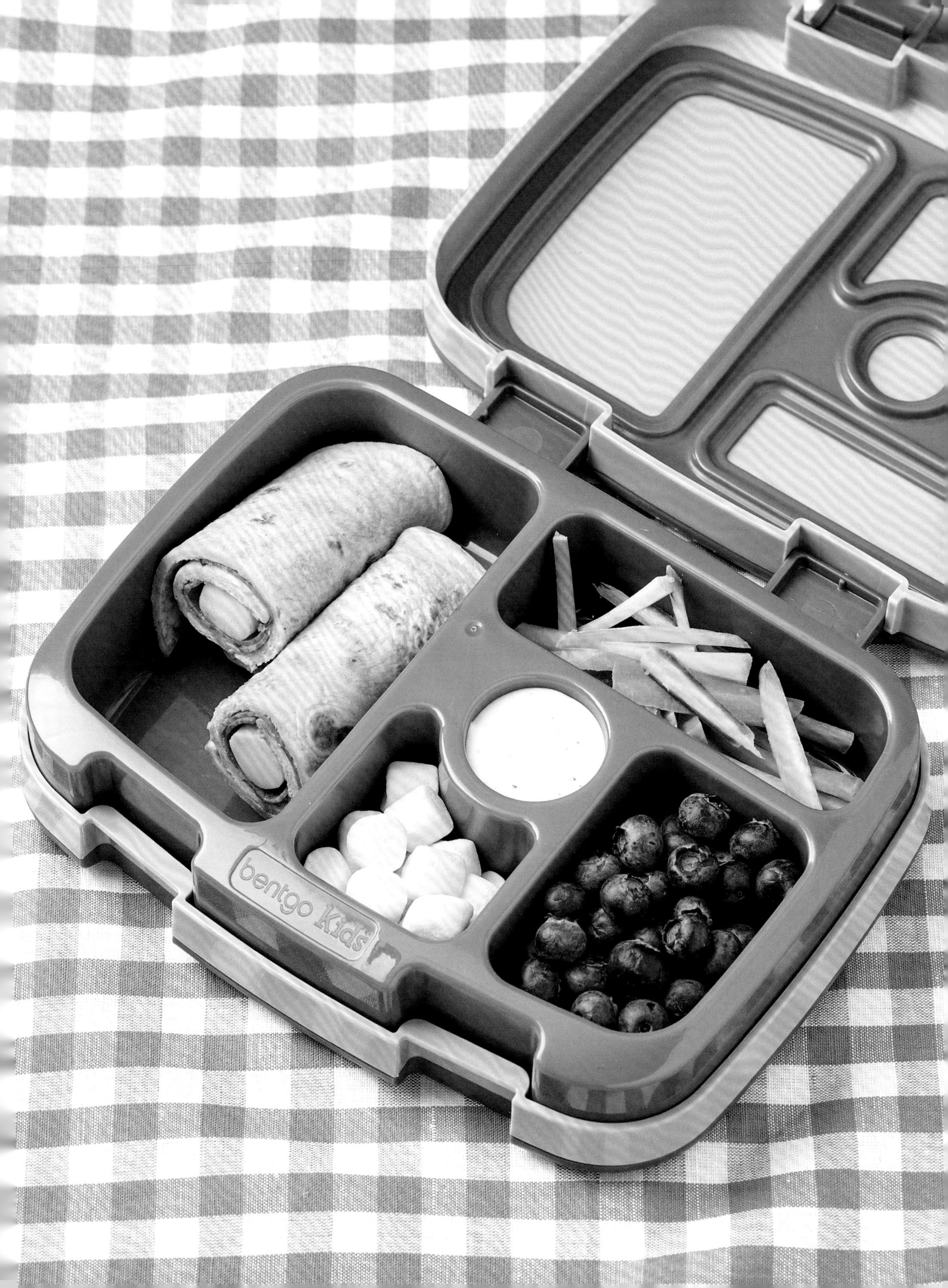
bentgo Kids

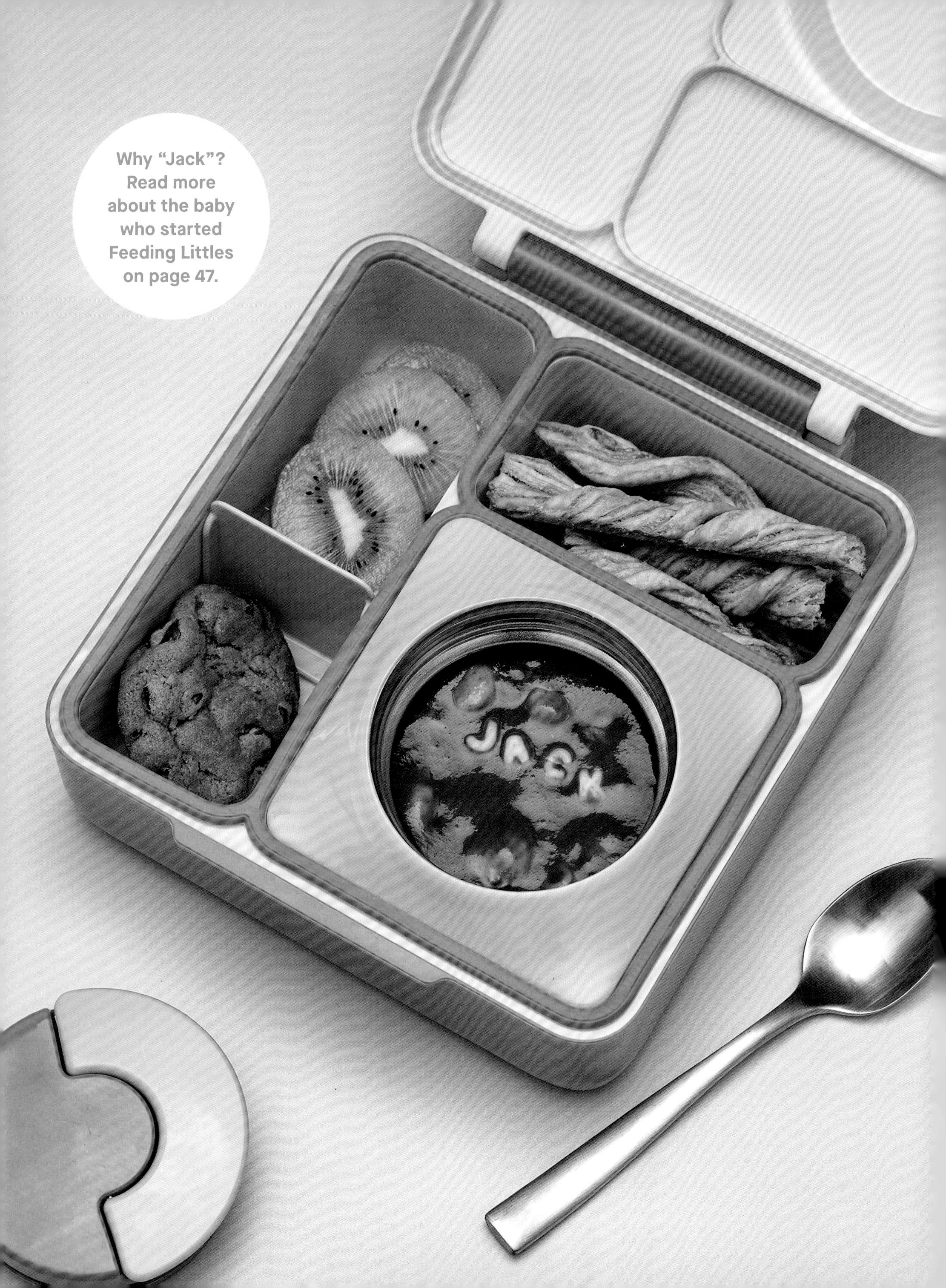

Why "Jack"? Read more about the baby who started Feeding Littles on page 47.

Alphabet Soup

Who doesn't love alphabet soup? This is another hot food option that is comforting on a cold day. If you're eating this as an adult and are not into alphabet soup, try minestrone, clam chowder, potato leek, or another favorite flavor.

Alphabet soup

Kiwi rounds

Cheese twists

Chocolate chip cookie

PREP TIP Follow your insulated container's instructions for sending hot food like soup. Don't forget to send a spoon!

ALLERGY TIPS

WHEAT: Use a gluten-free soup and send cheese snacks made without grains (Whisps, Moon Cheese). Send a gluten-free cookie or another dessert.

DAIRY: The cheese twists are a main source of protein for this meal, especially if your soup is low in protein. Try another non-dairy source of protein like cubed chicken, edamame, or salted kidney beans. Use a dairy-free cookie.

TODDLER TIP This might be a good lunch to wait on if your toddler still struggles with spoon skills. Consider serving it at home first.

PICKY EATING TIP Your child might love the novelty of these letters and might even try to find their name in the soup. Just a small amount of novelty can go a long way.

VEGETARIAN SWAP Some alphabet soup contains meatballs, so choose a brand that is vegetarian.

CONTAINER: OmieLife OmieBox

Broccoli Cheese Soup

Broccoli cheese soup might be the first way your child enjoys eating broccoli. Cheese helps cut the sometimes bitter taste of broccoli, and this soup is a warm and filling option you might have never thought to send to school.

Broccoli cheese soup

Strawberries

Whole-grain baguette strips

Oat bites

PREP TIPS

To prep the bread, simply cut the whole-grain baguette into long strips or use sliced bread to make strips.

Since this lunch contains both hot and cold foods (soup and strawberries), it's recommended to follow the container's instructions to heat up the warm compartment and send ice packs with the lunch box to keep the cold food cold. It sounds counterintuitive, but this is what was recommended by the manufacturer for lunches that have both hot and cold food. (Note: This only works with containers designed for both hot and cold purposes.)

ALLERGY TIPS

WHEAT: Send gluten-free bread and gluten-free soup (most broccoli cheese soup has flour in it).

DAIRY: Try dairy-free broccoli cheese soup or cream of broccoli soup.

TODDLER TIP

This might be a good lunch to wait on if your toddler still struggles with spoon skills, although broccoli cheese soup is thicker and stays on a spoon better than a thin soup.

PICKY EATING TIP

Show your child how to turn the bread strips into dippers by dunking them in the soup.

CONTAINER: OmieLife OmieBox

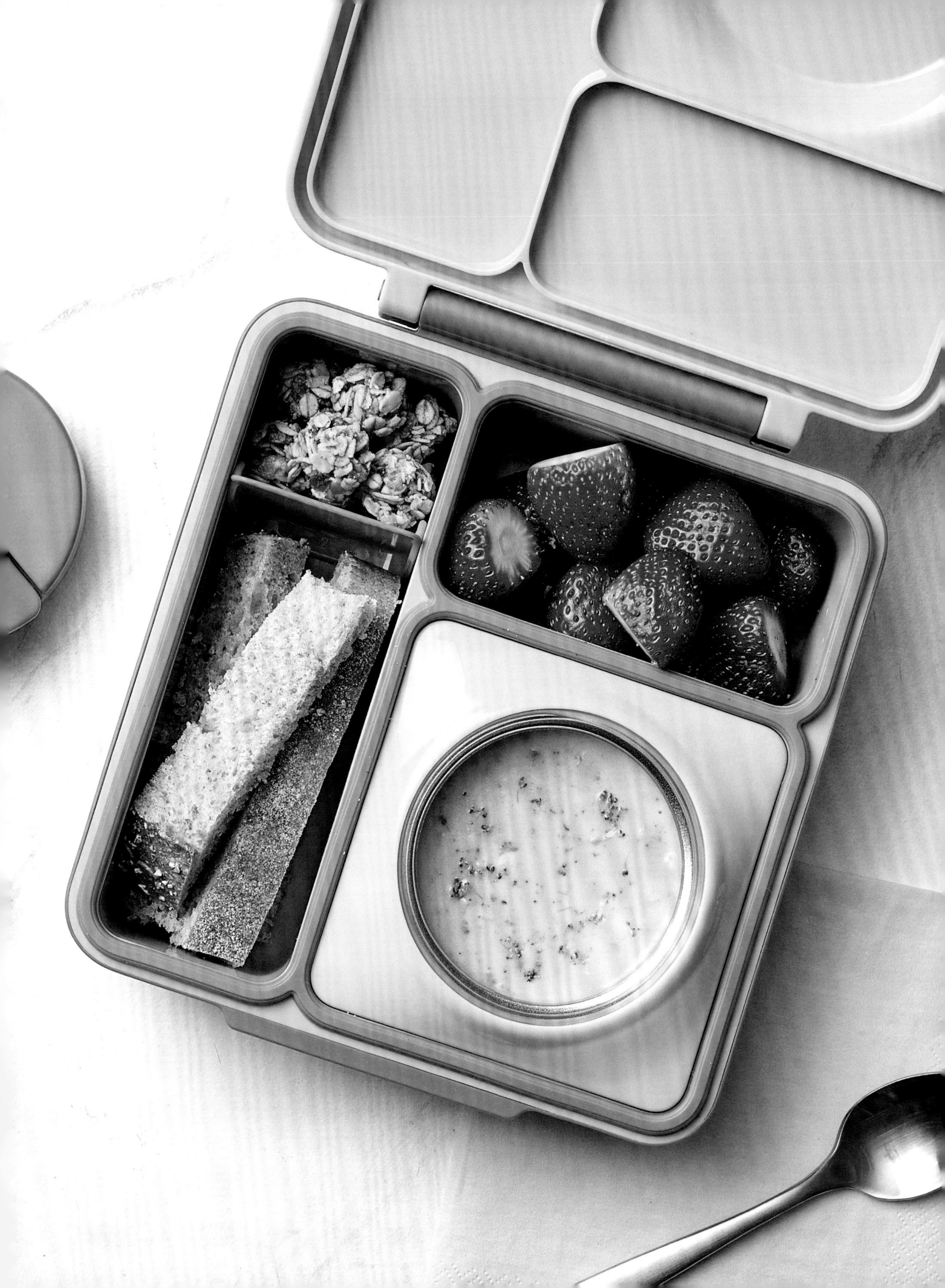

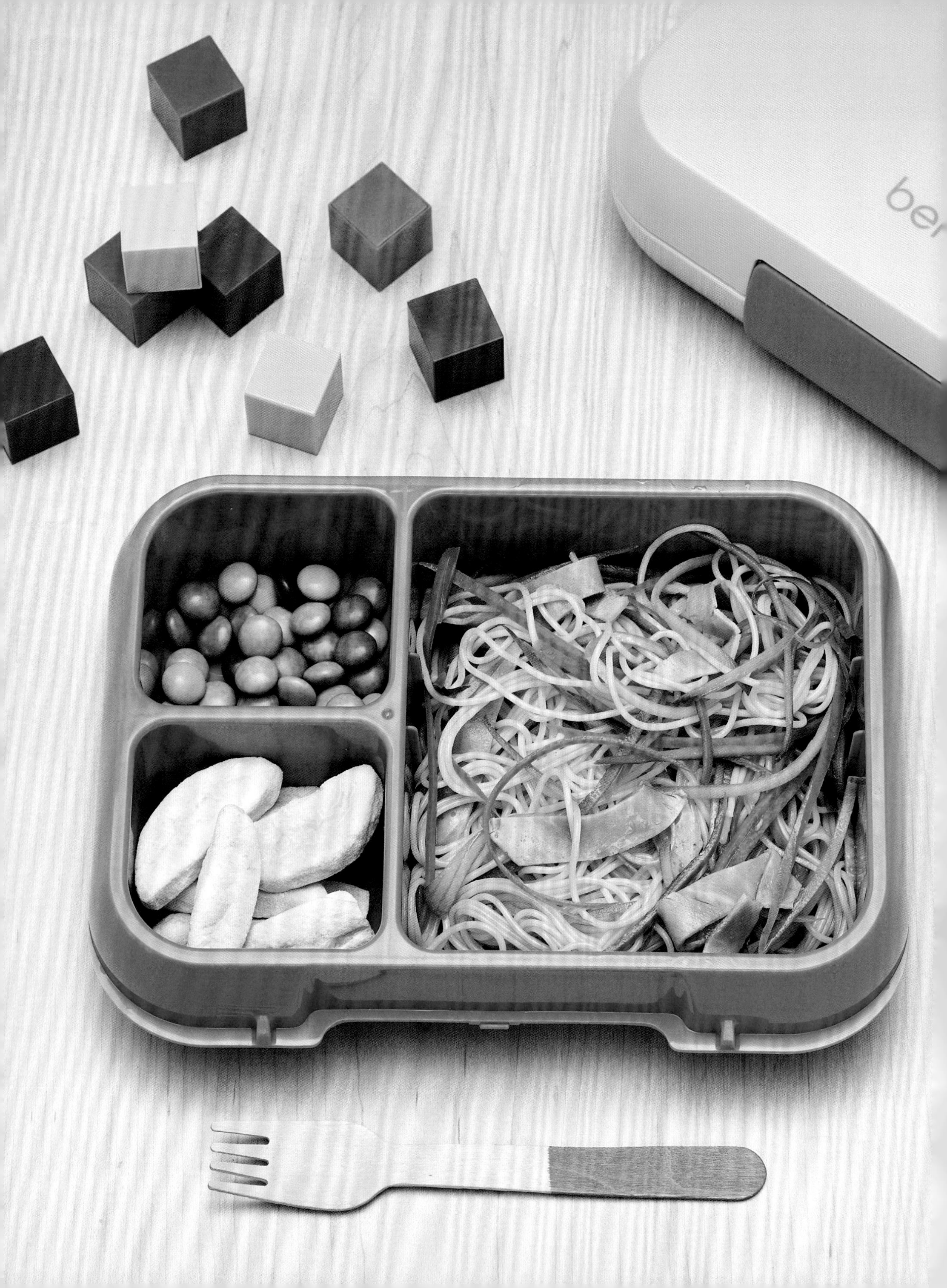

Cold Mixed Noodles

Our employee Yingzi loves making her spin on Chinese cold mixed noodles, *liang ban mian*, for her kids' lunches. It only requires a few simple ingredients and is really tasty—we all gobbled it up during the photo shoot for this book!

Angel hair pasta topped with sliced deli ham, shredded carrot/cucumber, and sesame oil

Freeze-dried mango

Chocolate-coated candies

PREP TIP

Use leftover angel hair pasta to prep this easily before school. Slice the ham and use a handheld julienne peeler (or mandoline) to create long, thin pieces of carrot and cucumber. Top with sesame oil—that's it! Super easy yet flavorful.

ALLERGY TIPS

DAIRY: No Whey Chocolate makes a good Top Nine–free, gluten-free chocolate-coated candy. Check out our Allergy Guide QR code (page 42) for more product recommendations.

WHEAT: Use gluten-free angel hair pasta (or other gluten-free long, thin pasta). Since many gluten-free noodles don't taste great as leftovers, this might be a good lunch to make at home so the noodles can be cooked fresh.

SESAME: Sesame oil makes up much of the flavor and mouthfeel of this dish. If that's not an option, try garlic olive oil or a sesame-free sauce (ponzu, soy sauce, coconut aminos). Perilla seed oil might be a nice alternative, since it has a similar flavor to sesame.

TODDLER TIP

This lunch is already modified for safety for toddlers. If you don't feel comfortable sending chocolate-coated candy, send another fruit or vegetable side.

PICKY EATING TIP

If you have a reluctant eater, get yourself a handheld julienne vegetable peeler. Using this tool is an extremely easy way to quickly prep vegetables for stir-fries or noodle dishes, and it creates thin, long strips that might be less intimidating for kids than large pieces of veggies.

VEGETARIAN SWAP

Use a thinly sliced omelet instead of ham.

CONTAINER: Bentgo Pop

Latkes and Brisket

Our employee Stacy's family celebrates Hanukkah and likes to send leftover latkes with brisket for school lunch the next day. They're really good eaten cold!

Potato pancakes/ latkes

Leftover brisket, shredded

Applesauce

Carrot chips

Dairy-free chocolate coins

"I CAN'T EVEN" TIP Use frozen latkes instead of homemade ones. Cook them per package instructions before adding them to your child's lunch box.

ALLERGY TIPS

WHEAT: Prepare gluten-free latkes. A quick online search will bring up a lot of recipes!

EGG: Make egg-free latkes. You'll find lots of recipes online.

TODDLER TIP This lunch is already modified for safety for toddlers. Show them how to dip the latkes in the applesauce!

PICKY EATING TIP Don't be discouraged if your child doesn't like your family's special or cultural foods yet. Holiday meals are really overwhelming to kids, especially reluctant eaters. You might find foods, flavors, and rituals comforting, but they're still learning about them. Give them time—they'll get there!

VEGE-TARIAN SWAP Send a hard-boiled egg or cheese instead of meat.

CONTAINER: **Bentgo Kids Chill**

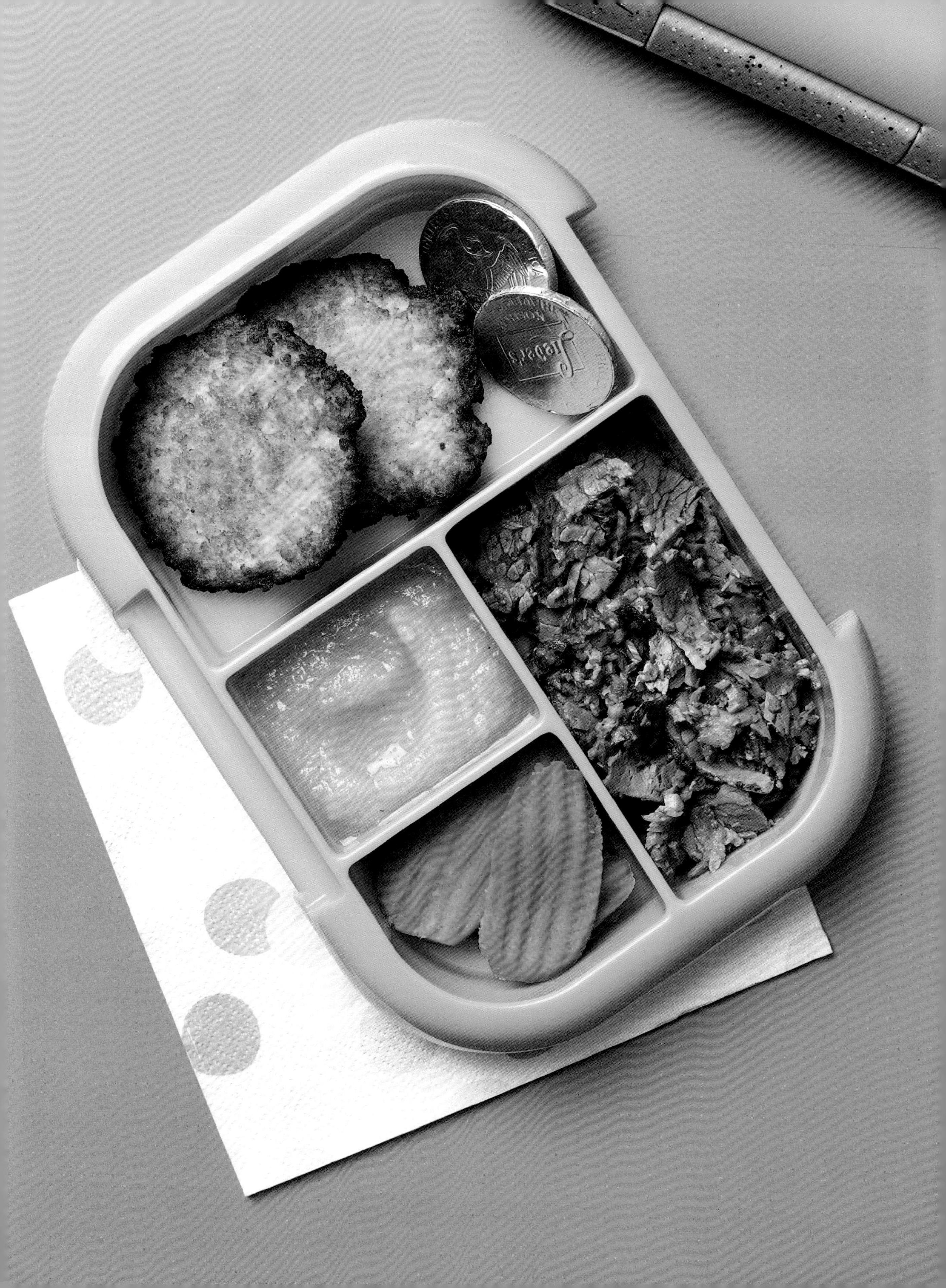

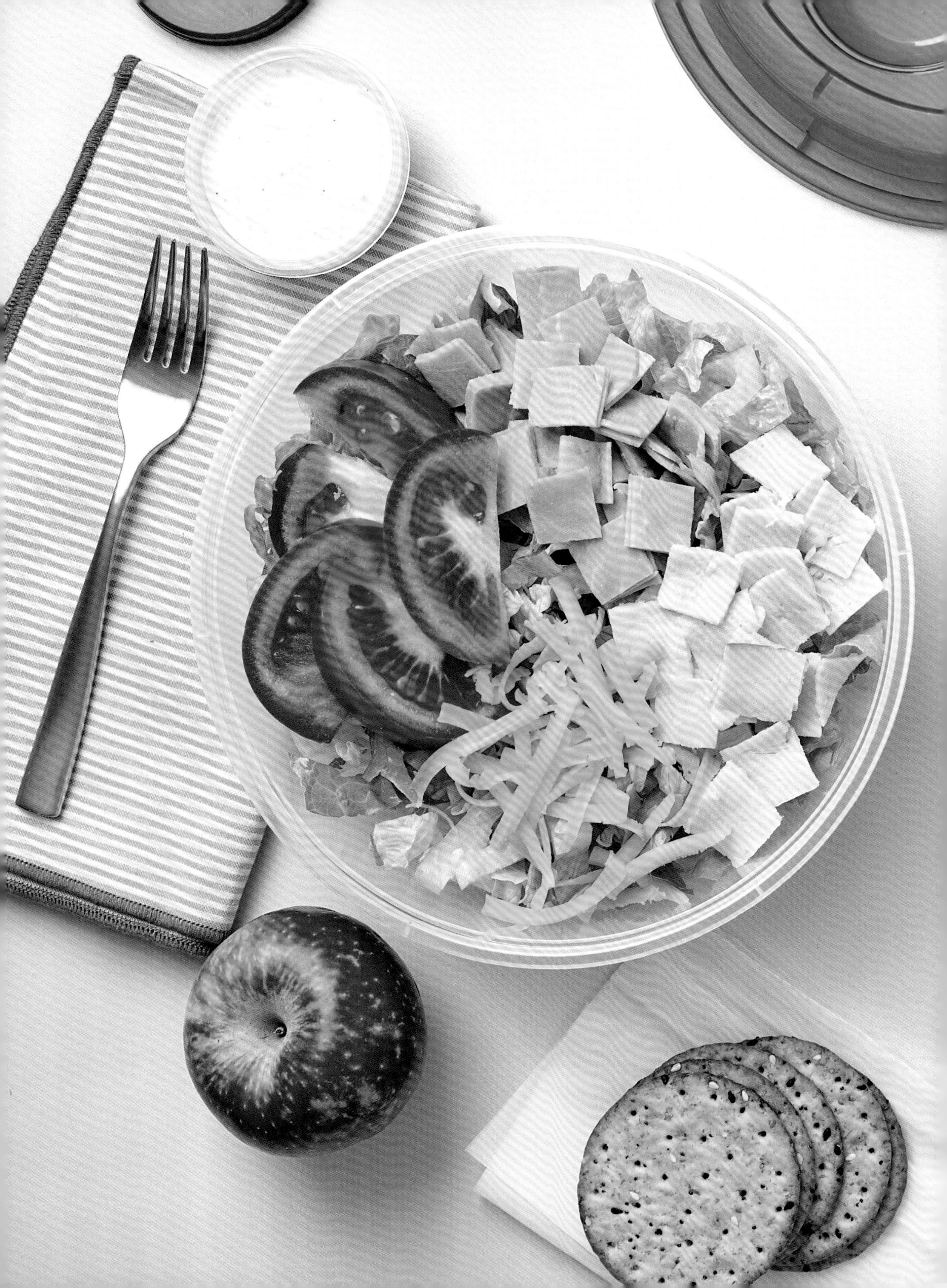

Chef Salad

Salads and . . . kids? Yes! Some kids really enjoy salads and love eating them at lunch, especially as they get older and have the skills (and desire) to eat a salad as a meal. Just make sure to serve a carbohydrate source, like whole-grain crackers, to round out the meal.

Build your own chef salad—lettuce, chopped ham and turkey, shredded cheese

Hearty whole-grain crackers

Apple

Ranch dressing

PREP TIP This container has a cup for dressing that stays on top and it's perfect for shaking up the salad once you dress it.

ALLERGY TIPS

WHEAT: Send gluten-free crackers or chips.

DAIRY: Omit cheese and send olives or guacamole (in an individual container) instead, or use your favorite dairy-free cheese.

TODDLER TIP Salad might be a tough lunch for your toddler, although it's great to serve it as a side dish! Start with crunchy lettuce that's easier for them to feel in their mouth, and as they get more skilled at chewing it, graduate up to any kind of leafy green! The more toddlers see salads on their plate and yours, the more likely they are to eat them one day.

PICKY EATING TIP Dressing makes all the difference with salads. Your child might not enjoy most veggies, but give them a salad with ranch dressing or Caesar salad dressing and they might be game. Since this salad makes up most of the meal, try it at home first to ensure that they can enjoy something like this for lunch.

VEGETARIAN SWAP Top with hard-boiled egg, tofu, garbanzo beans, tempeh, or a plant-based deli "meat" instead of turkey and ham.

CONTAINER: Bentgo Easyboxes Salad-to-Go Container and EcoSoul Compostable Resealable Bag

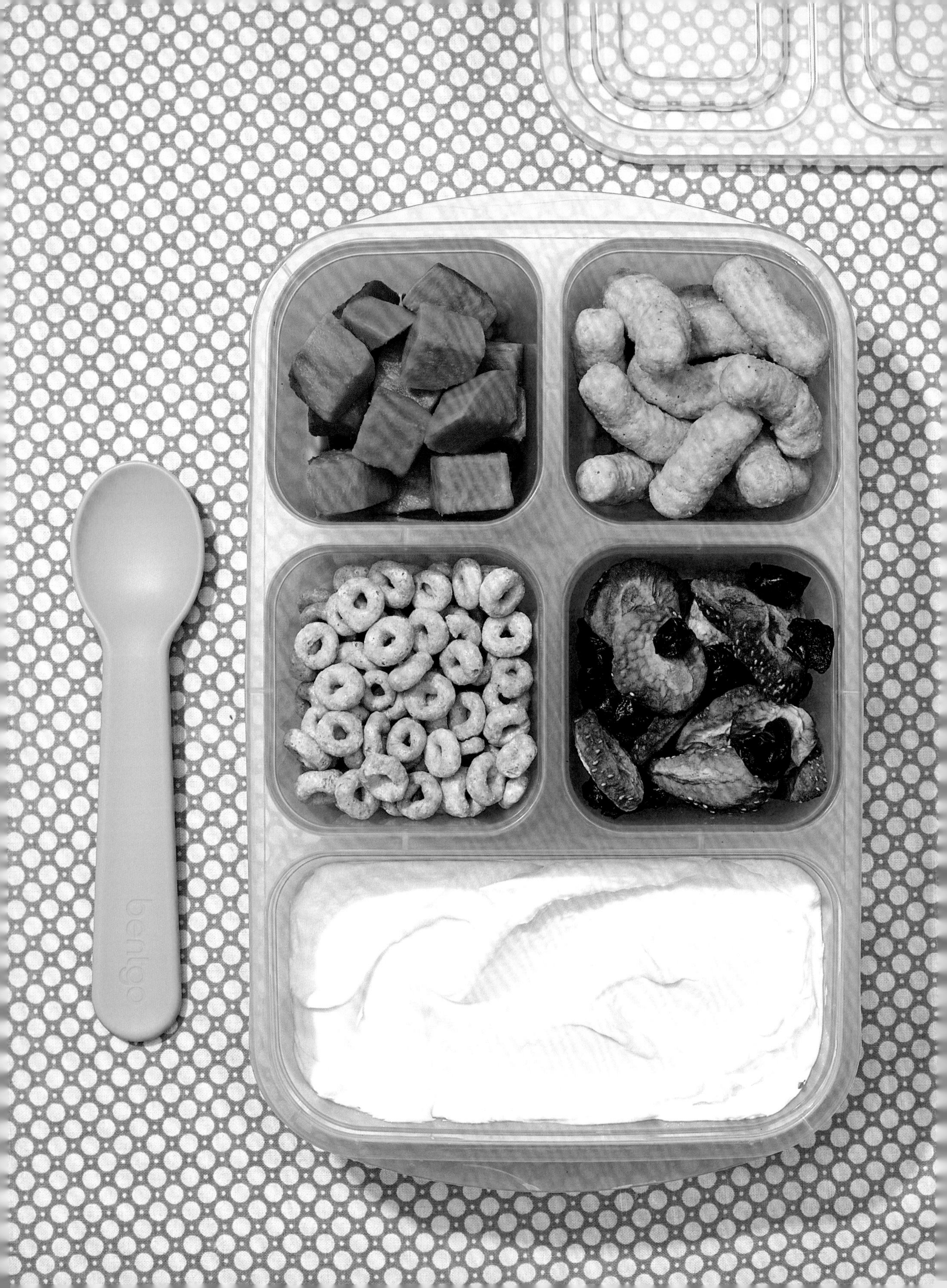
bentgo

Cereal and Yogurt

This is another toddler-favorite lunch that's still yummy for our older diners and a great option for kids who love crunch. Cheerios or another whole-grain cereal are a great source of iron and can lend some familiarity to a big day at school. Your child can mix the fruit into the yogurt or keep it separate, and even the puffed peanut butter snack is great dipped in yogurt!

Dry cereal
(Cheerios)

Greek yogurt
(sweetened or unsweetened)

Freeze-dried strawberries and craisins mix

Roasted sweet potato cubes

Peanut butter puffed snack
(Bamba)

PREP TIP

If you buy unsweetened Greek yogurt, you can use it in so many ways. Add it to boxed mac and cheese (instead of using fluid milk in the same quantity), stir it into mashed potatoes, put it in smoothies, or use it in a pinch as a sour cream replacement. When it's time to serve it on its own, sweeten it, if desired, with honey or maple syrup.

ALLERGY TIPS

PEANUTS: Omit Bamba or serve another peanut-free puff.

WHEAT: Many people in the gluten-free community cannot tolerate Cheerios. Use a safe-for-you cereal instead.

DAIRY: Use dairy-free yogurt instead of Greek yogurt.

TODDLER TIP

This lunch is toddler-ready. Just make sure that the craisins are soft and easy to chew.

PICKY EATING TIP

Your kid might be very particular about which types of cereal they like, and that's OK. Send their favorite instead. As they get used to this lunch, they might be OK branching out to another brand or flavor.

CONTAINER: Bentgo Easyboxes 5-Compartment Meal Container (formerly EasyLunchboxes brand)

Build-Your-Own Soft Taco

Taco night at Megan's house always involves a few different ingredients in bowls on the table so that everyone can assemble their dinner themselves. Her kids *love* making their own soft tacos and have a monumentally better track record of eating them when they get to make their tacos independently.

Sliced leftover chicken

Pinto beans

Small-medium tortillas

Shredded cheese

Chopped tomato

Freeze-dried raspberries

Individually packaged guacamole cup

PREP TIP If you make extra ingredients for taco night dinner, throw them in your kid's lunch box. Poof, lunch is done.

"I CAN'T EVEN" TIP Use precooked chicken or store-bought rotisserie chicken instead of making it at home.

ALLERGY TIPS **WHEAT:** Use corn tortillas (or any gluten-free tortilla of your choice).

DAIRY: Omit cheese or send dairy-free cheese.

TODDLER TIP Your toddler might eat all these components on their own without assembling a taco, and that's OK! They're basically eating a deconstructed taco.

PICKY EATING TIP Don't forget your child's favorite topping, like guacamole, sour cream, or salsa. Serve it in a separate container for a little fun and novelty.

VEGETARIAN SWAP Omit chicken—this is a complete meal without it.

CONTAINER: Yumbox Original

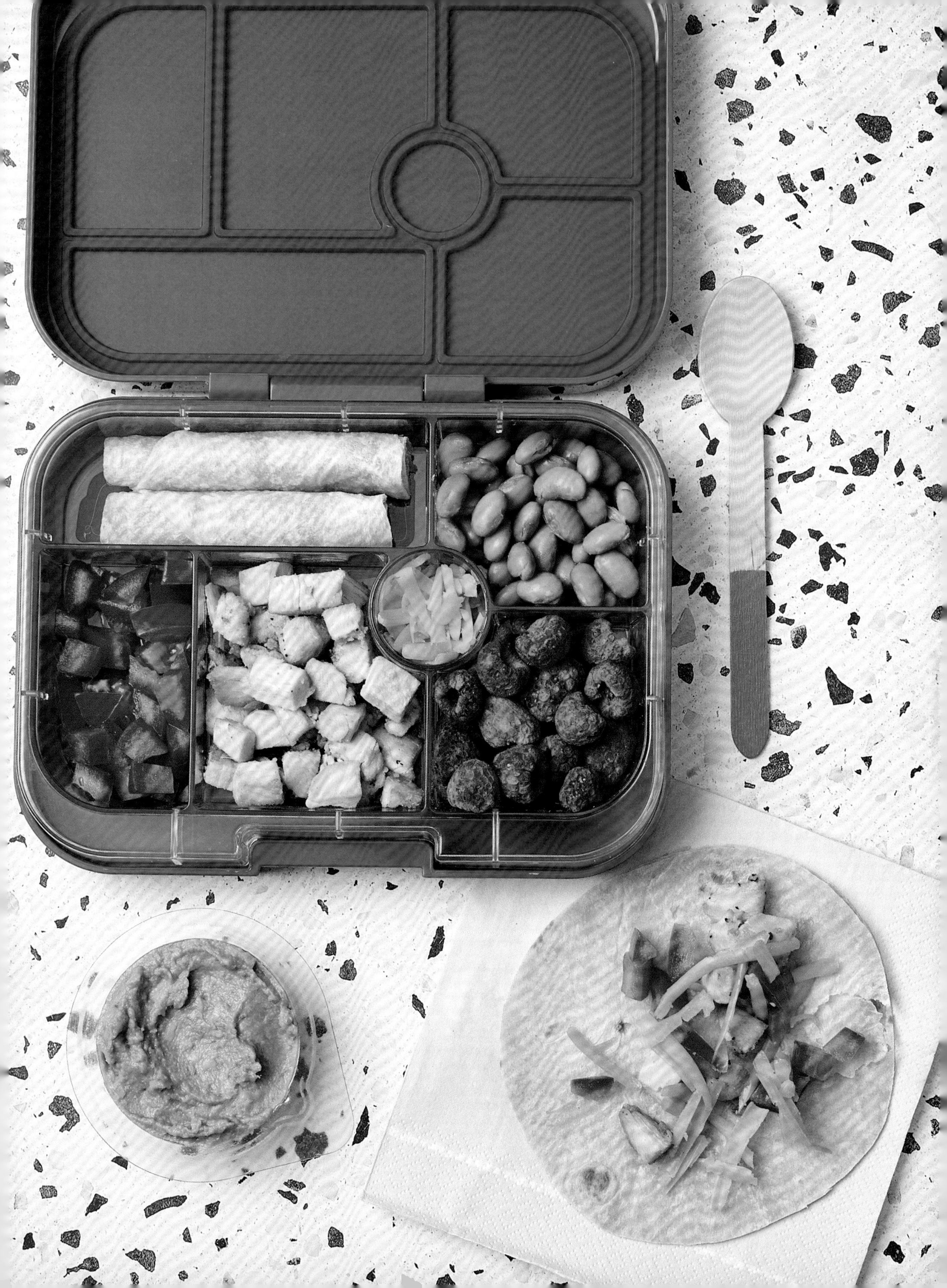

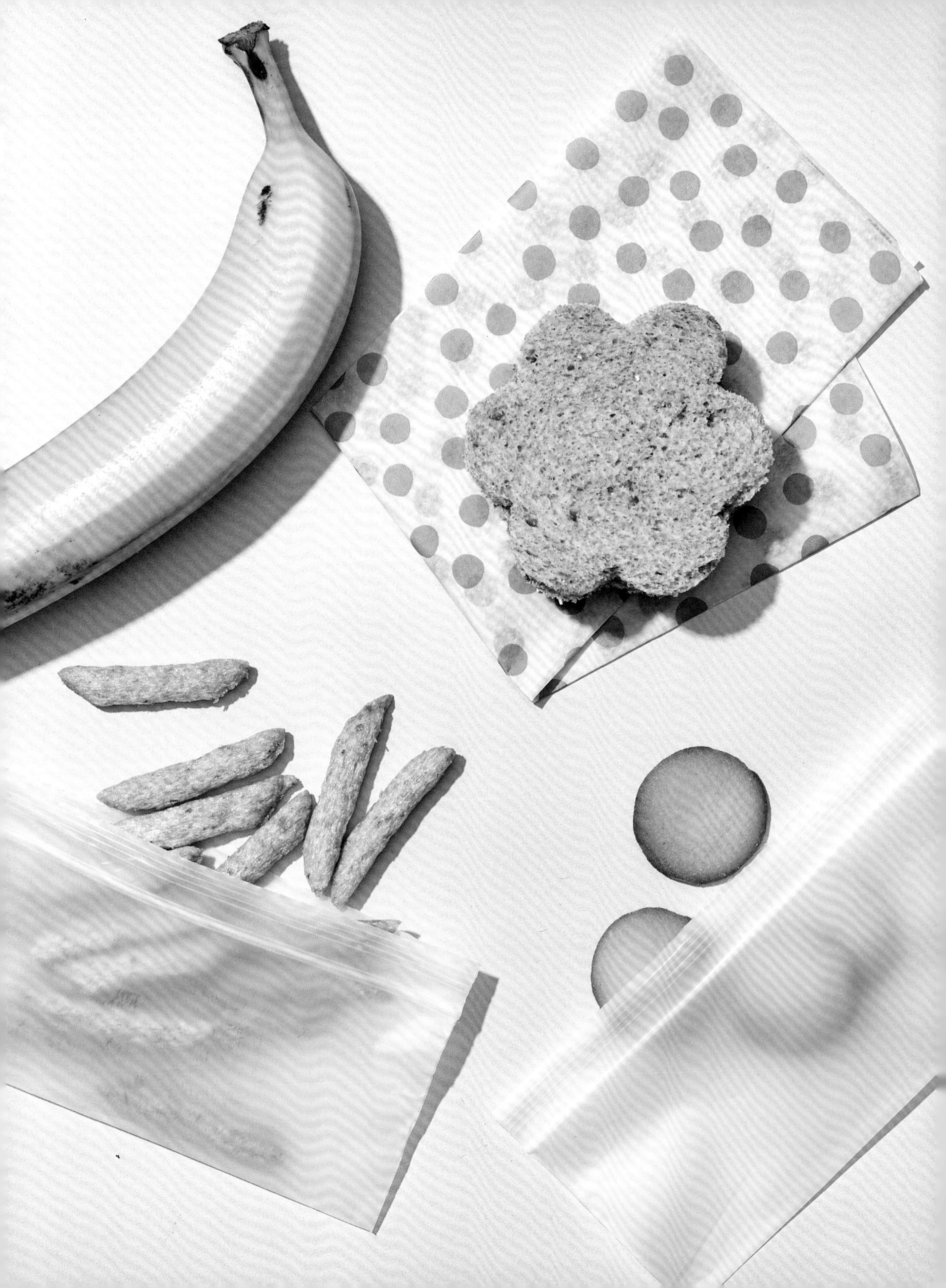

Cookie Cutter Sandwich

Remember how we promised you no making food into shapes in this book? Well, we do have *one* shape here, but we're showing it to make a point: Cookie cutter sandwiches go over really well with kids. It's a technique we use when we're not sure if our kid will be into a sandwich we send or if they're going through a picky phase. It doesn't take longer than cutting it with a knife—just use any cookie cutter you have on hand. And *no,* you never ever, ever have to do this if you really aren't into it, but we're telling you . . . it can work like magic.

Almond butter and mixed fruit jelly on whole-grain bread, cut with a cookie cutter

Whole banana

Snap pea crisps

Nilla wafers

PREP TIP

This lunch is fully shelf-stable and doesn't require refrigeration, meaning it's a great option to send on a field trip or outing where ice packs are not an option.

ALLERGY TIPS

Nilla wafers contain a lot of allergens. For wheat-, dairy-, and soy-free wafers, use Kinnikinnick wafers. If you're also egg-free, use a crunchy cookie from Partake Foods (gluten-free and Top Nine–free). See page 42 for the QR code for our Allergy Guide.

WHEAT: Use gluten-free bread instead of whole-wheat bread. Serve a gluten-free cookie or another gluten-free dessert.

DAIRY: Some snap pea crisp brands may contain milk or milk derivatives. Send freeze-dried broccoli instead (Trader Joe's has this).

TREE NUTS: Use sunflower seed butter, granola butter, or soy butter instead of almond butter.

TODDLER TIP

Cookie cutters are not only fun, but they can also help toddlers eat sandwiches because they slightly flatten the bread and create great spots to bite. Cookie cutters also offer different shapes along the edges that help make picking up the sandwich more interesting to the brain and more engaging for your child.

PICKY EATING TIP

The next time you go to a store that sells cooking gear, let your child pick out a few cookie cutter shapes they like. They will get a kick out of seeing their favorite letter or animal in their lunch box.

CONTAINER: EcoSoul Compostable Resealable Bags and Yumbox Sandwich Paper

Leftover Baked Ziti

You might notice that we don't have a lot of hot options in this book. The reason is twofold: (1) when polled, most of our audience sends cold lunches all or the majority of the time, and (2) it's hard to keep hot lunches hot until lunchtime. Insulated containers made for hot food can do a good job if the food is saucy and has a lot of liquid, but if it's dry it will almost definitely be cool (and potentially unsafe) by lunchtime. This baked ziti, prepped with some extra sauce, is something that can stay warm until it's time for your kiddo to eat it because it has so much sauce.

Leftover vegetarian baked ziti
(served hot)

Raw zucchini,
crinkle cut

Garlic bread slices

Fun-size candy

PREP TIPS

Use a handheld crinkle cutter to add some texture and fun to the zucchini. If you happen to also have a baby at home, crinkle-cutting food before you cook it makes it easier for new eaters to grip! You won't regret buying one.

Check out page 204 for tips on how to use this container with both hot and cold food.

ALLERGY TIPS

WHEAT: Use gluten-free noodles when making the baked ziti and send gluten-free garlic bread.

DAIRY: Use dairy-free cheese or omit cheese and combine pasta, ground meat, and sauce with Italian seasoning, and salt and pepper. Send bread toasted with olive oil or plant-based butter. Serve dairy-free chocolate.

TODDLER TIP

Your child might need help opening a hot-food-item container, as they're often sealed really tightly. Give their teacher a heads-up at drop-off that day if you don't usually send hot foods.

PICKY EATING TIP

Many kids love fruit, but some don't—and this lunch doesn't contain fruit! (OK, technically tomatoes are fruits, but culinarily they're veggies.) Our School Lunch Formula contains both a fruit and a veggie, so our kids are exposed to both, but if you are out of fruit or just don't want to serve it, that's fine too.

CONTAINER: OmieLife OmieBox

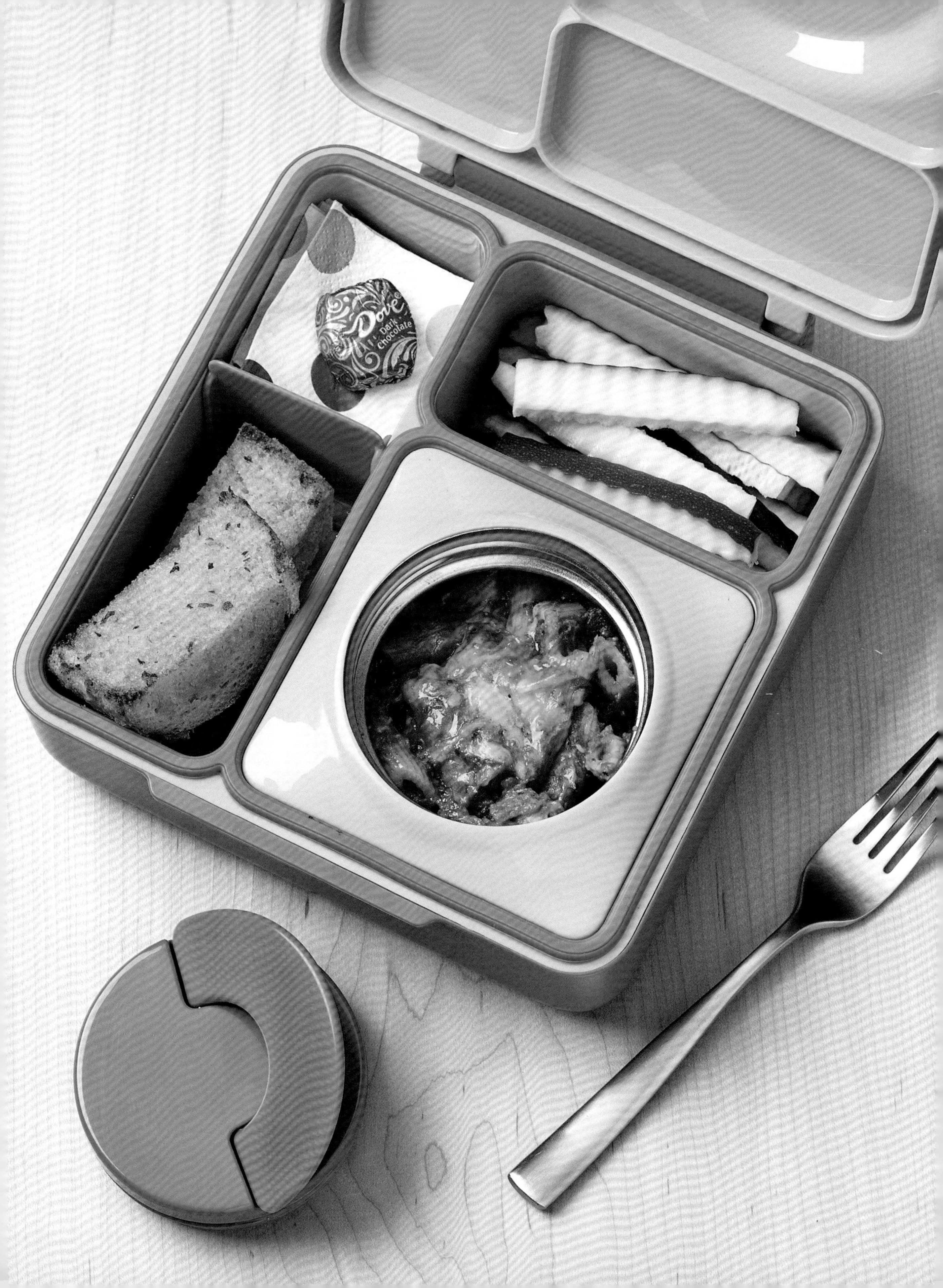
Dove
Dark Chocolate

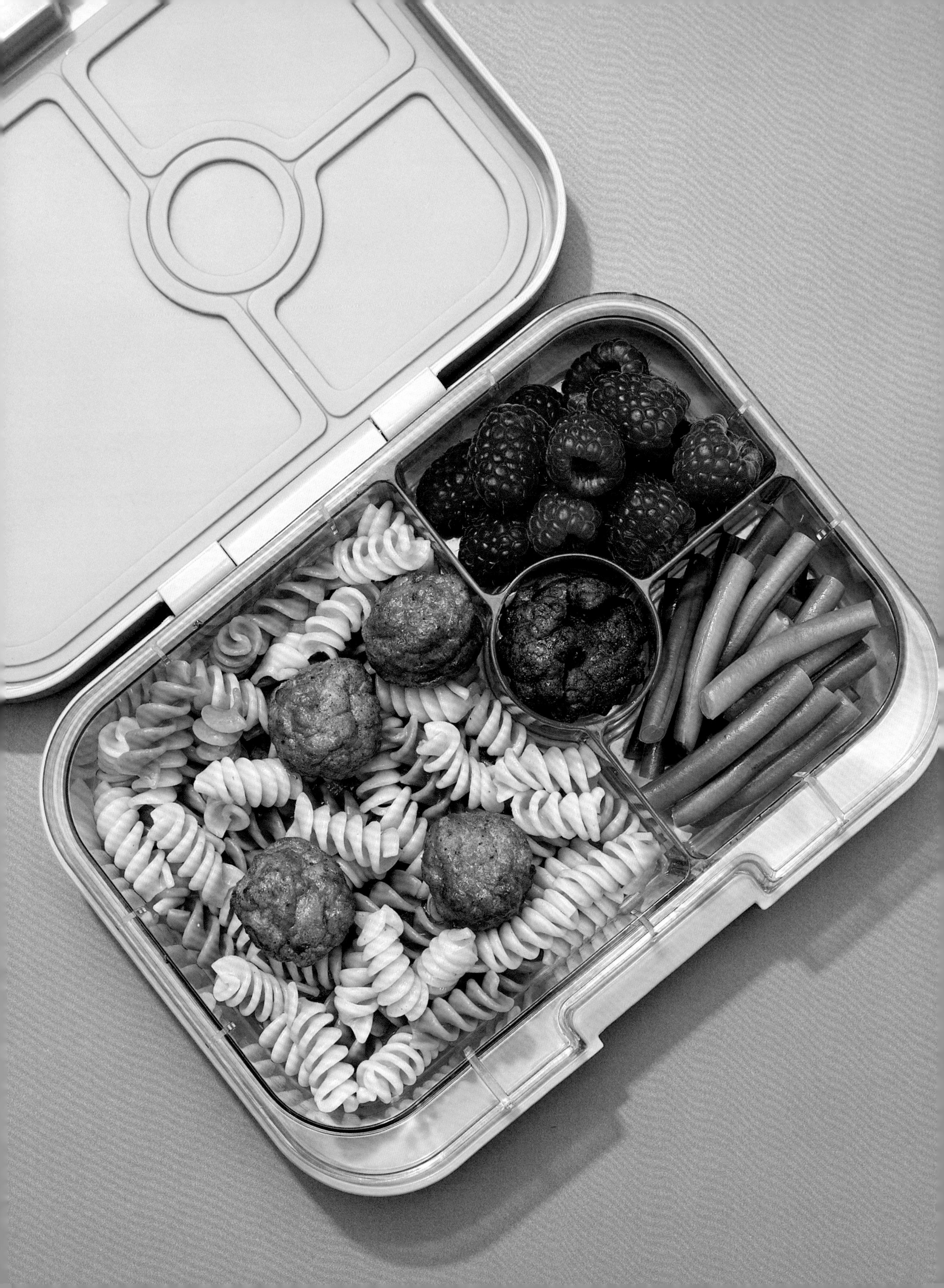

Meatballs and Spiral Pasta

Meatballs are beloved by kids and adults worldwide, and there are *so* many different meatball options in stores today. Fresh or frozen, beef, chicken, or plant-based—the possibilities are endless. We especially love Trader Joe's fresh chicken meatballs (gluten- and dairy-free), but any favorite meatball will do. You can also make some from scratch if desired.

Leftover beef or chicken meatballs

Leftover spiral pasta

Raspberries

Leftover steamed green beans

Chocolate grahams

PREP TIP

Take leftover meatballs, pasta, and cooked green beans from dinner and pop them into your child's lunch box, along with the other components of this lunch.

ALLERGY TIPS

Many commercial brands contain a range of allergens. Partake Foods makes a gluten-free and Top Nine–free graham cracker, and Kinnikinnick makes a gluten-free and allergy-friendly graham cracker.

WHEAT: Use gluten-free noodles, meatballs, and graham crackers.

DAIRY: Use dairy-free meatballs.

TODDLER TIP

To make these meatballs easier to eat, cut them into quarters.

PICKY EATING TIP

This is a pretty simple lunch when it comes to flavors. If your child is struggling with picky eating, they might appreciate these simple and straightforward foods. While adults may want seasonings and sauces, this might hit the spot for your kiddo.

VEGETARIAN SWAP

Use plant-based meatballs.

CONTAINER: Yumbox Panino

Pita and Baba Ghanoush

If your child likes hummus, they may enjoy baba ghanoush, a dip made from eggplant and sesame seeds that is popular in Mediterranean cuisine. This is the only eggplant dish that made its way into this book, and it's a delicious and less intimidating way to enjoy what can sometimes be an overwhelming food to particular eaters.

Baba ghanoush

Soft pita wedges

Garbanzo beans

Sliced feta

Sliced red apple

Cucumber slices

PREP TIP After cutting the apples, spritz them with lemon juice to keep them from browning. Note: We used two different silicone muffin cups in this lunch to help separate the different foods and prevent them from getting soggy. Just make sure to pack the cupcake liners nicely with other foods so they don't fly around in your child's lunch box.

ALLERGY TIPS

WHEAT: Use gluten-free pita instead of wheat-based pita.

DAIRY: Omit feta cheese or use a dairy-free feta.

SESAME: Serve tzatziki instead of baba ghanoush.

TODDLER TIP Serve applesauce or thinly cut apples instead of apple wedges to reduce choking risk.

PICKY EATING TIP Little silicone cupcake liners make this lunch fun and visually appealing to a reluctant eater. They might enjoy packing this with you, since these silicone liners are something they may not have seen before.

CONTAINER: Bentgo Kids Stainless Steel

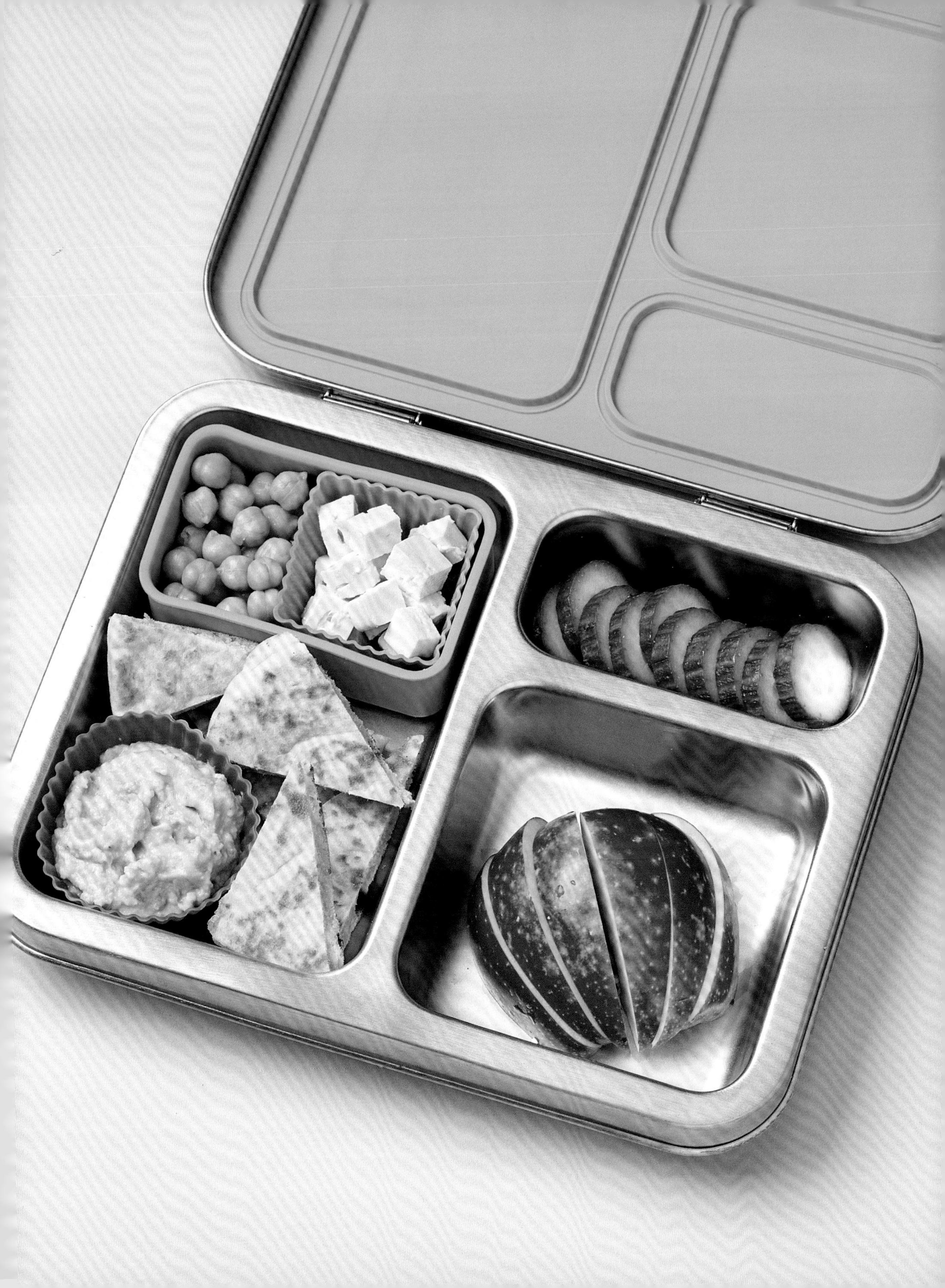

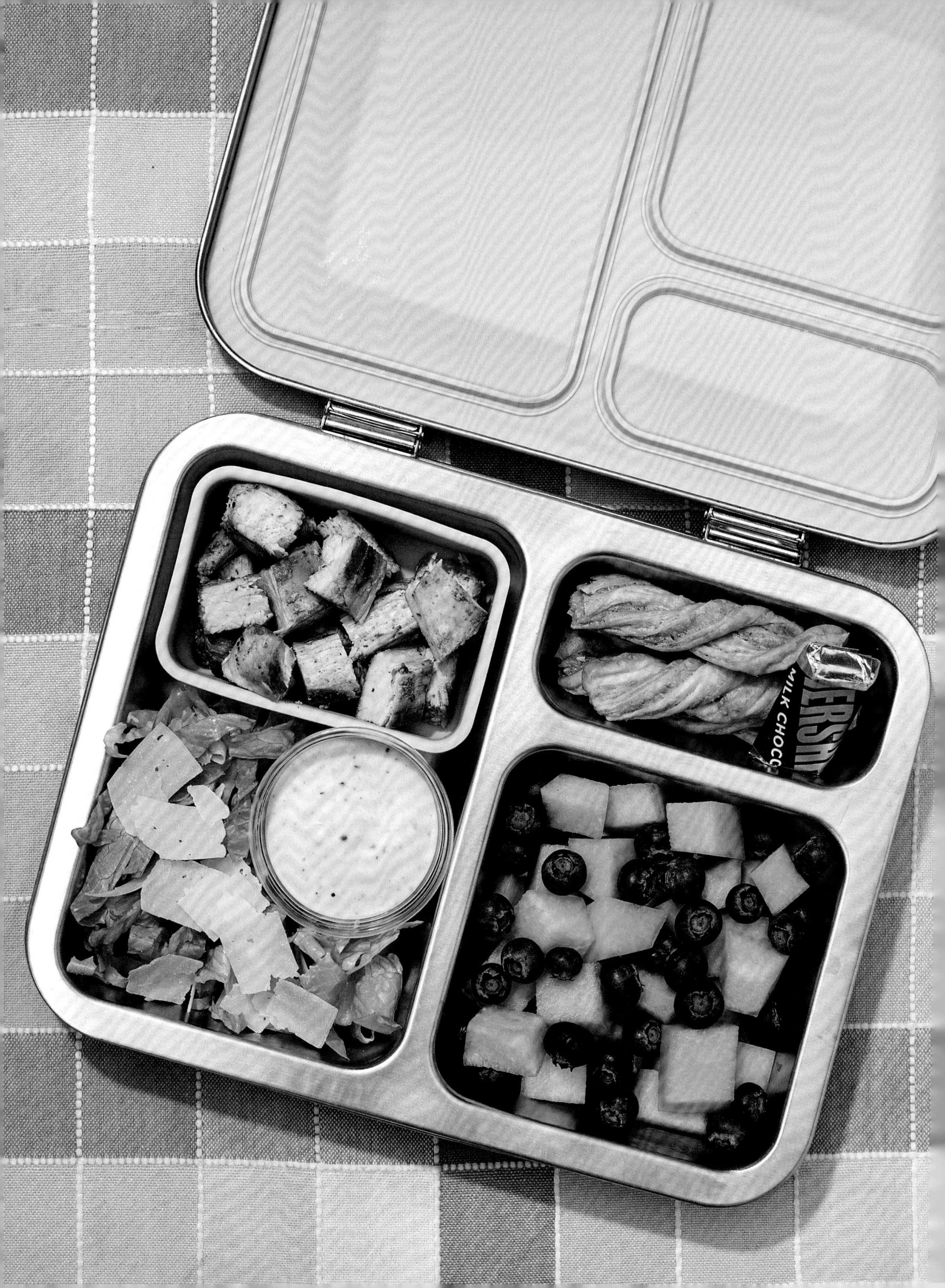
MILK

Chicken Caesar Salad

As we mentioned in the write-up for our Chicken Caesar Wrap lunch (page 162), we consider Caesar salad to be a "gateway salad." The flavors are appealing and mild, and they help kids learn to love eating green salads. Megan has sent this lunch many times with her girls in elementary school, and every time they love it. Just make sure there's enough room in the container to mix the salad components. The Bentgo Kids Stainless Steel comes with a silicone liner, so they just take it out, dump the chicken on the lettuce, and dress the salad.

Caesar salad
(romaine topped with shaved Parmesan and Caesar dressing on the side)

Diced leftover grilled chicken

Chopped cantaloupe and blueberries

Cheddar twists
(Trader Joe's brand shown; sub with croutons or whole-grain bread)

Fun-size chocolate

CONTAINER: Bentgo Kids Stainless Steel

PREP TIP

Make sure to separate the cheese twists (or croutons or other types of bread) from the lettuce, as they can get soggy.

ALLERGY TIPS

WHEAT: Use gluten-free crackers or croutons instead of cheese twists.

DAIRY: Omit Parmesan and use dairy-free Caesar dressing (like a "Paleo" brand). Use dairy-free crackers instead of cheese twists. Serve dairy-free chocolate.

EGG: Use an egg-free Caesar dressing.

SOY: Use a soy-free Caesar dressing.

TODDLER TIP

Assembled salads can be a difficult food for toddlers to eat because these salads require good fork and chewing skills. This might be something your toddler loves to eat deconstructed (as shown), dipping the lettuce into the dressing.

PICKY EATING TIP

If ranch is a preferred dressing, try that first instead of Caesar. It doesn't matter that it's not a "real" Caesar salad—the goal is to help your reluctant eater become comfortable with eating salad, period, and a preferred dressing can encourage that.

VEGETARIAN SWAP

Send chickpeas or cubed tofu instead of grilled chicken.

Mini Bagels and Lox

Smoked salmon on a bagel might not be the most obvious kid-friendly food, but some kids absolutely love it. Plus, this book was written for eaters of all ages, so we wanted to make sure to include it because it's a favorite of many people on our team!

Mini bagel, veggie cream cheese, and lox

Blackberries

Raspberries

Green bell pepper pieces

Sunflower seeds

PREP TIP

Does your kid like capers, those salty, tiny green buds that taste kind of like olives? Nestle some of those on top of the cream cheese before adding the lox for a little flavor boost.

ALLERGY TIPS

WHEAT: Use gluten-free bagels.

DAIRY: Use dairy-free cream cheese.

FISH: Substitute deli turkey for lox.

TODDLER TIP

To make this even safer for young toddlers, quarter the blackberries lengthwise and add some crackers or puffs instead of the sunflower seeds.

PICKY EATING TIP

If lox is an absolute "no" for your particular eater, remove it and send a plain bagel with cream cheese instead. It can take a while for kids to enjoy the strong flavor of fish. Try not to get frustrated—their taste preferences will hopefully evolve over time.

VEGETARIAN SWAP

Remove the lox and send a slice of tomato instead.

CONTAINER: Bentgo Kids

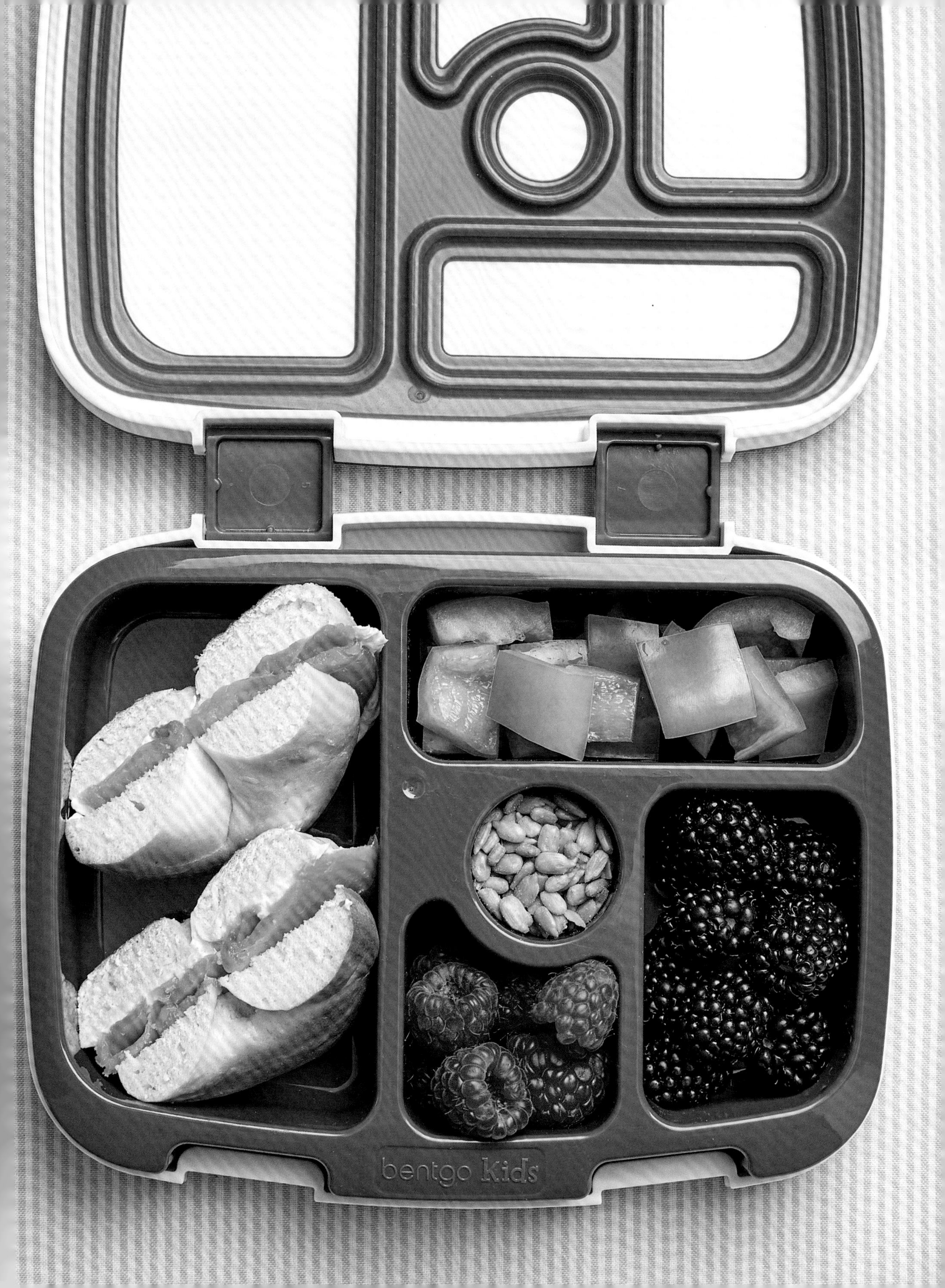
bentgo Kids

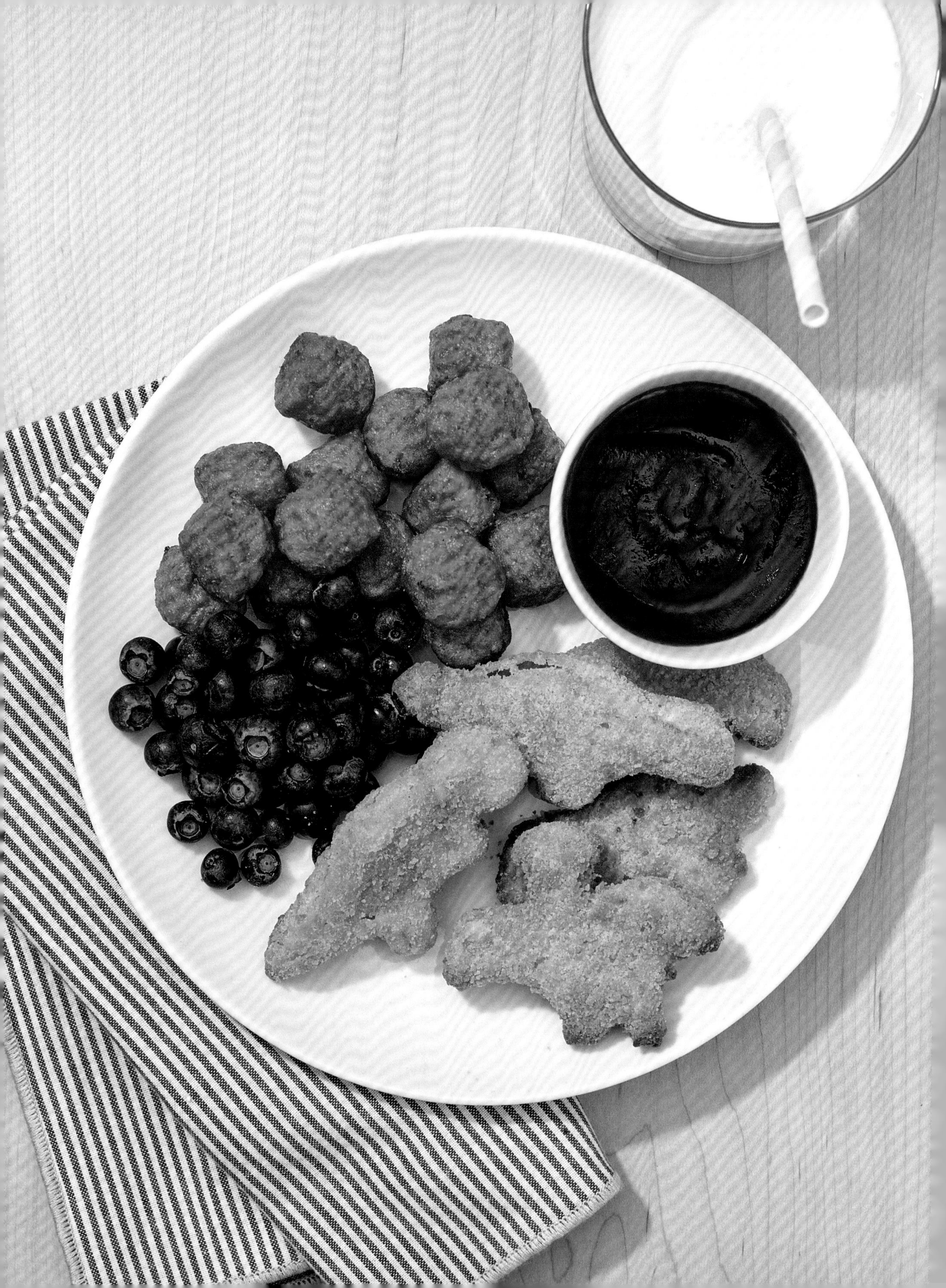

Nuggets and Sweet Potato Tots

You might eat lunch at home most days or want inspo for something to enjoy on the weekends. Enter Megan's favorite home lunch creation: air-fried nuggets and sweet potato tots paired with blueberries and a dipping sauce! There's a good mix of carbs, protein, and fat, plus some vitamins A and C from the sweet potato and fruit.

Air-fried nuggets
(from frozen)

Air-fried sweet potato tots
(from frozen)

Blueberries

BBQ sauce on side

Milk
(optional)

PREP TIP

Air-fry nuggets and tots on the same tray at 375°F for about five minutes. Turn them over, then continue air-frying them for another three to five minutes. Watch closely to make sure they don't burn.

ALLERGY TIPS

WHEAT: Use gluten-free nuggets and gluten-free BBQ sauce. Make sure your tots are also wheat-free.

DAIRY: Make sure your tots and nuggets are dairy-free. Use dairy-free milk or serve water. You can add flavor to water with fruit (strawberries, lemon, etc.).

TODDLER TIP

Toddlers tend to love this lunch. Don't be surprised if it becomes your favorite "I Can't Even" meal for busy nights or when you have a babysitter!

PICKY EATING TIP

Nuggets are a picky eater favorite because the breading makes them easy to chew and has a consistent texture and flavor. If your kid loves nuggets, try serving other types of breaded meats and veggies—it might help them "bridge" to a new food!

VEGETARIAN SWAP

Use a plant-based nugget instead of chicken nuggets.

CONTAINER: Just a white plate

Hummus and Cheddar Sandwich

Hummus lover at home? Try this delicious vegetarian sandwich. Red pepper hummus adds a little extra flavor, but you can always try traditional hummus instead.

Red pepper hummus, lettuce, tomato, and cheddar sandwich on whole-grain bread

Pitted cherries

Dried blueberries

Pretzel nuggets

PREP TIP

Put hummus on both pieces of bread to help the sandwich stick together a little better.

ALLERGY TIPS

WHEAT: Use gluten-free bread and gluten-free pretzels.

DAIRY: Use avocado spread instead of cheese (or a dairy-free cheese).

SESAME: Use avocado spread or a tahini-free dip instead of hummus.

TODDLER TIP

Freeze-dried blueberries can be super crunchy and hard, depending on the brand you buy. Make sure to check them before sending—if you can squish them between your fingers, your toddler can chew them!

Quarter cherries lengthwise to reduce choking risk.

PICKY EATING TIP

If your child is used to turkey sandwiches, try slowly bridging to this type of sandwich by adding hummus first. Then try a slice of cheese or a layer of hummus. Small, incremental changes can help a particular eater learn to enjoy new foods.

CONTAINER: Bentgo Kids Stainless Steel

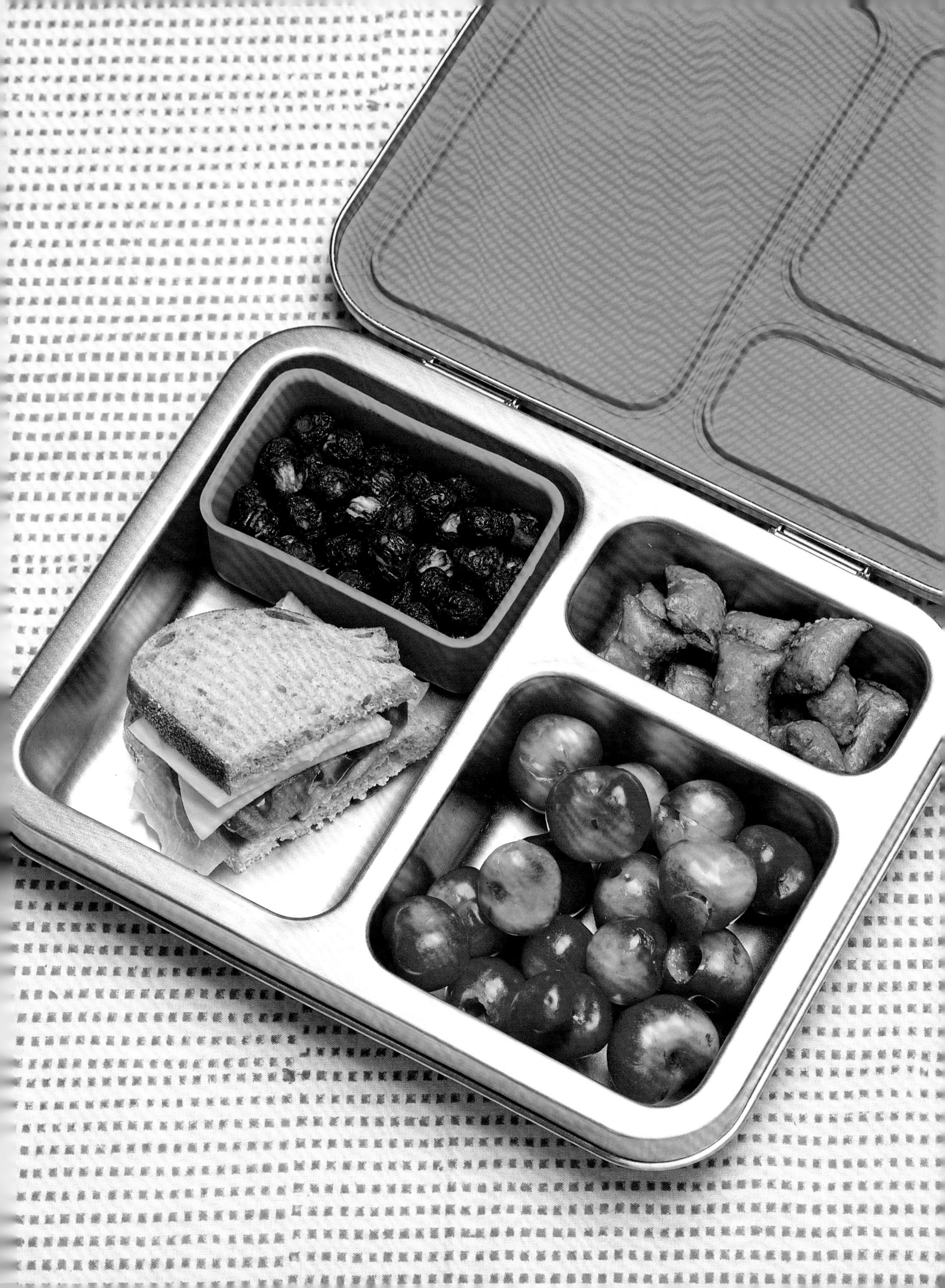

Acknowledgments

Just as it takes a village to raise a child, it also takes a village to take a book from concept to reality.

This project was a true labor of love for Feeding Littles, Rodale, the photography and food-styling team, and every single soul whose creativity, attention to detail, and love were poured into these pages. We are forever grateful for the ingenuity and thoughtfulness that every single one of you put into this project.

To Dervla Kelly, our incredible editor and fearless leader, thank you for believing in this book and for fighting so hard to spearhead this project. We love your passion for supporting families and offering them tools that will help them thrive in this busy, chaotic world. Thank you for allowing us to be our creative, outspoken selves, while also providing much-needed guidance. We are forever grateful for your wisdom and clarity.

To the entire Rodale team, including Katherine Leak, Abby Duval, Sarah Feightner, Jenny Davis, Allison Fox, Odette Fleming, and Ray Arjune, we are so grateful for your ability to think outside the box and create a truly unique, beautifully designed product. You thought of everything and helped us get this book to print under an extremely tight deadline. We know it wasn't easy, and we have so much appreciation for the work you do!

To our agent, Alyssa Reuben, thank you for pushing to make this dream a reality. When our first book launched, you told us it wouldn't be our last, even though we didn't know if we could do it again. You were so right. Thank you for believing in us when it was hard for us to believe in ourselves.

To the photography team, Carla Choy and Merisa Libbey, we have so much gratitude for the sheer grit you put into this project. Our photo shoot should have been a week long, and it was just three and a half days. You came up with ideas we never would have thought of, and it's so clear in these pages how much love and attention went into the photographs. You are rock stars!

To Hadas Smirnoff, our beloved food stylist (on our third project together), you are an incredible gift to this world! You work so hard and say yes to even the most challenging tasks, and you are an absolute genius at what you do. We literally could not have done this without you.

To Ali Maffucci, our co-author on our first book, *Feeding Littles & Beyond,* thank you for teaching us all you know about publishing. You are so generous with your wisdom, time, and resources, and we are so thankful for your encouragement to write this book.

To our special contributors, Susie Allison (@busytoddler), Kathlena (@theallergychef), and Marianne Richmond (@mariannerichmondwriter), *thank you.* Susie, you have always been a mentor to us, and your contribution to this book as an educator is so helpful to parents entering the new world of school lunch. You are an absolute gem and an incredible mom, teacher, businesswoman, wife, and friend. Kathlena, your dedication to this book is *astounding.* You spent days poring through these lunches, offering so many insightful suggestions. You are brilliant, and we so respect the work you've put into this book to help allergy/free-from families. And to Marianne, an author and mama we've so respected for the past decade—to have your words in this book is an enormous honor. Your book *If I Could Keep You*

Little describes exactly what it's like to be a parent: the bittersweet juxtaposition of wanting them to stay little while desperately hoping to watch them grow. Your contribution to this book is so, *so* special to us.

To our wonderful models, Eli, James, Genesis, Journey, Ellie, Liv, Dash, Grace, Audrey, Jack, Melia, Cole, Brody, Riley, Lennon, Gavin, Hannah, Mia, Prescott, and Elise, thank you for adding life and vitality to these pages. You represent the real-life kids who will be using this book, and it was so fun having your energy and spirit to guide us on photo-shoot days!

To the companies who contributed their products to this book, thank you so much for your generosity. Thank you Bentgo, EasyLunchboxes, PlanetBox, Yumbox, LunchBots, PackIt, Mabel's Labels, EcoSoul, Responsible Products, Stasher, OmieLife, and Lille Home. It was so fun trying out your wonderful products and featuring them in this book!

To the Feeding Littles team who has been instrumental in this entire process, we are so grateful for each and every one of you. Jessica Rhyan, you were an absolute workhorse during this photo shoot. We are amazed by your dedication and work ethic. Sarah Bonelli, we are so grateful for your design eye and creativity. You helped our vision come to life in such tangible and beautiful ways, and you always thought three steps ahead during this process. Yingzi Vraves, you are so creative and practical, both at the same time. Thank you for your immense input on this project. Leah Case, you are the silent hero, holding down the fort from afar and working so hard on every stage of this process. We so appreciate everything you do and can't wait to celebrate this with you! Stacy Kaplan, we literally could not have done this without you. Your attention to detail (and love for very tedious tasks) saved us so many times, and your leadership has been invaluable. You took on the very tough job of procuring and organizing all the lunch boxes, the food, and the schedule for the photo shoot, and you pushed this project forward on days we were tired or overwhelmed. Thank you forever for your help with this.

To our amazing Feeding Littles followers and supporters, we appreciate your encouragement more than you will ever know. Because of you, we are able to live out our professional dreams. It is such a privilege to do what you love every day, and we don't take it for granted.

To Sarah, Chris, and baby Jack, saying "thank you" will never be enough. The legacy you have created in Jack's memory reaches further and wider than we will ever comprehend. Thank you for turning your immense sadness into something beautiful and for continuing to champion Feeding Littles along every step of the way.

From Judy

There are so many people who have shared in this vision and have helped this book become a reality.

First, to the children and families throughout our Feeding Littles community and in my private practice, thank you. You are the teachers I celebrate every day!

To several parents who have helped in remarkable ways, thank you. And especially to one parent in particular: Kristina—a mom to a twenty-nine-week-old preemie, who was one pound, ten ounces at birth. As he grew, her son disliked everything food related—the smell, texture, and taste of food. I was his occupational therapist and feeding specialist who visited him within his home every week until he turned three years old. Then came Feeding Littles' online courses for parents, and Kristina's wish for me to share my work with the world came true! Axel is now seven years old and eats everything his family eats. Kristina, thank you for being my friend throughout this process and for continuing our friendship today.

To Megan McNamee, thank you. You're a breath of fresh air and optimism in your creations of daily lunches that you share with our followers over Instagram. The true inspiration behind *Feeding Littles Lunches*, you have been making lunches for your kids and sharing them for more than eight years through our Feeding Littles Instagram platform. You've created a unique way of making lunches so that they're easy for parents to prepare and fun and desirable for children to eat. You show that lunches don't have to be fancy, and most important, kids don't need to feel ashamed if they don't eat their food.

Megan, you have an incredible gift of teaching parents that food is food, that tomorrow is another day, and no matter how hard you try, kids sometimes just get the best of you. And when you least expect it, they surprise you and show you that your hard work has paid off. This is your book of love to parents, and to anyone who eats lunch! You are a gift of compassion and guidance to parents everywhere. I am so lucky to call you my business partner, co-author of our *New York Times* bestselling cookbook, and most important, my friend.

I am truly blessed to have an incredibly supportive family, Louie, Prescott, and Elise. Thank you for sharing in my passion and supporting my journey and for putting up with all the special requests that have come along with this voyage. You are my life's best achievements.

From Megan

To my parents, Mike and Michele, and my sister, Jessica, thank you for your immense support of my career from the very beginning. You walked me through organic chemistry exams, training at LA County Hospital, graduate studies, and my first job. You were there when I decided to make the jump to a full-time entrepreneur, even though it was scary. You have always had my back, and I love you.

To my many wonderful friends, thank you for being so excited for this book. You have been my emotional support on days when I was delirious from typing or editing. You are all so special to me.

To the incredible professionals who have taught me so much, thank you. Elyse Resch and Evelyn Tribole, you are high on my gratitude list. *Intuitive Eating* has changed the world, and we have you to thank for that.

To my husband, Greg, I am so grateful for you. You encouraged me to do this project and have celebrated every milestone along the way. You push me to become a better business owner, mom, wife, and human. I am forever appreciative of your wisdom, humor, and companionship.

To my beloved babies, Hannah and Mia, thank you for turning my world upside down when you were born. Thank you for teaching me that the most important thing in the world is doing life with you. These lunches might be photographed for the world to see, but the heart of this book lies in the private daily ritual of us packing lunches together so that you feel safe, loved, and taken care of while you're away from me. I love that your friends now want to eat *your* lunches, and I hope that you can use this book with your families one day.

And finally, to Judy, thank you for being you. Thank you for going along with my crazy ideas and encouraging me when I need it most. Yes, we are business partners, but you've always been a mentor to me. You have taught me all you know and have given me so much compassion and encouragement when I ran with it. Your expertise is woven into everything we do at Feeding Littles, and I feel so lucky to have been connected to you by baby Jack a decade ago. I can't believe we wrote another book! You should be so proud of the legacy you have created.

Index

D

E

F

About the Authors

JUDY DELAWARE is an occupational therapist who helps children with medical, developmental, and sensory issues learn to eat a wider variety of foods.

MEGAN McNAMEE is a registered dietitian nutritionist who specializes in maternal/child nutrition, disordered eating prevention, and food sensitivities.